CURRENT CLINICAL NEUROLOGY

Daniel Tarsy, MD, SERIES EDITORS

Neurological and Psychiatric Disorders: *From Bench to Bedside,* edited by *Frank I. Tarazi and John A. Schetz, 2005*

Status Epilepticus: *A Clinical Perspective,* edited by *Frank W. Drislane, 2005*

Thrombolytic Therapy for Acute Stroke, Second Edition, edited by *Patrick D. Lyden, 2005*

Movement Disorders Emergencies: *Diagnosis and Treatment,* edited by *Steven J. Frucht and Stanley Fahn, 2005*

Inflammatory Disorders of the Nervous System: *Pathogenesis, Immunology, and Clinical Management,* edited by *Alireza Minagar and J. Steven Alexander, 2005*

Multiple Sclerosis: Etiology, Diagnosis, and New Treatment Strategies, edited by *Michael J. Olek, 2005*

Parkinson's Disease and Nonmotor Dysfunction, edited by *Ronald F. Pfeiffer and Ivan Bodis-Wollner, 2005*

Seizures in Critical Care: *A Guide to Diagnosis and Therapeutics,* edited by *Panayiotis N. Varelas, 2005*

Vascular Dementia: *Cerebrovascular Mechanisms and Clinical Management,* edited by *Robert H. Paul, Ronald Cohen, Brian R. Ott, Stephen Salloway, 2005*

Atypical Parkinsonian Disorders, edited by *Irene Litvan, 2005*

Handbook of Neurocritical Care, edited by *Anish Bhardwaj, Marek A. Mirski, and John A. Ulatowski, 2004*

Handbook of Stroke Prevention in Clinical Practice, edited by *Karen L. Furie and Peter J. Kelly, 2004*

Clinical Handbook of Insomnia, edited by *Hrayr P. Attarian, 2004*

Critical Care Neurology and Neurosurgery, edited by *Jose I. Suarez, 2004*

Alzheimer's Disease: *A Physician's Guide to Practical Management,* edited by *Ralph W. Richter and Brigitte Zoeller Richter, 2004*

Field of Vision: *A Manual and Atlas of Perimetry,* edited by *Jason J. S. Barton and Michael Benatar, 2003*

Surgical Treatment of Parkinson's Disease and Other Movement Disorders, edited by *Daniel Tarsy, Jerrold L. Vitek, and Andres M. Lozano, 2003*

Myasthenia Gravis and Related Disorders, edited by *Henry J. Kaminski, 2003*

Seizures: *Medical Causes and Management,* edited by *Norman Delanty, 2002*

Clinical Evaluation and Management of Spasticity, edited by *David A. Gelber and Douglas R. Jeffery, 2002*

Early Diagnosis of Alzheimer's Disease, edited by *Leonard F. M. Scinto and Kirk R. Daffner, 2000*

Sexual and Reproductive Neurorehabilitation, edited by *Mindy Aisen, 1997*

Neurological and Psychiatric Disorders

From Bench to Bedside

Edited by

Frank I. Tarazi, PhD, MSc

Department of Psychiatry and Neuroscience Program,
Harvard Medical School, Boston, MA;
Laboratory of Psychiatric Neuroscience,
McLean Hospital, Belmont, MA

John A. Schetz, PhD

Department of Pharmacology and Neuroscience,
University of North Texas Health Science Center,
Fort Worth, TX

Foreword by

John L. Waddington, PhD, DSc

Department of Clinical Pharmacology,
Royal College of Surgeons in Ireland,
Dublin

HUMANA PRESS ✳ TOTOWA, NEW JERSEY

Due diligence has been taken by the publishers, editors, and authors of this book to assure the accuracy of the information published and to describe generally accepted practices. The contributors herein have carefully checked to ensure that the drug selections and dosages set forth in this text are accurate and in accord with the standards accepted at the time of publication. Notwithstanding, as new research, changes in government regulations, and knowledge from clinical experience relating to drug therapy and drug reactions constantly occurs, the reader is advised to check the product information provided by the manufacturer of each drug for any change in dosages or for additional warnings and contraindications. This is of utmost importance when the recommended drug herein is a new or infrequently used drug. It is the responsibility of the treating physician to determine dosages and treatment strategies for individual patients. Further it is the responsibility of the health care provider to ascertain the Food and Drug Administration status of each drug or device used in their clinical practice. The publisher, editors, and authors are not responsible for errors or omissions or for any consequences from the application of the information presented in this book and make no warranty, express or implied, with respect to the contents in this publication.

This publication is printed on acid-free paper. ∞
ANSI Z39.48-1984 (American Standards Institute) Permanence of Paper for Printed Library Materials.

Cover design by Patricia F. Cleary

Production Editor: Robin B. Weisberg

For additional copies, pricing for bulk purchases, and/or information about other Humana titles, contact Humana at the above address or at any of the following numbers: Tel.: 973-256-1699; Fax: 973-256-8314; E-mail: humana@humanapr.com, or visit our Website: http://humanapress.com

Photocopy Authorization Policy:

Printed in the United States of America. 10 9 8 7 6 5 4 3 2 1

eISBN: 1-59259-856-0

Library of Congress Cataloging-in-Publication Data

Neurological and psychiatric disorders : from bench to bedside / edited by
Frank I. Tarazi, John A. Schetz.
    p. ; cm. -- (Current clinical neurology)
  Includes bibliographical references and index.
  ISBN 1-58829-369-6 (hardcover : alk. paper)
  1. Neuropsychiatry. I. Tarazi, Frank I. II. Schetz, John A. III. Series.
  [DNLM: 1. Mental Disorders. 2. Nervous System Diseases. WL 140 N4919
2005]
RC341.N397 2005
616.8--dc22

                                                    2004015772

Dedication

To the countless colleagues and organizations that have helped us realize this book project and to our families for their everlasting support and encouragement.

Series Editor's Introduction

The disciplines of neurology and psychiatry have had a long and complicated relationship for many years. Although both specialties deal with the brain, scientific and clinical approaches to this complex organ have differed widely during the past century. However, beginning in the 1960s both fields saw an enormous growth in understanding the role of neurotransmitters in normal and abnormal brain function and, as a result, an important convergence of scientific inquiry took place. During this time, dopamine was recognized to be a neurotransmitter rather than a precursor of norepinephrine, dopamine replacement therapy was discovered to be an effective treatment for Parkinson's disease, and dopamine receptor-blocking drugs were found to be effective for the treatment of schizophrenia and other psychotic disorders. The era of biogenic amines was launched and dopamine, norepinephrine, and serotonin came under intensive study with the strong expectation that further insights into the pathophysiology and treatment of other neurological and psychiatric disorders would be forthcoming.

Fast forwarding to the present, *Neurological and Psychiatric Disorders: From Bench to Bedside* brings us up to date on the role of the biogenic amines in the pathophysiology and treatment of a core group of neurological and psychiatric disorders. However, the early notion that manipulation of a single neurotransmitter could produce profound and lasting therapeutic effects for any of these conditions was clearly simplistic. As pointed out by Drs. Tarazi and Schetz, many pharmacological treatments provide relief for only one or several symptoms in a particular disorder. This includes even Parkinson's disease where there is much more to the story than simple dopamine deficiency. Other neurotransmitters including but not limited to γ-aminobutyric acid, glutamic acid, and acetylcholine as well as a variety of neuropeptides and other small molecules also play a key role in these diseases. More also needs to be understood about the complex neuronal circuits and pathways between basal ganglia, limbic system, and cerebral cortex, which appear to underlie normal and abnormal motor, emotional, and cognitive functions.

Neurological and Psychiatric Disorders: From Bench to Bedside provides much more than an overview of the neurobiology of a group of neurological and psychiatric disorders. The chapters are uniformly very well organized to provide a broad, comprehensive and systematic review of the epidemiology, pathophysiology, molecular biology, genetics, neuropathology, brain imaging, clinical features, and pharmacological and nonpharmacological treatments of several mental illnesses, that will serve as a valuable core of information for physicians, scientists, advanced students, and health care professionals in this area. A unique bonus in this volume is the very sophisticated psychiatric approaches to neurological disorders and neurological approaches to psychiatric disorders, which are provided, in the individual chapters. Finally and most importantly, this book should also serve to promote future interdisciplinary research which will further the understanding of these disorders.

Daniel Tarsy, MD
Parkinson's Disease and Movement Disorders Center
Beth Israel Deaconess Medical Center
Harvard Medical School, Boston, MA

Foreword

In the 1970s I had the privilege of meeting the long-serving British Prime Minister Harold Wilson at a degree-conferring ceremony, in his capacity as chancellor of the University of Bradford, United Kingdom. Our brief conversation gave no hint of what was to come: within a short period he had unexpectedly resigned as prime minister, engendering enormous intrigue and controversy. Only many years later, on his death, was it confirmed that he had developed Alzheimer's disease and that his resignation from office appeared to reflect some insight and concern that his mental abilities were not what they were. This is in striking contrast to a generation later when, in the 1990s, former US President Ronald Reagan wrote his poignant letter to the American people informing them that he was leaving public life to face the challenges of Alzheimer's disease.

Subsequently, a series of high-profile individuals in the United States have revealed and spoken publicly of their conditions, including Charlton Heston (Alzheimer's disease) and Michael J. Fox (Parkinson's disease). In the United Kingdom, the leading English soccer team, Manchester United, signed a new goalkeeper, Tim Howard, who speaks openly of having Tourette's syndrome. This new public openness in relation to neurological and psychiatric disorders, which had been faced previously in secrecy and even shame, has served both to help de-stigmatize such disorders and to indicate the need for increasing research thereon. Perhaps no individual in the public eye helped to focus attention on neuroscience as a route to improved treatment modalities than did Christopher Reeve. Prior to his recent untimely death, Reeve's passionate advocacy of neuroscience research as an imperative for his own salvation and that of others affected similarly exemplified the individual adversities that give real, highly personalized meaning to "from bench to bedside."

Here, Drs. Frank Tarazi and John Schetz have assembled a team of expert authors to give an authoritative, contemporary overview of the field. In sport, teams usually have to play to a manager's tactical plan. The editors have proceeded similarly with their team of authors to good effect, focusing on the extent to which the "holy grail" of a bench-to-bedside research trajectory has been realized. Introductory chapters describe, at an accessible level, the principles underpinning research in this area: first, the neural principles of neurological and psychiatric disorders, from laboratory methods to clinical neuroimaging techniques and the insights that they can provide; second, the pharmacotherapeutic principles that underpin treatment, from receptorology to applied issues that govern the most effective use of medications. Thereafter, chapters describe our current understanding of major disorders in neurology (Alzheimer's disease, Huntington's disease, Parkinson's disease) and psychiatry (schizophrenia, autism spectrum disorders, Tourette's syndrome and tic disorders, obsessive-compulsive disorder, unipolar depression, bipolar disorder, attention deficit hyperactivity disorder). It should be noted that these chapters indicate how contemporary neuroscience reveals the arbitrariness of this somewhat artificial separation into "neurological" and "psychiatric" disorders; these may more reflect historical artifact and professional territory than indicate fundamental distinctions in terms of scientific understanding and human suffering.

To achieve their bench-to-bedside perspective, the editors have prevailed on their authors to adopt a uniform structure for each chapter. This leads the reader from the relevant brain pathways, molecular mechanisms and targets, through genetics and animal models, to clinical epidemiology, phenomenology, and treatment issues. Unusually, at the end of each chapter is a useful glossary of medical terminology that constitutes an additional aid to clarity and accessibility. Through these innovations, the editors and authors have marshalled concisely the most up-to-date information pertaining to major neurological and psychiatric disorders that constitute some of our most serious public health problems. Although not yet fully realized, this volume documents that the bench-to-bedside research trajectory is no longer a "holy grail" but a realistic goal toward which considerable progress has been made.

John L. Waddington, PhD, DSc,
Department of Clinical Pharmacology,
Royal College of Surgeons in Ireland,
Dublin

Preface

The neurological and psychiatric disorders discussed in *Neurological and Psychiatric Disorders: From Bench to Bedside* are commonly treated with pharmacotherapies that target brain dopaminergic, serotonergic, or noradrenergic systems, either individually or in combination. Additional treatment strategies, including psychiatric, psychosocial, psychosurgical, and electrical/magnetic therapies are also available either as monotherapies or to augment drug treatments. Pharmacotherapies for neurological and psychiatric disorders are thought to be primarily palliative, and often they are prescribed to provide relief for only one of a range of symptoms encountered for each disorder. For example, antipsychotic drugs are prescribed for the treatment of agitation in Alzheimer's disease, aggression and self-injury in autism, mania in bipolar disorder, motor dysfunction in Huntington's disease, motor tics in Tourette's syndrome, and psychosis in schizophrenia. Antidepressant drugs are employed in the treatment of depression in unipolar and bipolar depression and obsessive behaviors in obsessive–compulsive disorder. Such a range of treatments for different symptom modalities for different disorders owes to either the direct or indirect dysfunction of dopaminergic, serotonergic, and noradrenergic system(s). In addition, there is considerable overlap in selected portions of the extended brain pathways related to the pathophysiology and treatment of certain of these disorders. *Neurological and Psychiatric Disorders: From Bench to Bedside* provides the reader with a full appreciation for all such factors as they relate to preclinical research and to clinical diagnosis and treatment of the neurological and psychiatric disorders.

Neurological and Psychiatric Disorders: From Bench to Bedside aims to provide comprehensive and systematic coverage of the basic and clinical aspects of the core neurological and psychiatric disorders that are commonly taught to doctorate- and postdoctorate-level students. Until now, many texts were needed to cover the preclinical and clinical aspects of different disorders in sufficient breadth and depth to allow for MDs, PhDs, and PharmDs to master their qualifying (board) exams, and, at the same time, effectively and safely practice their future health care professions. Having a single text will not only facilitate cross-discipline teaching and learning by providing a uniform instructional platform, but will also satisfy student concerns about the costs and variable coverage generated by the need for multiple texts. The editors and contributing authors undertook a collaborative effort to produce such a textbook, which is based on the syllabus and content of an advanced graduate-level course concerning the neurological basis of diseases and disorders and their treatment that Dr. Schetz developed and continues to teach. The primary editorial responsibilities and the recruitment of authoritative authors for the chapters on the individual disorders were divided evenly between the editors:

Dr. Tarazi recruited authors for and edited the chapters on attention deficit hyperactivity disorder, bipolar disorder, Huntington's disease, Parkinson's disease, and schizophrenia, and Dr. Schetz recruited authors for and edited the chapters on Alzheimer's disease, autism, obsessive–compulsive disorder, Tourette's syndrome, and unipolar depression.

Neurological and Psychiatric Disorders: From Bench to Bedside opens with two introductory chapters that reintroduce the reader to the neural and pharmacotherapeutic principles of neurological and psychiatric disorders. These chapters also discuss theoretical and methodological parameters relevant to the appropriate interpretation of pharmacodynamic, pharmacokinetic, neuroanatomical, and imaging data presented throughout. Subsequent chapters provide a standard minimum content concerning each disorder along with a uniformity that is intended to promote not only the comparing and contrasting of the disorders discussed throughout, but also the cross-discipline training many health care industry experts believe is lacking. The standard minimum uniform content for each disorder can be divided into the following nine categories:

1. Incidence/prevalence
2. Etiology and general description
3. Molecular targets and mechanisms of action
4. Brain structures and pathways, and neurotransmitter systems
5. Animal models
6. Signs and symptoms in humans (diagnostics, markers, comorbidities, subclassifications)
7. Genetics
8. Treatments (pharmacological and other types of therapies)
9. Related medical terminology

Thus, the objective is to promote a systematic, comprehensive, and advanced understanding of each disorder from molecules to human behaviors. Our intended audience includes graduate- and postgraduate-level physicians and scientists, preclinical and clinical research scientists, and pharmacists with an intermediate to advanced understanding of neuroscience and pharmacology.

We extend our deepest gratitude to the chapter authors for their outstanding scholarly contributions. A special thanks goes to our advisors and mentors who have over the years generated in us an intense and perpetual desire to challenge ourselves and to instill in the next generation of young scientists, physicians and pharmacists the excitement and satisfaction that we experience from working in the health care profession and answering the call to public service. In particular, we wish to recognize the kind and astute influences that Dr. Ian Creese and Dr. Ross J. Baldessarini have had on Dr. Tarazi and that Dr. William G. Luttge, Dr. David R. Sibley, and Dr. Harel Weinstein have had on Dr. Schetz.

Frank I. Tarazi, PhD, MSc
John A. Schetz, PhD

Contents

Color Plates

Color plates 1–5 appear in an insert preceding p. 51.

Contributors

MATTHEW J. ALBERT, BA • Department of Psychiatry, University of Rome
at San Andrea Hospital and Centro Lucio Bini, Rome, Italy

EVDOKIA ANAGNOSTOU, MD • Seaver and New York Autism Center
of Excellence, Department of Psychiatry, Mount Sinai School
of Medicine, New York, NY

CHRISTOPHER BAETHGE, MD • Department of Psychiatry, McLean Hospital,
Harvard Medical School, Boston, MA; Department of Psychiatry,
Free University of Berlin, Berlin, Germany

ROSS J. BALDESSARINI, MD • Mailman Research Center, Department
of Psychiatry, McLean Hospital, Harvard Medical School, Boston, MA

SABINA BERRETTA, MD • Laboratory of Translational Neuroscience, McLean
Hospital, Department of Psychiatry, Harvard Medical School, Boston,
MA

JULIE A. BLENDY, PhD • Department of Pharmacology, University of Pennsylvania
School of Medicine, Philadelphia, PA

SUSAN E. BROWNE, PhD • Department of Neurology and Neuroscience, Weill
Medical College of Cornell University, New York, NY

EUGEN DAVIDS, MD • Departments of Psychiatry and Psychotherapy,
University of Essen, Essen, Germany

WAYNE K. GOODMAN, MD • Department of Psychiatry, University of Florida
College of Medicine, Gainesville, FL

STEPHAN HECKERS, MD • Schizophrenia and Bipolar Disorder Program
and Functional Neuroanatomy Laboratory, McLean Hospital,
Department of Psychiatry, Harvard Medical School, Boston, MA

ERIC HOLLANDER, MD • Seaver and New York Autism Center of Excellence,
Department of Psychiatry, Mount Sinai School of Medicine,
New York, NY

DAVID S. HUSTED, MD • Department of Psychiatry, University of Florida
College of Medicine, Gainesville, FL

MARC J. KAUFMAN, PhD • Brain Imaging Center, McLean Hospital,
Department of Psychiatry and Neuroscience Program, Harvard
Medical School, Boston, MA

ROBERT A. KING, MD • Child Study Center, Yale University School
of Medicine, New Haven, CT

ALEXIA E. KOUKOPOULOS, MD • Department of Psychiatry, University
of Rome at San Andrea Hospital and Centro Lucio Bini, Rome, Italy

JAMES F. LECKMAN, MD • Child Study Center, Yale University School
of Medicine, New Haven, CT

IRWIN LUCKI, PhD • Department of Psychiatry, University of Pennsylvania School of Medicine, Philadelphia, PA

MARK P. MATTSON, PhD • Laboratory of Neurosciences, Gerontology Research Center, National Institute on Aging; Department of Neurology, Johns Hopkins University School of Medicine, Baltimore, MD

JOHN A. SCHETZ, PhD • Department of Pharmacology and Neuroscience, University of North Texas Health Science Center, Fort Worth, TX

NATHAN A. SHAPIRA, MD, PhD • Department of Psychiatry, University of Florida College of Medicine, Gainesville, FL

JAMES E. SWAIN, MD, PhD • Child Study Center, Yale University School of Medicine, New Haven, CT

DANIEL TARSY, MD • Parkinson's Disease and Movement Disorders Center, Beth Israel Deaconess Medical Center, Harvard Medical School, Boston, MA

FRANK I. TARAZI, PhD, MSc • Laboratory of Psychiatric Neuroscience, McLean Hospital, Department of Psychiatry, Harvard Medical School, Boston, MA

LEONARDO TONDO, MD • Department of Psychology, University of Cagliari, and Centro Lucio Bini, Stanley Medical Research Center, Cagliari, Sardinia

JOHN L. WADDINGTON, PhD DSc • Department of Clinical Pharmacology, Royal College of Surgeons in Ireland, Dublin, Ireland

THOMAS WICHMANN, MD • Department of Neurology, Emory University School of Medicine, Atlanta, GA

KEHONG ZHANG, MD, PhD • McLean Hospital, Department of Psychiatry, Harvard Medical School, Boston, MA

I Introduction

1

Neural Principles of Neurological and Psychiatric Disorders

Frank I. Tarazi and Marc J. Kaufman

Summary

Recent progress in understanding the neurobiology and pharmacology of brain neurotransmitters and their neural circuits and pathways has been remarkable and serves as the foundation for in-depth preclinical research on neurological and psychiatric disorders. Most of the neurotransmitter receptors have been cloned and their anatomical localization and distribution have been clarified using advanced neurochemical methods. Novel discoveries have greatly stimulated clinical studies in the neuropathophysiology and neurogenetics of brain disorders. Sophisticated developments in neuroimaging techniques have yielded revolutionary insights into the complexity of maldevelopment or dysfunction of neuronal elements in neurological and psychiatric disorders, and have assisted in the rational design of novel neuropsychotropic agents for improved treatment of these disorders.

Key Words: Brain pathways; dopamine; emission tomography; magnetic resonance; neuroimaging; norepinephrine; serotonin.

1. INTRODUCTION

Nerve cells in the brain (neurons) communicate with each other via chemical substances (neurotransmitters) that are released from synaptic terminals. Once released, these neurotransmitters target adjacent neurons and alter cellular activities and functions of influenced neurons. Neurons and neurotransmitters can be organized into specialized circuits and signaling pathways. Neural circuits can be as simple as one synapse and one neurotransmitter or very complex and involve different synapses, multiple neurotransmitters, and extend across different brain regions. Preclinical and clinical evidences strongly suggest that abnormal development of brain neurons and malfunctions of brain circuits significantly contribute to the development of different neurological and psychiatric disorders. Subsequently, drugs developed for treatment of these disorders tend to restore neurotransmission and normalize neuron–neuron communications. Advances in histochemical and autoradiographic techniques have improved the detailed charac-

From: *Current Clinical Neurology: Neurological and Psychiatric Disorders:
From Bench to Bedside*
Edited by: F. I. Tarazi and J. A. Schetz © Humana Press Inc., Totowa, NJ

terization of the anatomical localization of different neurotransmitter receptors, and the quantification of their levels in laboratory animals and in postmortem human tissue. Additionally, sophisticated imaging techniques have helped to identify specific brain regions associated with particular modes of behaviors and permitted the direct visualization of neurotransmitter receptors in healthy subjects and diseased patients. This chapter introduces some of the key brain neurotransmitters and brain pathways as well as neurochemical and neuroimaging techniques that greatly enriched our knowledge of the neural principles of neurological and psychiatric disorders.

2. BRAIN NEUROTRANSMITTERS

Three major brain neurotransmitter systems—dopamine (DA), norepinephrine (NE), and serotonin—are intimately involved in the pathophysiology, neuropathology, and pharmacotherapy of neurological and psychiatric disorders discussed in following chapters.

2.1. Dopamine

For the longest time, DA was considered an intermediate molecule in the biosynthesis of other catecholamines including epinephrine and NE. In mid-1950s, Arvid Carlsson and his colleagues proposed a prominent biological role for DA as an independent neurotransmitter. These seminal proposals were the impetus for explosive advances in DA research. Several clinically relevant contributions had emerged from the study of DA systems, including the role of these systems in the pathophysiology and treatment of attention deficit hyperactivity disorder (ADHD), Huntington's chorea, Parkinson's disease, schizophrenia, Tourette's syndrome, and other tic disorders *(1)*.

2.1.1. DA Pathways

DA neurons of the mammalian central nervous system (CNS) are organized into four major subsystems: (a) the *nigrostriatal* system: neurons project from the substantia nigra pars compacta, also called A_9 neurons, to the caudate-putamen (CPu). This system accounts for 70% of the total brain content of DA, and its degeneration makes a major contribution to the pathophysiology of Parkinson's disease; (b) the *mesolimbic* system: originates in the ventral tegmental area, also called A_{10} neurons, and projects to different components of the limbic system including the nucleus accumbens, lateral septal nuclei, amygdala, hippocampus, and the entorhinal cortex; (c) the *mesocortical* system: arises from cell bodies in ventral tegmental area and project to cerebral cortex, particularly to mesioprefrontal areas; and (d) the *tuberinfundibular* neuroendocrinological system: neurons arise in the arcuate and other nuclei of the hypothalamus and end in the median eminence of the inferior hypothalamus, in which DA exerts regulatory effects in the anterior pituitary, and serves as a prolactin inhibitory factor *(2)*.

2.1.2. DA Synthesis and Metabolism

DA is synthesized from L-tyrosine, which is converted to L-3,4-dihydroxyphenylalanine (L-DOPA) in a reaction catalyzed by the enzyme tyrosine hydroxy-

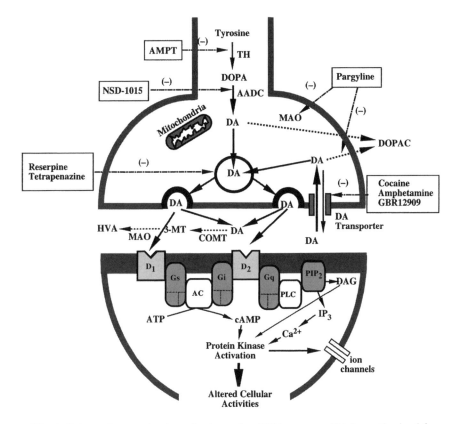

Fig. 1. Schematic organization of a dopamine (DA) synapse. DA is synthesized from L-tyrosine, which is converted to L-3,4-dihydroxyphenylalanine (L-DOPA) by tyrosine hydroxylase. DA is produced by decarboxylation of L-DOPA and stored in membrane-enclosed presynaptic vesicles, and subsequently released by depolarization in the presence of calcium by membrane fusion (exocytosis). DA stimulates its D_1-like and D_2-like postsynaptic receptors; the receptors activate different subtypes of G proteins and coupled effector enzymes to produce second-messenger molecules, which alter the functional activities of the cell. DA can be inactivated by active transport back into the presynaptic terminals or it can be metabolized to 3,4-dihydroxy-phenylacetic acid and homovanillic acid (*see* text for details). As shown, several drugs have the ability to block the synthesis, storage, reuptake, and degradation of DA.

lase (TH) using molecular oxygen and tetrahydrobiopterin (BH_4) as cofactors (Fig. 1) *(3)*. DA is formed from L-DOPA via removal of a side chain carboxyl group in chemical reaction catalyzed by the enzyme L-amino acid decarboxylase (AADC). TH is the rate-limiting enzyme that controls overall rate of formation of DA. Phosphorylation of TH by protein kinases activates the enzyme and subsequently enhances synthesis of DA. Inhibitors of TH, such as α-methyl-*p*-tyrosine (AMPT), deplete levels of endogenous DA. In contrast, inhibitors of AADC, most notably

the mammalian brain with specialized cortical executive functions. Disturbances in NE neurotransmission have been clinically associated with depression, as well ADHD, schizophrenia, and other disorders of attention and cognition *(3)*.

2.2.1. NE Pathways

The nuclei of origin for the central NE system are in the pons and medulla *(4)*. These nuclei consist of three main groups:

1. *locus coerulus (LC) complex*: This is the most prominent NE nucleus. Axons of LC project to several telencephalic and diencephalic regions, including several areas of cerebral cortex, hippocampus, amygdala, septum, thalamus, and hypothalamus;
2. *lateral tegmental system*: Axons of this system project caudally to the spinal cord and terminate in the intermediolateral cell columns of the thoracic and upper lumbar cord. The rostral projections of this system make up the ventral NE bundle, which terminates in the hypothalamus and other diencephalic structures; and
3. *dorsal medullary group*: Fibers of this system project to nucleus of tractus solitarius in the medulla, dorsal vagal complex, and other primary motor and visceral nuclei of the cranial nerves. Sympathetic ganglia and chromaffin cells of adrenal medulla represent major populations of peripheral NE-containing neurons *(4)*.

2.2.2. NE Synthesis and Metabolism

NE is synthesized from DA in a reaction catalyzed by dopamine β-hydroxylase (DβH) using copper, oxygen and ascorbic acid as cofactors. Because NE and DA share a similar anabolic pathway, TH is also the rate-limiting enzyme that controls overall rate of formation of NE. Synthesis of NE can be blocked by TH inhibitors or by DβH inhibitors, such as FLA63 *(3)*.

NE is stored in membrane-enclosed presynaptic vesicles, and it is released into the synaptic cleft by Ca^{2+}-mediated exocytosis. It is inactivated by active reuptake into presynaptic terminals via NE transporters or by degradation. Degradation of NE starts with either deamination or *O*-methylation. MAO can catalyze the breakdown of NE into 3,4-dihydroxyphenylglycoaldeshyde (DHPGA), which is further metabolized into two intermediates 3,4-dihydroxyphenylglycol (DHPG) or 3,4-dihydroxymandelic acid (DHMA). DHPG and DHMA are further *O*-methylated into 3-methoxy-4-hydroxyphenylglycol (MHPG) and vanillymandelic acid , respectively. NE can be metabolized by COMT to give normetanephine, which is later deaminated to 3-methoxy-4-hydroxyphenylglycolaldehyde (MHPGA). MHPGA is further broken down by aldehyde dehydrogenase to a major metabolite MHPG *(3)*.

2.2.3. NE Receptor Subtypes

NE receptor proteins are also characterized by having seven relatively hydrophobic TMS segments, as well as a functionally critical third intracytoplasmic loop that couples to G proteins. NE receptors are subdivided into α-adrenergic (α_1 and α_2) and β-adrenergic (β_1, β_2, and β_3) subfamilies. Although β-adrenergic receptor subtypes are expressed at variable levels in different areas of the brain, they apparently do not play a prominent role in the treatment of several neurological and psychiatric disorders, and consequently, they are not emphasized here *(5,6)*.

2.2.3.1. α_1 RECEPTORS

These receptors are divided into two subtypes: α_{1A} and α_{1B}. α_{1A} receptors are highly expressed in hippocampus, pons-medulla and spinal cord, whereas α_{1B} receptors are mainly detected in cerebral cortex, thalamus, hypothalamus, and cerebellum. Both receptors are equally distributed in the striatum. Both α_{1A} and α_{1B} receptor activation results in generation of second messengers inositol 1,4,5-trisphosphate and diacylglycerol and activation of Ca^{2+} channels.

2.2.3.2. α_2 RECEPTORS

α_2 receptor family were originally divided into two subtypes (α_{2A} and α_{2B}). Subsequently, two additional members (α_{2C} and α_{2D}) were included in the family. Autoradiographic and *in situ* studies showed that α_{2A} receptors are expressed in substantial levels in amygdalo–hippocampal area, the central and basolateral nuclei of the amygdala, and dorsolateral nucleus of the thalamus. The α_{2A} receptor protein and mRNA are highly expressed in locus coerulus, indicating that this receptor subtype serves as a somatodendritic autoreceptor in NE neurons. Other α_2 receptors are found in dentate gyrus, substantia nigra pars reticulata and hippocampal CA_1 region. α_2 receptors decrease the activity of adenylyl cyclase, whereas α_2 autoreceptors inhibit the release of NE by increasing K^+ conductance which hyperpolarizes NE neurons *(5)*.

2.3. Serotonin

Serotonin or 5-hydroxytryptamine (5-HT) was initially isolated from chromaffin cells of the intestinal mucosa. Only 1 to 2% of total body 5-HT is found in the mammalian CNS. Biochemical abnormalities in 5-HT synthesis and degradation have been linked to various forms of mental illness including bipolar disorder, depression, obsessive–compulsive disorders, and schizophrenia *(3)*.

2.3.1. 5-HT Pathways

There are nine major groups of 5-HT containing neurons known as B1–B9. These groups are mainly localized in the raphe nuclei and reticular region of the lower brain stem. The 5-HT neurons of the brain stem are divided into caudal and rostral systems. The caudal system consists of B1–B4 groups and projects from median and paramedian groups of the medulla and caudal pons to the spinal cord. The rostral 5-HT system comprises the B5–B9 cell groups, and they are associated with the raphe nuclei of the rostral pons and mesencephalon, as well as the caudal linear nucleus, the nucleus pontis oralis, and the supralemniscal region *(7)*.

The rostral 5-HT system gives rise to two distinct ascending projections termed the ventral and dorsal pathways. The ventral ascending pathway originates from group B6–B8 cells and innervates basal ganglia, limbic system, and cortex. A major part of the ventral pathway enters the medial forebrain bundle and innervates the medial habenula, thalamus, and hypothalamus. Other fibers innervate the dorsal and ventral striatum, amygdala, hippocampus, septal nucleus, olfactory cortex, and all regions of cerebral cortex. The dorsal ascending pathway originates from group cells B7 and B8 and innervates mesencephalic gray as well as inferior and superior colliculi *(7)*. Two additional 5-HT systems have been identified in the brain. One system projects to cerebellum and terminates in the cerebellar cortex and deep cerebellar nuclei, and the other system innervates locus coeruleus, dorsal tegmental nucleus, nucleus solitarius, reticular formation, and several cranial nerve nuclei.

2.3.2. 5-HT Synthesis and Metabolism

The first step in synthesis of 5-HT is the hydroxylation of the amino acid tryptophan to yield 5-hydroxytryptophan (5-HTP) in a reaction catalyzed by tryptophan hydroxylase *(3)*. 5-HTP is then converted by AADC to 5-HT. Tryptophan hydroxylase, the rate-limiting enzyme that controls the synthesis of 5-HT, requires molecular oxygen and BH_4 cofactor. It can be activated by phosphorylation, proteolysis and Ca^{2+} phospholipids. Once 5-HT is synthesized, it is stored in vesicles and released into the synaptic cleft by exocytosis. Released 5-HT can be inactivated by active reuptake into the presynaptic terminals via 5-HT transporters. Excessive synaptic 5-HT undergoes deamination by monoamine oxidase to yield 5-hydroxyindolaldehyde, which is rapidly oxidized by the enzyme aldehyde dehydrogenase to form 5-hydroxyindolacetic acid , the major metabolite of 5-HT. 5-hydroxyindolacetic acid is then transported by an acid transport system out of the brain and into cerebrospinal fluid *(3)*.

2.3.3. 5-HT Receptors

5-HT receptor family is more heterogenous than DA and NE receptor families as it includes a large number of members *(8)*. 5-HT receptors are currently classified as: 5-HT_1 subfamily (includes subtypes A, B, D, E, and F), 5-HT_2 subfamily (includes types A, B, and C), and separate 5-HT_3, 5-HT_4, 5-HT_5 (and its subtypes 5-HT_{5A} and 5-HT_{5B}), 5-HT_6, and 5-HT_7 receptors. There are additional "orphan" 5-HT that are not well characterized *(8)*. All in all, there are probably 18 5-HT receptor subtypes. With the exception of 5-HT_3 receptor, which is a ligand gated channel, all of the other 5-HT receptor subtypes have the characteristic seven TMS segments, are coupled to G-proteins and initiate multiple signal transduction mechanisms. 5-HT_{1A}, and 5-HT_{2A} remain the most pharmacologically and functionally characterized 5-HT receptor subtypes *(8)*.

2.3.3.1. 5-HT_{1A} Receptors

Rat and human 5-HT_{1A} receptors show 99% sequence homology in their seven TMS domains. They are expressed in high densities in hippocampus, lateral septum, amygdala, frontal and entorhinal cortices. 5-HT_{1A} receptors are also found in median and dorsal raphe nuclei indicating a somatodendritic autoreceptor role for these receptors. 5-HT_{1A} receptor stimulation inhibits cAMP production, decreases Ca^{2+} conductance and increases K^+ conductance. The development of 5-HT_{1A} selective agonists (8-OH-DPAT, ipsapirone) and antagonists (SDZ 216-525, WAY-100135) helped to characterize the behavioral and physiological functions of these receptors. Administration of 5-HT_{1A} agonists induces hyperphagia, hypothermia and other behaviors predictive of anxiolytic-like activity. 5-HT_{1A} agonists can also produce resting tremor, muscular rigidity, lateral head weaving, and excessive salivation. Recent evidence suggests that 5-HT$_{1A}$ agonism contributes to improved treatment of schizophrenia and other psychotic disorders *(9)*.

2.3.3.2. 5-HT$_{2A}$ RECEPTORS

5-HT$_{2A}$ receptors are highly expressed in different areas of cerebral cortex, hippocampus, olfactory nuclei, and parts of the basal ganglia. In the frontal cortex, 5-HT$_{2A}$ receptors are the dominant 5-HT receptor subtype. These receptors mediate neuroexcitation in cortical pyramidal neurons, raphe cell bodies, and NAc neurons. Additionally, 5-HT$_{2A}$ receptor activation stimulates phospholipase C leading to the hydrolysis of phosphatidylinositol and elevation of intracellular Ca^{2+}. The agonist (α-methyl-serotonin) and the antagonists (ketanserin, ritanserin and LY-53857) are among the most selective agents in terms of their 5-HT$_{2A}$ receptor affinities. 5-HT$_{2A}$ receptors exhibit unique regulatory mechanisms to stimulation or blockage because they are downregulated after repeated treatment with either 5-HT$_{2A}$ agonists or antagonists.

3. NEUROTRANSMITTER LOCALIZATION AND VISUALIZATION

Several neurochemical techniques have been discovered and successfully implemented in examining the localization and quantification of different neurotransmitter receptors and their gene expression in CNS. The following section describes some of the most common of these techniques.

3.1. In Vitro Receptor Autoradiography

Autoradiography is the labeling of different receptors and cellular components with specific radioactive ligands. This method uses frozen tissue sections that are sliced in a cryostat and mounted on gelatin-coated slides. Following incubation with the appropriate radioligand in specific incubating buffers, sections are washed to remove unbound radioligand, air-dried, and then are placed against radioisotope sensitive films or dipped in liquid photographic emulsion. After appropriate exposure time, films or emulsions are developed and the generated autoradiograms are processed for image analysis. Optical densities of brain regions of interest are commonly determined using computerized image analysis systems. The amount of radioactivity can be calculated by using standard precalibrated amounts of radioactivity that are placed adjacent to tissue sections and exposed identically. A standard curve generated from optical densities of standards is used to quantify optical densities produced by radiolabeled tissue *(10,11)*.

Autoradiographic techniques provide an advantage over homogenate binding because different radioligands can be used to evaluate and compare multiple receptors in adjacent brain sections generated from the same experimental animal. This technique has been useful in defining the receptor and transporter targets of different psychotropic drugs and in studying the effects of surgical and chemical brain lesions on the expression of selected neurotransmitter receptors and transporters *(10,11)*.

3.2. In Vivo Receptor Autoradiography

In this method, the radioligand of choice is injected systemically into a live animal. The radioligand enters the vascular circulation, crosses blood–brain barrier, and binds to the receptor of interest *(12)*. The animal is then sacrificed, the brain is sliced, and radiolabeled brain sections are processed for autoradiography and image analysis, as described above. Several neurotransmitter receptors including dopamine receptors have been successfully labeled using in vivo technique. Additionally, this method provides a means of measuring transmitter levels or receptor occupancy under controlled experimental conditions. Despite its technical simplicity, the analysis of the results generated from this method is more complex than that of in vitro autoradiography. Several factors such as blood levels of radioligand, its metabolism, and biodistribution must be factored in the analysis *(12)*.

3.3. Immunocytochemistry

Immunocytochemistry (ICC) provides information on the location and density of protein targets of interest using a specific antigen–antibody reaction labeled with a tag suitable for light or electron microscopy *(13)*. Fluorescein and alkaline phosphatase are commonly used for light microscopy detection, whereas ferritin and colloidal gold are used for electron microscopy detection. There are two types of antibodies. The first, "polyclonal antibodies" can be produced by injection of antigenic substance of choice repeatedly into a host (most often rabbit). However, these antibodies often lack the high degree of selectivity and they can be heterogenous from batch to batch. The production of the second type, "monoclonal antibodies," overcame most of these shortcomings. In this method, cells from the spleen of the mouse that have been sensitized to a specific antigen are fused with tumor cells to produce hybrid cells or "hybridoma." The antibody-producing cells are isolated, cloned, and then screened for their antibody characteristics. Only cells with viable and selective immunoreactivity are maintained and grown in culture medium *(14)*. The generated antibodies can be directly labeled with a tag and then applied to tissue section. They can be also applied unlabeled in the form of antiserum to the tissue to localize the antigen, then the reaction in visualized by a labeled second antibody that has been prepared to the immunoglobulin of the first antibody (e.g., fluorescence-labeled goat-antirabbit immunoglobulin G) *(13)*.

Additionally to its ability to map the neuronal localization of neurotransmitter and neuropeptide receptor proteins and related synthesizing enzymes, ICC can analyze the effects of psychotropic drugs on neurotransmitter and neuropeptide systems. ICC can be also employed to localize chemicals in subsets of neurons or within subcellular structures in a single neuron.

3.4. In Situ Hybridization

In situ hybridization (ISH) is a histochemical technique that detects the location and levels of mRNA molecules encoding proteins essential to neuron functions such as enzymes, ion channels, receptors, and peptides *(15)*. ISH can be also used to quantify psychotropic drug-induced alterations in regional mRNAs expression. It provides an advantage over other methods of RNA detection, such as Northern blots, because the morphology and integrity of nucleic acids within nerve cells remain intact *(15)*.

The ISH method commonly uses fixed tissue slices. First, the sliced fixed tissue is mounted on gelatin-coated slides. The tissue is then dehydrated, delipidated, and rehydrated before being covered with hybridization buffer, which contains a probe for the targeted nucleic acid. The probe can be one of three types: complementary DNA (cDNA), RNA, or oligonucleotide probes *(16)*. These probes are produced either by cloning procedures (cDNA and RNA) or manufactured by automated DNA synthesizers (oligonucleotides). They can be labeled with different isotopes (^{32}P, ^{35}S, ^{125}I) or a nonradioactive label. The labeled probe is hybridized (typically overnight), and the tissue is then washed, dehydrated, and dried before being exposed, together with precalibrated standards to X-ray films. Hybridization signal is either examined autoradiographically with a computerized image analyzer as detailed above, or evaluated microscopically after the sections are dipped in photographic emulsion, exposed, developed, and stained *(15,16)*.

4. BRAIN CIRCUITS AND PATHWAYS

Knowledge of complex maps of neuronal circuits and pathways provides profound insights into how the brain and nervous system function. There is significant convergence and divergence of circuits and pathways between different brain regions that ensure efficient flow of neuronal information and its transformation into motor commands, emotional behaviors, and cognitive functions. In this section, we examine the anatomical organization of three functional circuits that exemplify the sophisticated architecture of the brain.

4.1. Basal Ganglia-Thalamocortical Circuitry

The basal ganglia consist of five interconnected subcortical nuclei that span the telencephalon, diencephalon, and mid-brain. These nuclei include the caudate putamen (CPu), globus pallidus (GP), subthalamic nucleus (STN), substantia nigra *pars* compacta, and substantia nigra *pars* reticulata (SNpr) *(17,18)*. The medium spiny neurons are the principle neurons in the CPu and contain the inhibitory neurotransmitter γ-aminobutyric acid (GABA). The medium spiny neurons receive the bulk of the incoming excitatory glutamatergic input from the cerebral cortex and a heavy dopaminergic input from substantia nigra *pars* compacta. These neurons, which constitute the only striatal output, send their projections via two major pathways. The *direct* or *striatonigral* pathway, in which the striatal neurons project directly to the SNpr, and the *indirect* or *striatopallidal* pathway, in which striatal neurons project to GP, then to STN and terminate in SNpr (Fig. 2). The two striatal pathways and projections from the GP to STN are GABAergic in nature. The STN, which receives an excitatory glutamateric input from the cortex, provides an excitatory output to both GP and SNpr. The SNpr sends GABAergic projections to the

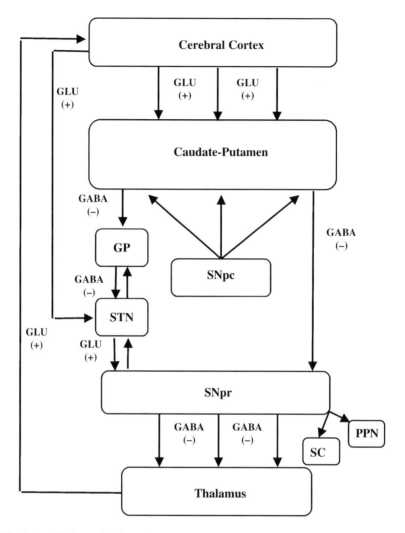

Fig. 2. Detailed organization of basal ganglia-thalamocortical circuitry. GABA, γ-amino-butyric acid, inhibitory [–] neurotransmitter; GLU, glutamic acid, excitatory [+] neurotransmitter; GP, globus pallidus; PPN, pedunclopontine nucleus; substantia nigra pars compacta [SNpc] and substantia nigra pars reticulata [SNpr]; STN, subthalamic nucleus; SC: superior colliculus (*see* text for details).

ventral anterior, ventral lateral, and mediodorsal thalamic nuclei, which in turn provide an glutamatergic input to the cerebral cortex (Fig. 2). SNpr also provides less prominent projections to superior colliculus and pedunclopontine nucleus.

The basal ganglia are involved in the programming and initiation of movement, particularly slow movements, and in motor memory and retrieval. DA plays a complex role within the basal ganglia as it appears to have a net excitatory effect on the direct pathway and an inhibitory effect on the indirect pathway. Therefore, DA can initiate programmed movement by stimulating the direct pathway, which activates thalamocortical projections and subsequently motor cortex, or can inhibit programmed movement by suppressing the activity of the indirect pathway and inhibiting activity of thalamocortical projections and their cortical inputs. The relative and balanced responsiveness of striatonigral and striatopallidal neurons to cortical glutamatergic input, nigral dopaminergic input, and the orchestrated interaction between different neurotransmitter receptors in the basal ganglia-thalamocortical circuitry determine the functional and behavioral outcome of the basal ganglia. Disorders of the basal ganglia may produce uncontrollable and involuntary movements as in Huntington's disease or restricted and rigid movements as in Parkinson's disease *(19)*. Additionally, abnormalities in the basal ganglia nuclei and/or their projecting targets have been linked to schizophrenia and motor extrapyramidal side effects associated with classical antipsychotic drug treatment *(1)*.

4.2. The Limbic System

The limbic system is the primary circuit of the brain that mediates feelings and emotionally significant stimuli *(20)*. The original circuitry, proposed by James Papez and also known as the Papez circuit, is comprised of cingulate gyrus, the parahippocampal gyrus, and the hippocampal formation, which includes the hippocampus, dentate gyrus, and the subiculum. Papez proposed that the hippocampal formation processes information from the cingulate gyrus and conveys it to the mammillary bodies of the hypothalamus via the fornix (the main fiber bundle that communicates the outflow of hippocampus). In turn, the mammillary bodies of the hypothalamus provides information to cingulate gyrus via anterior thalamic nuclei (Fig. 3) *(21)*. In the expanded limbic circuit proposed by Paul MacLean, several additional brain structures are included such as parts of the hypothalamus, the septal area, nucleus accumbens, orbitofrontal cortex, and the amygdala (Fig. 3). The amygdala is composed of many nuclei that are reciprocally connected to the hypothalamus, hippocampal formation, neocortex and thalamus. More recent clues indicated that the amygdala is the part of the limbic system being specifically involved in mediating emotional feelings, whereas the hippocampus, the mammillary bodies, and anterior thalamic nuclei are more involved in cognitive forms of memory storage *(21,22)*. Maldevelopment of neuronal connectivity between different components of limbic brain structures, and subsequent dysfunction in information processing within the limbic system and among closely associated structures and regions may contribute to the pathophysiology of several neurological and psychiatric disorders, as detailed in the following chapters.

4.3. The Cortico-Striato-Pallido-Mescencephalic Circuitry

Cortico-striato-pallido-mescencephalic circuitry also mediates cognitive and affective behaviors. This circuit is implicated in the pathophysiology of schizo-

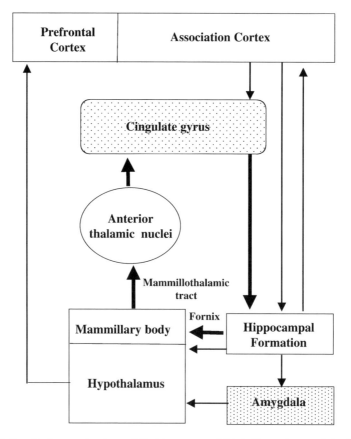

Fig. 3. Detailed organization of limbic system. Thick lines show original circuit. Fine lines show expanded circuit. The hippocampal formation includes hippocampus, subiculum and entorhinal cortex. The hippocampal formation projects via fornix to hypothalamic regions and via reciprocal connections to association cortex. Hypothalamic-cortical projections are indicated. (Diagram modified from ref. *21.*)

phrenia and Parkinson's disease, and it is modulated by several classes of drugs used for treatment of different neurological and psychiatric disorders *(23)*. An important brain region of this circuitry is the medial prefrontal cortex (mPFC), which can be subdivided into distinct subregions including the medial precentral, anterior cingulate, prelimbic and infralimbic cortices. These subregions receive afferents from the mediodorsal thalamic nuclei and basolateral amygdala. All of these areas receive dopaminergic afferents from the DA neurons in the ventral tegmental area (VTA). The mPFC sends projections to nucleus accumbens in addition to caudate putamen. These projections are topographically organized within the different subregions and each of these projections has distinct targets in different parts of striatum.

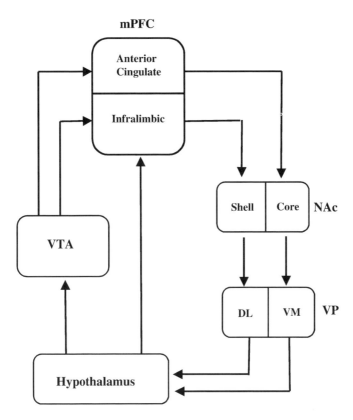

Fig. 4. Detailed organization of cortico-striato-pallido-mescencephalic circuitry. DL, dorsolateral; mPFC, medial prefrontal cortex; NAc, nucleus accumbens; VM, ventromedial; VP: ventral pallidum; VTA, ventral tegmental area (*see* text for details).

The nucleus accumbens integrates information from the mPFC, hippocampus, and amygdala, before transmitting signals to the hypothalamus and frontal cortex. The nucleus accumbens is subdivided into two compartments: the core and the shell. The core and shell receive separate excitatory glutamatergic projections from the MPC with the core receiving inputs from the anterior cingulate mPFC and the shell receiving projections from the infralimbic mPFC. The core of the nucleus accumbens projects to brain regions associated with the basal ganglia (e.g., the subthalamic nucleus, entopeduncular nucleus, and substantia nigra), although the shell projects to brain regions more closely involved with the limbic system (e.g., lateral hypothalamus and VTA). The nucleus accumbens also sends inhibitory GABAergic projections to the ventral pallidum (VP), with the core projecting to the dorsolateral part of the VP and the shell projecting to the ventromedial part of VP. The VP in turn sends GABAergic projection to the hypothalamus and VTA. This circuitry is schematically presented in Fig. 4.

5. NEUROIMAGING METHODS

The past decade has seen a tremendous increase in utilization of neuroimaging technology for research into neurological and psychiatric disorders. The most commonly used methods are emission tomographic techniques including positron emission tomography (PET) and single photon emission computed tomography (SPECT), and magnetic resonance techniques including imaging (MRI), functional imaging (fMRI), and magnetic resonance spectroscopy (MRS).

Each of these techniques is relatively noninvasive and has a high safety margin for most patients/research subjects. Each technique also has important advantages and limitations in terms of sensitivity, spatial or temporal resolution, safety, and cost. This section briefly describes PET, SPECT, MRI, fMRI, and MRS methods and applications in neurological and psychiatric diagnosis and research. Although detailed technical descriptions are beyond the scope of this section, references are provided that will allow interested readers to learn more about the technical foundations for these methods.

5.1. Emission Tomography

PET and SPECT imaging are routinely used to study brain and other organ system blood flow, metabolism (glucose uptake or oxygen utilization), drug pharmacodynamics, and pharmacokinetics, neurotransmitter synthesis and release, receptor distribution and density (DA, 5-HT, NE, their transporters, and other receptor systems), enzyme function, and BBB transport in healthy and diseased patients. PET and SPECT imaging utilize chemical probes containing radioactive atoms (radionuclides) to allow detection of these biological phenomena (Table 1). Some probes are identical to endogenous molecules of biological interest that have had a radioactive atom (radioisotope) substituted in for a stable (nonradioactive) atom (e.g., the PET probe [^{15}O]water). Others, such as (^{18}F)fluorodeoxyglucose ([^{18}F]FDG), a glucose analog used to detect glucose uptake into brain and other tissues, are biologically active molecules with an added radioactive atom that does not alter biological activity . Some probes are synthetic compounds that have been developed to study specific phenomena; for example, (^{99m}Tc)hexamethylpropyleneamine oxime ([^{99m}Tc]HMPAO; a SPECT cerebral blood flow tracer). Radionuclide probes most often are administered intravenously, although other routes can be used. Once administered, these probes accumulate at sites in the body containing high concentrations of receptors or other types of association sites at which they have high affinity, or in regions in which blood flow or metabolism are increased. Their chemical nature determines probe tissue distribution patterns.

The process of radioactive decay generates the signals detected from these probes. Radioactive atoms are unstable and have a nuclear excess of protons that decay to form more stable nuclei. The decay process generates photons that can be detected by PET and SPECT scanners. The decay rate of a radioactive atom is referred to as its half-life, or the time it takes half the substance to decay to the more stable, nonradioactive material. Radionuclide half-lives differ substantially (Table 1)

Table 1
PET, SPECT, and MR Isotope Characteristics and Typical Uses

Technique	Isotope	Half-life (minutes)	Spatial resolution (meters)	Temporal resolution (seconds)	Typical uses
PET	^{15}O	2^a	$.001–.005^b$	10–30	CBF & CMR
	^{11}C	20^a	$.001–.005^b$	10–30	Receptor and transporter distribution, density, and pharmacodynamics, dopamine neurotransmission
	^{18}F	110^a	$.001–.005^b$	10–30	CMR (deoxyglucose uptake), dopamine synthesis, receptor distribution, density, and pharmacodynamics
SPECT	^{99m}Tc	360^a	$.005–.010^b$	60+	CBF, dopamine transporter distribution
	^{123}I	780^a	$.005–.010^b$	60+	Receptor & transporter distribution, density, pharmacodynamics
	^{133}Xe	7560^a	$.005–.010^c$	60+	CBF
MRI/fMRI/MRS	^{1}H	Stable	$.0001–.010^c$	$.05–300+^c$	Anatomy, fMRI, CBF, neuronal, glial and mitochondrial function, GABA and glutamate turnover
MRS	^{13}C	Stable	$.01^c$	$300+^c$	Intermediary metabolism, neuronal and glial function, GABA and glutamate turnover
MRS	^{17}O	Stable	$.01^c$	$300+^c$	CBF & CMR
MRS	^{19}F	Stable	$.01^c$	$300+^c$	Therapeutic drug (e.g., SSRI) distribution and pharmacodynamics
MRS	^{31}P	Stable	$.01^c$	$300+^c$	CMR (ATP, PCr), phospholipid turnover, pH determination
MRI/fMRI	^{157}Gd	Stable	$.001^c$	$.05–1+^c$	BBB patency, lesion enhancement, fMRI, smart contrast agents

[a] radioactive, with ionizing radiation exposure.
[b] does not include anatomical image coregistration errors.
[c] magnetic field strength-dependent.

ATP, adenosine triphosphate; BBB, blood–brain barrier; CBF/CMR, cerebral blood flow/metabolism; fMRI, functional magnetic resonance imaging; GABA, γ-aminobutyric acid; PET, positron emission tomography; MRI, magnetic resonance imaging; MRS, magnetic resonance spectroscopy; PCr, phosphocreatine; SPECT, single-photon emission computed tomography; SSRI, selective serotonin reuptake inhibitor (e.g., fluoxetine and fluvoxamine).

and range from about 2 minutes (^{15}O) to several days (^{133}Xenon). PET radionuclides generally have shorter half-lives than SPECT probes and must be generated (by a cyclotron) in proximity to the PET scanner, so that radiochemistry preparatory steps occur rapidly and radionuclides can be administered within the first few half lives after probe generation (e.g., <6 minutes for ^{15}O). Thus, PET probes can be more difficult to work with than SPECT probes. However, their shorter half-lives are considered advantageous in studies requiring multiple assessments over short time frames because some can be administered several times during the course of a single study. SPECT radionuclides with longer half-lives tend to offer much more flexibility in terms of preparatory steps and can even be prepared remotely from the administration site. However, their slower decay rates mean that subjects may experience higher radiation doses.

Although PET and SPECT radionuclide decays both result in γ-ray (photon) emissions, hence the term "emission" tomography, their decay and detection processes differ. PET radionuclide decay involves ejection of a positively charged electron (positron) from the nucleus. After traveling a short distance, the positron collides with an electron creating an "annihilation event" that produces two high-energy photons. These photons travel away from the collision site in the opposite (antiparallel) direction and are detected by two photon-sensitive crystals placed at opposite sides of PET camera circular sensor arrays. PET camera detectors are electronically linked and only register photons activating opposing crystals within a short time window (on the order of nanoseconds) as reflecting true radionuclide decay events. This detection scheme is termed "coincidence detection" and it ensures high sensitivity by reducing the likelihood that noncoincident photons, which can be generated as a result of random noise, photon scatter, or other events, contribute to PET images. Photon paths identified as originating from coincident photons are registered and their summation is used to form multidimensional images of radionuclide localization. The fact that multiple (as opposed to single) image planes are acquired and can be used for image construction makes this a tomographic, as opposed to a planar, imaging technique. Images can be filtered or otherwise corrected for confounding processes, such as attenuation or scatter, prior to final image generation.

In SPECT, radionuclide decay occurs when the extra nuclear proton attracts an orbital electron by a process termed electron capture, to form a metastable nucleus. This generates energy (80–160 keV) that is emitted in the form of a single γ-ray (photon). SPECT cameras use the collimation (definition: to make straight or parallel) process for image formation. Collimators contain many parallel narrow, channels that open to crystal photon sensors. Photons traveling parallel paths pass through the collimator and are registered and treated similarly to those in PET studies, with similar filtering and reconstruction methods applied to generate SPECT images. However, because collimators eliminate signals from photons traveling nonparallel paths, some photons are unregistered and their signal is lost. Another source of signal loss in SPECT occurs when photons originally maintaining trajectories parallel to collimator holes are diverted by interactions with soft tissue components. These "scattered" photons are excluded from image formation. The inverse problem also occurs when photons originally traveling in nonparallel paths are diverted into parallel paths to provide incorrect image localization information. Photon energy levels are substantially lower for SPECT (80–160 keV) than for PET radionuclides (511 keV), and SPECT photons can undergo more attenuation as they pass through tissues (via absorption or scattering) than PET radionuclides, further lowering SPECT image generation efficiency vs PET. Thus, SPECT is a less efficient image generation technique and tends to have lower spatial resolution and than PET. However, SPECT radionuclides have longer half-lives than PET radionuclides and thus can be handled more easily and synthesized remotely from the study site. Furthermore, SPECT typically costs less than half of PET. These advantages in part account for SPECT's widespread use.

Although both PET and SPECT are highly sensitive for detecting low concentrations of radionuclide-labeled probes (subnanomolar concentrations), this sensitivity requires sampling times on the order of multiple seconds to minutes, so that sufficient quantities of radioactive decays can occur and photon counts be accumulated for image formation. Although this temporal resolution is more than adequate to study many physiological processes, it presents some limitations in studies of processes that occur at rates on the order of one to several seconds. Additionally, neither PET nor SPECT produce high-resolution anatomical images of tissues under study. Their spatial resolution, on the order of millimeters, is adequate for many purposes, though some applications require image coregistration with high-resolution anatomical images (e.g., computed axial tomography [CT], or MRI) to precisely determine radionuclide localization. The image coregistration process itself has limitations and thus the spatial resolution of anatomically coregistered PET/SPECT images can approach but not equal that afforded by CT or MRI *(24–26).*

5.2. Magnetic Resonance

MRI, formerly referred to by the acronym NMR (nuclear magnetic resonance), is actually a family of techniques whose signals are generated as a consequence of several fundamental phenomena that when linked, permit structural imaging, fMRI, and chemical imaging (also known as MRS). The nuclear part of NMR refers to the fact that the technique is limited to molecules containing atoms with odd numbers of protons and/or neutrons, which possess net nuclear magnetic moments. MR-detectable atoms include hydrogen (^{1}H–protons and ^{2}H–deuterium), helium (^{3}He), lithium (^{7}Li), carbon (^{13}C), oxygen (^{17}O), fluorine (^{19}F), sodium (^{23}Na), phosphorus (^{31}P), and potassium (^{39}K). Thus, most atoms present in molecules of biological interest can be visualized with MR techniques. Moreover, all of these atoms are stable, nonradioactive isotopes, so, as noted above, MR studies are conducted without exposure to ionizing radiation. Thus, MRI techniques are inherently safer than those utilizing ionizing radiation (e.g., PET, SPECT, and CT imaging). This difference is especially important in repeated measures studies requiring multiple image acquisition sessions.

The magnetic part of NMR refers to the fact that when MR-visible atoms are placed in strong magnetic fields, their molecular spins become quantized into higher and lower energy states, oriented antiparallel and parallel to the main magnetic field (B_o), respectively. These spins behave like small gyroscopes and rotate around the B_o axis. As B_o increases, the energy difference between higher and lower spin states (determined by the Boltzmann constant) increases such that at sufficiently large B_o, a few excess spins drop down into the lower energy state and become unpaired. These unpaired spins serve as tracers for the rest of the paired (MR-invisible) spins in the substance of interest. For hydrogen atoms (^1H, protons) studied at 1.5 Tesla (1.5 T, equivalent to about 30,000 times the earth's magnetic field at Asian, European, and North American latitudes), roughly 10 out of every 1 million protons have unpaired spins in the lower energy state and are observable in MR studies. This is the reason that MR techniques are relatively insensitive (can detect micromolar or higher concentrations) when compared to PET or SPECT imaging.

In MR studies, once tracer spins have been generated by placing an object into a large magnetic field, a radiofrequency (RF) pulse at the resonance (larmor) frequency (determined by the nucleus under study and the field strength of the magnet, e.g., 63.87 MHz for protons at 1.5 T) is broadcast into the object. This is the resonance part of NMR. Tracer protons spinning at the resonance frequency absorb RF pulse energy and are boosted to the higher energy spin orientation (antiparallel to B_o). After the RF pulse is turned off, tracer spins begin relaxing back to the lower energy state, shedding their excess energy by *resonating* RF signals at the larmor frequency. Thus, MR can in some ways, like PET and SPECT, be considered an emission technique. Each MR-visible atom spins at a different resonance frequency at a given magnetic field strength, making it possible to selectively detect substances containing any MR-visible atom by choosing the resonance frequency at which to broadcast and absorb RF energy.

During relaxation, tracer spins rotate around the main magnetic field axis and their emitted energy is detected with highly sensitive antennas (e.g., volume, surface, or phased array coils) tuned to the larmor frequency. These antennas detect two different types of relaxation behaviors, longitudinal relaxation, also known as spin-lattice or T1 relaxation, and transverse relaxation, also known as spin–spin or T2 relaxation. Longitudinal relaxation is the process by which higher energy state tracer spins release their absorbed energy to the environment as they return to the lower energy state. Transverse relaxation is the process by which higher energy state tracer spins exchange energy with other local spins either within the same molecule or with other molecules in the object, as the entire spin ensemble comes to equilibrium. The parameters T1 and T2 reflect the times it takes half of the excited spins to return to equilibrium either with the main magnetic field (B_o) or with other spins in the object of interest, respectively, and T2 generally is much shorter than T1. MRI measures water relaxation behavior (T1 and T2) that is modulated in complex ways by its interactions with proteins and lipids in brain or other tissues. By timing image acquisitions to more heavily represent T1 or T2 behavior or their combination, one can acquire "T1-weighted," "T2-weighted," or "proton density" images, respectively. These image types offer different forms of tissue contrast. For example, in T1-weighted images (used to study normal anatomy), gray matter looks gray and white matter looks white, whereas in T2-weighted images (used to assess brain pathology), abnormal tissue is highlighted as bright or white. By manipulating image acquisition timing and thus T1 and T2 contrast, it is possible to study brain structure (and function) with many image contrast variations.

5.3. fMRI Techniques

5.3.1. Blood Oxygen Level-Dependent (BOLD) fMRI Technique

Perhaps the most well-known fMRI technique used in studies of neurological and psychiatric disorders is called BOLD fMRI. This technique is, as its acronym suggests, sensitive to changes in brain oxygenation that occur in response to focal activations associated with sensations, movements, thoughts, or their combinations. When brain is activated, local metabolism and blood flow increase to provide extra oxygen and glucose. However, by design, more oxygen is delivered than required to support increased metabolic demand, and this leads to oxygen oversupply and a net reduction in content of the endogenous MR contrast agent, deoxyhemoglobin (deOHb). Because the iron atom at the active site of deOHb (unbound to oxygen) is paramagnetic and distorts local magnetic fields (changing water T1 and T2), a reduced deOHb content improves local magnetic field homogeneity and increases image intensity. BOLD images obtained during activation are subtracted from baseline images, revealing areas of deOHb washout, which appear bright. BOLD imaging can be conducted at high speeds (~1 second) permitting dynamic studies of brain function. This speed, combined with the fact that BOLD data can be overlaid on sequentially acquired high resolution anatomical (MRI) images, makes fMRI optimal for localization studies of brain function.

However, although BOLD is extremely fast, versatile, and popular, the BOLD signal response is a complex and convoluted measurement of dynamic blood flow, volume, and oxygenation changes *(27)*, and it is difficult to determine absolute changes in any of these parameters with BOLD fMRI. Additionally, at conventional magnetic field strengths (~1.5 T), BOLD acquisition parameters strongly influence whether fMRI signals reflect intravascular events in large vessels (somewhat remote from activated neurons, typical of gradient echo acquisitions) or in small vessels (closer to the site of neuronal activation, typical of spin echo acquisitions). However, as magnet field strength increases, BOLD measurements tend to reflect extravascular events occurring within tissues. This fact, along with improved temporal and spatial resolution that can be obtained with stronger magnets, has driven an instrumentation trend toward the development of high field MRI scanners (>3.0 T). An excellent discussion of advantages and disadvantages of higher magnetic field strength scanning is presented by Kim and Garwood *(28)*.

In addition to BOLD contrast, other contrast mechanisms are used in fMRI studies. Some studies involve intravenous administration of contrast agents containing a chelated form of the lanthanide metal gadolinium, which is strongly paramagnetic and potently increases water T1 and T2 relaxation and alters image intensity. These agents are used clinically to determine blood brain barrier patency, but also can be infused dynamically to determine cerebral blood volume (CBV) and its responses to drugs or other challenges. Newer contrast agents containing novel paramagnetic atoms or particles (e.g., superparamagnetic iron oxide particles) also are under development. Additionally, "smart contrast agents" containing molecular structures that respond to specific biological processes are being developed *(29)*.

5.3.2. Arterial Spin Labeling (ASL) fMRI Technique

Active manipulation of the magnetization and relaxation properties of water flowing through blood vessels is the basis for the ASL fMRI technique, which generates images of blood flowing through vessels *(30)*. With this technique, the magnetization of blood water is altered by scan pulses and the resultant image is subtracted from a normal image taken from the same plane, revealing a blood flow image. This method is used to study brain blood flow abnormalities in many disorders and can be used dynamically to quantitatively assess blood flow responses to functional or chemical challenges.

5.3.3. Diffusion Tensor Imaging (DTI) Technique

Another scan type that is being used increasingly to identify and characterize white matter integrity and connectivity is DTI, which is a complex variant of diffusion weighted imaging. DTI applies multiple gradients over time to alter water magnetization in six or more directions, to identify three-dimensional water diffusion patterns. Water tends to diffuse more readily outside of or along neuronal or glial membranes (as opposed to within or across those membranes). As diffusion coherence, or anisotropy, increases, so does the DTI signal. The DTI signal is highest in white matter areas containing myelinated axons that form tightly packed water diffusion channels, through which water tends to diffuse unidirectionally. The technique is very sensitive to white matter disruption or damage, which reduces diffusion anisotropy and DTI signal.

5.4. Chemical Spectroscopy Techniques

5.4.1. Proton Spectroscopy

A chemical form of imaging, known as proton (^{1}H) spectroscopy (^{1}H MRS), is now widely used to study neurological and psychiatric disorders. Proton MRS studies (as well as MRS studies of other MR-visible nuclei including phosphorus, carbon, and so on) (Table 1) produce spectra containing several types of information including chemical environment (chemical shift and peak splitting) and concentration (peak amplitude) measures. MRS studies can acquire spectra from single brain cubes (voxels) and also can simultaneously acquire data from planar arrays of voxels using a technique called chemical shift imaging, which like imaging, applies combinations of gradients to localize spectral data from multiple voxels in two or three dimensions. The chemical shift (horizontal part of the spectrum at which a chemical peak occurs) of any particular functional group (e.g., methyl-, methylene-, or hydroxyl-) is determined by the magnetic field experienced by the hydrogen nucleus when it is in a large magnetic field. Electron-donating and -withdrawing groups produce more negatively and positively charged nuclei, respectively, and differentially alter chemical shift. Additionally, the hydrogen atoms attached to adjacent carbon atoms can magnetically couple with each other to induce peak splitting patterns in proton spectra.

In proton spectra, metabolites easily visualized include N-acetylaspartate (a marker for neuronal viability and perhaps mitochondrial function), choline-containing compounds (membrane phospholipids and other constituents), and a peak combining creatine and phosphocreatine (the latter of which is the high energy phosphorus storage form). Proton MRS also can be used to detect the main inhibitory and excitatory neurotransmitters GABA and glutamate. However, glutamate is both a neurotransmitter and an energy intermediate, and the neurotransmitter component is best assessed indirectly by measuring glutamine (the catabolite of glutamate neurotransmission, which is shuttled from glial to neuronal cells for resynthesis into neurotransmitter glutamate). MRS studies are the least sensitive of the techniques discussed in this chapter; sample volumes must be large (>1 cm^3) and sampling times are long (multiple minutes). Despite its limitations, the ability to acquire chemical information noninvasively makes MRS quite attractive for use in psychiatric and other types of brain research.

5.4.2. Other Forms of Chemical Spectroscopy

Other MRS forms also provide meaningful information on brain chemistry and metabolism, and can be used to quantify brain levels of therapeutic drugs (Table 1). For example, phosphorus spectroscopy (^{31}P MRS) detects both high-energy phosphate intermediates phosphocreatine and adenosine triphosphate (ATP), and can also be used to determine tissue pH and magnesium concentration. Fluorine spectroscopy (^{19}F MRS) can be used to detect the antidepressant fluoxetine in brain or other tissues, as well as other therapeutic compounds containing fluorine atoms. Lithium (^{7}Li) MRS has been used to determine brain lithium concentrations during therapeutic administration. Carbon spectroscopy (^{13}C MRS) can be used to detect signals from molecules involved in tissue metabolism including glucose, the neurotransmitters GABA and glutamate, as well as intermediary metabolism. Unfortunately, ^{31}P and ^{13}C MRS signals are only about 6 and 2% as strong, as the proton MRS signal, respectively. Thus, ^{31}P and ^{13}C MRS are even more limited in terms of spatial and temporal resolution than proton MRS. This has limited their use in psychiatric research to date. However, as noted previously, the MR sensitivity problem can be overcome in part by increasing magnet field strength. For further review of the advantages and disadvantages of higher strength magnets on MRS applications and for additional details on MR imaging methods and applications see Kim and Garwood *(28)* and Renshaw and colleagues *(31)*.

6. CONCLUSION

Principles of neural sciences represent a merger of molecular biology, neurochemistry, neuroanatomy, neurophysiology and embryology. Proper study of neurological and psychiatric disorders begins with the study of the brain. Understanding neuron–neuron communications and synaptic neurotransmission is necessary for considering how disruption of neural functions leads to brain disorders. Clinical treatment of these disorders has been greatly strengthened by novel insights into cellular neurobiology of neurons. Advanced neuroimaging techniques helped to identify brain regions and neural pathways that mediate normal emotional, cognitive, motivated, and motor behaviors, which are typically disturbed, at least in part, in patients diagnosed with neurological or psychiatric disorders.

ACKNOWLEDGMENT

This work was supported in part by NARSAD, NIH grants HM-68359, HD-043649 (FIT), and DA-017324 (MJK).

REFERENCES

1. Baldessarini RJ, Tarazi FI. Drugs and the treatment of psychiatric disorders. In: Hardman JG, Limbird LE, eds. Goodman and Gilman's The pharmacologic basis of therapeutics. 10th ed. New York: McGraw-Hill, 2001:485–520.
2. Baldessarini RJ, Tarazi FI. Brain dopamine receptors: A primer on their current status, basic and clinical. Harvard Rev Psychiatry 1996;3:301–325.
3. Cooper JR, Bloom EF, Roth RH. The biochemical basis of neuropharmacology. 8th ed. New York: Oxford University Press, 2003.
4. Lindvall O, Bjorklund A. Dopamine and norepinephrine containing neuron systems: their anatomy in the rat brain. In: Emson PC, ed. Chemical Neuroanatomy. New York: Raven Press, 1983:229–255.
5. Bylund DB, Eikenberg DC, Hieble JP, et al. International Union of Pharmacology nomenclature of adrenoceptors. Pharmacol Rev 1994;46:121–136.
6. Hieble JP, Ruffolo RR Jr. Functions mediated by b-adrenoceptor activation. In: Ruffolo RR Jr, ed. Progress in basic and clinical pharmacology, vol. 7, b-Adrenoceptors: molecular biology, biochemistry and pharmacology. Basel: Karger, 1991:1–25.
7. Tork I. Anatomy of the serotonergic system. Ann NY Acad Sci 1990;600:9–35.
8. Barnes NM, Sharp T. A review of central 5-HT receptors and their function. Neuropharmacology 1999;38:1083–1152.
9. Millan MJ. Improving the treatment of schizophrenia: focus on serotonin 5-HT$_{1A}$ receptors. J Pharmacol Exp Ther 2000;295:853–861.
10. Tarazi FI, Zhang K, Baldessarini RJ. Long-term effects of olanzapine, risperidone, and quetiapine on dopamine receptor types in regions of rat brain: implications for antipsychotic drug treatment. J Pharmacol Exp Ther 2001;297:711–717.
11. Tarazi FI, Campbell A, Yeghiayan SK, Baldessarini RJ. Localization of dopamine receptor subtypes in caudate-putamen and nucleus accumbens septi of rat brain: comparison of D$_1$-, D$_2$-, and D$_4$-like receptors. Neuroscience 1998;83:169–176.
12. Young AB, Frey KA, Agranoff BW. Receptor assays: in vitro and in vivo. In: Phelps M, Mazziotta J, Schelbert H, eds. Positron Emission Tomography and Autoradiography: Principles and Applications for the Brain and Heart. New York: Raven Press, 1986:73–111.
13. Sternberger LA. Immunocytochemistry. New York: Wiley, 1986.
14. Mudgett-Hunter M. Monoclonal antibodies. In: Fozzard H, Haber E, Jennings R, Katz H, Morgan H, eds. The Heart and Cardiovascular System. New York: Raven Press, 1986:189–201.

15. Eberwine JH, Valentino KL, Barchas JD. In Situ Hybridization in Neurobiology. New York: Oxford University Press, 1994.
16. Chesselet M-F. In Situ Hybridization Histochemistry. Neurobiology. Boca Raton: CRC Press, 1990.
17. Graybiel AM. Neurotransmitters and neuromodulators in the basal ganglia. Trends Neurosci 1990;13:244–254.
18. Gerfen CR. The neostriatal mosaic: multiple levels of compartmental organization. Trends Neurosci 1992;15:133–139.
19. Alexander GE, Crutcher MD. Functional architecture of basal ganglia circuits: neural substrates of parallel processing. Trends Neursci 1990;13:266–271.
20. LeDoux JE. The Emotional Brain. New York: Simon and Schuster, 1996.
21. Iversen S, Kupfermann I, Kandel ER. Emotional states and feelings. In: Kandel ER, Schwartz JH, Jessell TM, eds. Principles of Neural Science. 4th edition. New York: McGraw-Hill, 2000:982–997.
22. Aggleton JP. The contribution of the amygdala to normal and abnormal emotional states. Trends Neurosci 1993;16:328–333.
23. Deutch AY. Prefrontal cortical dopamine systems and the elaboration of functional corticostriatal circuits: implications for schizophrenia and Parkinson's disease. J Neural Transm 1993;91:197–221.
24. Malison RT. Positron emission tomography and single-photon emission computed tomography. Methods and applications in substance abuse research, In: Kaufman MJ, ed. Brain Imaging in Substance Abuse: Research, Clinical, and Forensic Applications. Totowa, NJ: Humana Press, 2001:29–46.
25. Volkow ND, Fowler JS, Wang GJ. Positron Emission Tomography and Single Photon Emission Computed Tomography in Substance Abuse Research. Seminars Nuclear Med 2003;XXXIII:114–128.
26. Fowler JS, Volkow ND, Wang G-J, Ding Y-S. 2-Deoxy-2-[^{18}F]Fluoro-D-Glucose and alternative radiotracers for positron emission tomography imaging using the human brain as a model. Seminars Nuclear Med 2004;XXXIV:112–121.
27. Logothetis NK, Wandell BA. Interpreting the BOLD signal. Ann Rev Physiol 2004;66:735–769.
28. Kim D-S, Garwood M. High-field magnetic resonance techniques for brain research. Curr Opin Neurobiol 2003;13:612–619.
29. Meade TJ, Taylor AK, Bull SR. New magnetic resonance contrast agents as biochemical reporters. Curr Opin Neurobiol 2003;13:597–602.
30. Wong EC, Buxton RB, Frank LR. Implementation of quantitative perfusion imaging techniques for functional brain mapping using pulsed arterial spin labeling. NMR Biomed 1997;10:237–249.
31. Renshaw PF, Frederick B, Maas LC III. Fundamentals of magnetic resonance. In: Kaufman MJ, ed. Brain Imaging in Substance Abuse: Research, Clinical, and Forensic Applications. Totowa, NJ: Humana Press, 2001:47–76.

2

Pharmacotherapeutic Principles of Neurological and Psychiatric Disorders

John A. Schetz

Summary

The pharmacotherapeutic management of neurological and psychiatric disorders relies primarily on the modulation of central nervous system (CNS) neurotransmission with drugs that intervene at chemical synapses. The receptors, transporters, and enzymes for the dopaminergic, serotonergic, and noradrenergic systems are the most common neuropsychiatric drug targets, because these neurotransmitter systems play a central role in the regulation of a range of cognitive and motor behaviors. The key to understanding or anticipating the clinical profile (dose–effect) of a particular drug is to have an appreciation for both its pharmacodynamic and pharmacokinetic properties.

Key Words: Psychiatric; neuroscience; pharmacology; pharmacodynamics; pharmacokinetics; synapse; G protein-coupled receptors; dose–effect; theory; disorder; neurotransmission.

1. INTRODUCTION

The appropriate, effective, and safe utilization of drugs in the treatment of disease requires a basic understanding of the dose–effect relationships of medications. Relating dose to effect requires a combined appreciation of pharmacodynamic concentration–effect relationships, or what drugs do to the body, and of pharmacokinetic dose–concentration relationships, or what the body does to or with drugs. For this reason, considerable attention is devoted to both the pharmacodynamic and pharmacokinetic aspects of drug therapies. The aim of this chapter is to provide a theoretical rationale that is necessary for appropriately interpreting the results of basic and clinical neuropharmacology studies and for understanding many of the drug treatment strategies commonly encountered in clinical neurology and psychiatry.

Approximately one-fourth of all drugs prescribed worldwide exert their therapeutic actions on CNS targets. Of the top five selling drugs in this category, three are antidepressants and two are atypical antipsychotics (1). The relative success of pharmacological intervention is highlighted further when one considers that these

From: *Current Clinical Neurology: Neurological and Psychiatric Disorders:*
From Bench to Bedside
Edited by: F. I. Tarazi and J. A. Schetz © Humana Press Inc., Totowa, NJ

drugs are treating an estimated 7–15% of the population who suffer from one or more of the neurological or psychiatric disorders discussed in this book. Currently, the biogenic amine neurotransmitter systems, and in particular dopaminergic, serotonergic, and noradrenergic receptors, transporters, and metabolic enzymes, cover the vast majority of neuropsychiatric drug targets. The reason for this is that the biogenic amine systems are key modulators of neuronal excitability, and the molecular components of these systems are located at chemical synapses, which are sites that are accessible to intervention by drugs.

2. THE CHEMICAL SYNAPSE
AS THE MAIN SITE OF DRUG INTERVENTION

Therapeutic approaches to modulating neuronal excitability at chemical synapses can be categorized as presynaptic and postsynaptic. Presynaptic strategies involve altering the levels of neurotransmitter in the synaptic cleft. This can be achieved by changing the amount of endogenous neurotransmitter released or available for release into the synaptic cleft, or by altering the amount of neurotransmitter taken back up (reuptake) into the presynaptic terminal. The dopaminergic synapse can be used as a specific example to illustrate these points (Fig. 1). For example, monoamine oxidase B inhibitors, such as selegiline, block dopamine (DA) degradation, which makes more DA available for release. Inhibitors of DA synthesis, such as α-methylparatyrosine, reduce the amount of DA available for release. Drugs like reserpine and tetrabenazine decrease vesicular-mediated release by blocking vesicular monoamine transporters, which prevents the storage of neurotransmitter into synaptic vesicles. Inhibitors of plasmalemmal DA transporters, such as buproprion or cocaine, block the reuptake of DA from the synapse, and thereby, keep levels of DA in the synaptic cleft high. Certain drugs, like the psychostimulant amphetamine, cause nonvesicular DA release by running the DA transporter in reverse. In some cases, receptors are located on presynaptic terminals that bind the neurotransmitter being released, e.g., a DA receptor located on a presynaptic dopaminergic terminal. When these so-called autoreceptors are stimulated they attenuate, and when blocked they facilitate, subsequent rounds of neurotransmitter release.

In contrast to presynaptic strategies, which alter the levels of endogenous neurotransmitter in the synaptic cleft, postsynaptic strategies modulate neurotransmission with chemical agents that act directly on postsynaptic receptors. For example,

---

Fig. 1. *(opposite page)* Schematic of a chemical synapse. The dopaminergic synapse is shown to illustrate the common points of drug intervention, which include presynaptic effects on dopamine synthesis, storage in synaptic vesicles, release and reuptake, and postsynaptic effects on postsynaptic dopamine receptors. Degradation is depicted as occurring at both presynaptic and postsynaptic sites, which reflects the different locations of the different metabolic enzymes (e.g., monoamine oxidases and catechol-*O*-methyltransferase *[2,3]*). *See* color insert preceding p. 51. (Copyright John A. Schetz, 2003.)

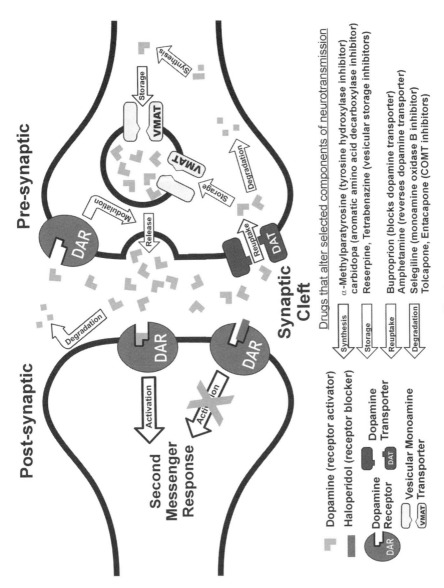

Fig. 1.

agonists, such as DA or the antiparkinsonian drug pergolide, directly activate DA receptors, whereas neuroleptic drugs like thioridazine and haloperidol block DA receptor activation.

3. CLASSIFICATION OF DRUGS ON THE BASIS OF THE RESPONSES THEY PRODUCE ON THEIR RECEPTORS

When a drug reversibly binds to the orthosteric (primary) site on its receptor one of four outcomes are to be expected: the receptor becomes activated, the receptor becomes partly activated, the receptor becomes inactivated, or the receptor is unable to be activated. Consequently, drugs are generally classified based on their actions. A drug is an agonist if it fully activates receptors, a partial agonist if it partly activates receptors, an inverse agonist if it inactivates receptors (and prevents them from being activated), or an antagonist if it only prevents receptors from being activated. For instance, the endogenous neurotransmitter DA is an (full) agonist of DA receptors, and the antiparkinsonian drug bromocriptine is a partial agonist at D_2 receptors. Antipsychotics like haloperidol and clozapine may be inverse agonists of D_2 DA receptors *(4,5)*, whereas L-741,626 is an (neutral) antagonist.

Receptor activation is a thermodynamic process, whereby agonist binding induces a conformational change in the receptor and converts it from the inactivated state (agonist low-affinity binding state) to the activated state (agonist high-affinity binding state). Typically, neutral antagonist binding is indifferent to the conformational (affinity) state of its receptor, because it must only occupy the orthosteric site rather than occupy and then induce a change in it. However, an inverse agonist is a special type of antagonist in that when it binds to a receptor in the activated state it converts it to the inactivated state. For this reason, inverse agonists reduce the basal levels of constitutive receptor activity, which corresponds to the (typically small) proportion of receptors that are in the activated state in the absence of agonist. Such distinctions in the molecular mechanisms of action of antipsychotic drugs that act on D_2-like dopamine and 5-hydroxytryptamine (5-HT)$_2$-like serotonin receptors may be critical to understanding their unique therapeutic profiles *(4,6)*.

Although most drugs bind directly to the orthosteric site of the receptor, other drugs bind at another (secondary) receptor site, called an allosteric site. Ligands that bind to the allosteric site are known as allosteric modulators, because they indirectly modulate the binding of primary ligands to the orthosteric site by remotely altering the orthosteric-binding site. The modulation is said to be positive if the modulator facilitates a primary ligand's interaction with the primary site or negative if the modulator attenuates its interaction with the primary site. The extent to which the allosteric site and the orthosteric site are coupled, or their cooperativity, can be weak or strong. Noncompetitive interactions, which result in a complete occlusion of the orthosteric site leading only to a decrease in the maximum density of sites with no change in affinity, are also allosteric in nature but they are a special case of neutral cooperativity. Within the DA receptor family, for example, a diverse range of allosteric mechanisms and corresponding allosteric sites exist for modulating the effects of endogenous and therapeutic agents *(7)*. For example, the endogenous tripeptide proline–leucine–glycine (PLG) is a positively cooperative allosteric modulator of agonist binding to D_2 DA receptors. Sodium ions are negatively cooperative allosteric modulators of agonist binding to D_2 DA receptors, and zinc ions are neutrally cooperative allosteric modulators of antagonist binding to D_4 DA receptors.

4. PHARMACODYNAMICS OF PHARMACOTHERAPIES

Chemical agents that have therapeutic actions are referred to as drugs. The term pharmacodynamics describes what drugs do to the body. Most drugs exert their actions on the body by interacting with specific sites called receptors. Consequently, pharmacodynamics deals with the interactions of drugs with their receptor sites. The most critical drug–receptor properties concern the strength of their attraction (binding affinity) and functional effects (potency) expressed in units of drug concentration, and the quantity of receptor in the target tissue (receptor density) or the maximal extent of a receptor's functional effect (efficacy). The density of receptor sites is typically expressed as moles receptor per amount of tissue, whereas the maximal functional effect, which relies in part on receptor density, is usually expressed as receptor activity per unit amount of tissue. The functional activity of a receptor can be measured by a variety of endpoints, ranging from changes in biochemical markers to behaviors.

Two coupled events occur when a drug interacts with its receptor. First the drug binds to its receptor, and second it mediates some functional effect that is transduced by the receptor. Although drug binding and receptor activation are coupled, they are mechanistically distinct molecular processes under the control of unique receptor microdomains and they can be influenced by different factors. Consequently, there may not be a direct one to one correspondence linking one process to the other.

4.1. Determination of Drug Affinity and Maximal Receptor Density: Ligand–Receptor Binding Interactions

The reversible (noncovalent) binding of a ligand with its receptor is a dynamic process, which is usually studied in one of two ways. The first way is to measure the kinetics of binding—the rate of approach to or departure from the equilibrium condition. The second way is to measure the free energy forces of binding under the equilibrium condition. It is helpful to review the general principles of receptor binding theory, in order to know what sorts of experiments to perform to extract kinetic and equilibrium properties of ligand–receptor binding interactions, and additionally, to know how to interpret the meaning of such properties in the context of drug therapies.

The theoretical construct that allows one to extract the properties that describe both kinetic and equilibrium types of ligand binding processes and the relationship between them is referred to as the mass action law. This law assumes that a ligand reversibly binds to a single homogenous population of receptor sites. Because the law is restricted to reversible reactions, which are those that can attain an equilibrium condition, the ligand–receptor interaction can be modeled as an equilibrium reaction. As with all equilibrium reactions, when equilibrium is achieved the rate of the forward and reverse reactions are equal; at equilibrium, the rate of ligand–receptor association equals the rate of ligand–receptor dissociation as shown in Eq. 1.

$$\text{Rate of association (forward reaction)} = \text{Rate of dissociation (reverse reaction)} \quad (1)$$

The rates at equilibrium can be expressed mathematically in terms of reactants and products as shown in Eqs. 2 and 3.

$$\text{Rate of association} = [\text{LIGAND}][\text{RECEPTOR}]k_{on} \quad (2)$$

$$\text{Rate of dissociation} = [\text{LIGAND·RECEPTOR}]k_{off} \quad (3)$$

in which

[LIGAND] is the ligand concentration expressed in units of Molarity (i.e., moles/liter)
[RECEPTOR] is the total receptor concentration expressed in units of Molarity
[LIGAND·RECEPTOR] is the ligand–receptor complex expressed in units of Molarity
k_{on} is the association rate constant for the binding of a ligand with its receptor expressed in units of $(s^{-1} M^{-1})$
k_{off} is the dissociation rate constant for the separation of ligand from its receptor expressed in units of s^{-1}

A mathematical model of receptor occupancy can thus be formulated from the theoretical expectation at equilibrium by substitution of the equalities in Eqs. 2 and 3 for those in Eq. 1 to yield Eq. 4.

$$[\text{LIGAND}][\text{RECEPTOR}] \, k_{on} = [\text{LIGAND·RECEPTOR}] \, k_{off} \quad (4)$$

Equation 4 can be rearranged such that all the concentration variables occur on one side of the equation and all rate constants occur on the other side as shown in Eq. 5. The ratio of the reactants (ligand and receptor) to products (ligand–receptor complex) thus equals the ratio of the rate of complex dissociation over the rate of reactant association.

$$([\text{LIGAND}][\text{RECEPTOR}])/[\text{LIGAND·RECEPTOR}] = k_{off}/k_{on} = K_D \quad (5)$$

These ratios are also equal to the equilibrium dissociation constant (K_D), which represents the concentration of ligand required to occupy half of the total number of receptors. The units of K_D are Molarity. A series of substitutions and algebraic manipulations to Eq. 5 *(8)* puts it in the general form of a rectangular hyperbola (Eq. 6) to yield Eq. 7.

$$y = ax/(b+x) \quad (6)$$

$$[\text{LIGAND·RECEPTOR}] = ([\text{RECEPTOR}][\text{LIGAND}])/(K_D + [\text{LIGAND}]) \quad (7)$$

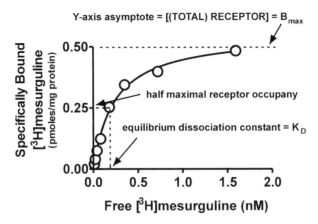

Fig. 2. Example of saturation isotherm data for [^{3}H]mesurguline equilibrium binding to cloned human serotonin 5-HT2C receptor expressed in COS-7 cells. A saturation isotherm experiment is conducted by keeping all conditions fixed while varying the concentration of radioligand. The K_D = 0.24 nM and Bmax = 0.5 pmoles/mg protein. (Copyright John A. Schetz, 2003.)

Separation of the dependent and independent variables allows for the graphing of the data and the extraction of the receptor-binding properties for a ligand that are the constants in the square hyperbola equation (e.g., a = [RECEPTOR] and b = K_D). In the laboratory, the amount of ligand that is specifically bound to its receptor ([LIGAND·RECEPTOR]) is measured as a function of various ligand concentrations ([LIGAND]), and then the [RECEPTOR] and K_D are solved for graphically (by applying a square hyperbolic math function). A common practice is to introduce a radioactive atom into the ligand (so that it can be detected), incubate various concentrations of this radiolabeled ligand in a solution containing a fixed amount of its receptor until equilibrium is reached, and then rapidly separate (so as not to disrupt the equilibrium condition) the radioligand bound to the receptor ([LIGAND· RECEPTOR]) from the unbound radioligand in solution ([LIGAND]). The radioactivity of the receptor-bound and (unbound) free radioligand is then quantified in a radioactivity counter. The resulting data obtained for such a saturation isotherm type of binding experiment is depicted in Fig. 2.

As can be seen from Eq. 5, the equilibrium dissociation constant can also be calculated by measuring the kinetic rates of ligand association and dissociation from its receptor as the binding reaction proceeds toward or away from the equilibrium condition. This can be accomplished by measuring the amount of radioligand bound to its receptor as a function of time. Kinetic determinations of K_D require two separate experiments (association and dissociation rates) for each K_D determination and provide no information on receptor density. Therefore, they are usually not the method of choice for determining equilibrium dissociation constant values.

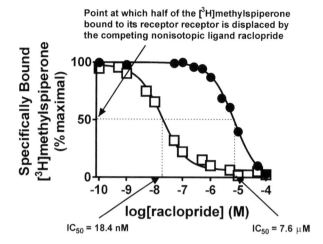

Fig. 3. Example of competition binding data for raclopride displacement of [³H]methyl-spiperone from cloned rat dopamine D_2 and D_4 receptors expressed in COS-7 cells. The IC_{50} is the concentration of competing ligand, which is needed to displace half of the radioligand occupying the receptors. Note that IC_{50} values are relative measures that are dependent on the concentration of radioligand employed in the experiment. In order to convert IC_{50} values to a concentration-independent equilibrium binding constant (K_i) a correction factor called the Cheng-Prusoff equation must be applied *(9)*. (Copyright John A. Schetz, 2003.)

Although saturation isotherms have the advantage that they are direct measures of affinity (K_D) and receptor density (B_{max}), relatively few radiolabeled ligands are available, and consequently the binding affinity for most ligands must be determined indirectly. The inhibition constant (K_i) is an indirect measure of a ligand's affinity for its receptor that is numerically equivalent to the equilibrium dissociation constant ($K_i = K_D$). In contrast to saturation isotherm experiments, in which the only ligand present is the radioligand, an inhibition type equilibrium binding experiment examines the ability of a nonisotopic ligand to compete with the radioligand for binding to the receptor site. The inhibition binding experiment is performed with a fixed concentration of radioligand and receptor vs increasing concentrations of competing ligand. An inhibition affinity constant for the nonisotopic ligand is derived from its IC_{50}, which is the concentration of nonisotopic (cold) ligand required to displace half of the total amount of radioligand bound to the receptor (Fig. 3). The semilog dose–response curves for competition experiments take on a sigmoidal appearance. The relative IC_{50} value extracted from the sigmoidal dose–response curve is then converted, by applying the Cheng-Prusoff transformation *(9)*, to an absolute affinity value (K_i) that is independent of radioligand affinity and concentration. The competitive form of the Cheng-Prusoff equation (Eq. 8) is a measure of receptor occupancy at equilibrium that obeys the law of mass action, i.e., it assumes that the nonisotopic ligand binds the same receptor in the same manner as the radioligand—a perfectly competitive inhibition at a single homogenous population of receptor sites.

$$K_i = IC_{50}/(1 + ([RADIOLIGAND]/K_D)) \tag{8}$$

The K_D value in Eq. 8 corresponds to the affinity of the radioligand and the K_i value corresponds to the affinity of the competing ligand.

If the interaction is truly competitive then the linear part of the sigmoidal inhibition curve will have a negative slope equal to unity (pseudo Hill slope = 1). More shallow slopes can indicate more than one type of receptor, more than one affinity state for a single receptor or a negatively cooperative allosteric interaction. Steeper slopes indicate a positively cooperative allosteric interaction. For example, agonists can bind different conformational states of the receptor (e.g., high- and low-affinity states) with different affinities, and in these cases, the apparent slope will be shallow. When the slope is different from unity the assumptions of the law of mass action are violated and a true K_i value cannot be determined. In practice many ligand–receptor interactions are not perfectly competitive, which is sometimes indicated by reporting a relative inhibition constant ($K_{0.5}$). If the difference between high- and low-affinity states are large enough (e.g., approx 100-fold) the binding curve will be clearly biphasic, and in these cases, the binding interaction can be described with a two-state model. A simple competitive binding model is usually not appropriate for determining the equilibrium dissociation constants for allosteric modulators, because they are by definition not acting at the same site on the receptor as the primary ligand-binding site. Instead Schild-type null pharmacological methods *(10)* or complex kinetic methods *(11)* must be used, in order to assign an equilibrium dissociation constant that accurately reflects the binding interaction of the allosteric modulator with its allosteric receptor site.

4.2. Determination of Ligand Potency and Efficacy: Ligand–Receptor Functional Interactions

Although the description of the binding of a ligand to a receptor provides information about the affinity of the ligand for its receptor, it lacks information about what sort of response the ligand induces in the receptor once it is bound. In order to accommodate a response component, additional terms, which describe factors that affect the functional response can be incorporated into the framework of the receptor occupancy model outlined above. For example, the Ariens equation *(12)* expresses receptor activity as a fraction, $A_{fraction}$, of the maximal activity, A_{max}, and equates this activity ratio to the fraction of ligand–receptor complex ([LIGAND·RECEPTOR]) and the total amount of receptors ([RECEPTOR]) as shown in Eq. 9.

$$A_{fraction}/A_{max} = (\alpha[LIGAND \cdot RECEPTOR])/[RECEPTOR] \tag{9}$$

The term α is a proportionality factor that is an expression of the efficiency of the coupling of the binding of the ligand with its receptor to its subsequent activation of a receptor response. This efficiency of coupling term is an acknowledgment that some agonists, known as partial agonists, promote less than the optimal coupling that is required to produce a full response. Consequently, even at maximal receptor occupancy the maximal response for a partial agonist will be less than for a full agonist. In other words, the amount of receptor occupancy is not directly proportional to the relative amount of response if the ligand is not a full agonist. The quantity α thus represents the intrinsic activity of a ligand, which is generally defined as equal to one for the endogenous agonist, 0 for an antagonist, and in between 0 and 1 for a partial agonist. Because the endogenous agonist is assumed to be a full agonist, xenobiotic agonists that produce a greater maximal response than the endogenous agonist can have an efficacy greater than unity.

Inverse agonists are a special case of negative efficacy. The negative value is owing to the fact that low levels of receptor can, under normal circumstances, assume the activated state in the absence of agonist. This basal agonist-independent activated state is known as constitutive activity. The concept of negative efficacy is a result of defining the basal state (agonist-independent activity) as the 0 or baseline value for agonist-stimulated activity. Because inverse agonists bind to the activated (high-affinity) state of the unoccupied receptor and convert it to the inactivated (low-affinity) state, they inhibit basal activity and are said to possess negative efficacy. In contrast to an inverse agonist, an antagonist has no effect on basal activity and because it also is incapable of stimulating the receptor to produce a functional response it is said to have no efficacy.

From Eq. 9 it can be seen that two important factors controlling the measured functional activity of receptors in response to ligand binding are receptor density ([RECEPTOR]) and stimulus–response coupling efficiency (intrinsic activity, α). Like Eq. 7, which describes a saturation binding reaction, Eq. 9 describing the functional response also can be expressed in the form of a rectangular hyperbola (Eq. 6) to yield Eq. 10.

$$A_{fraction} = (\alpha \, A_{max}[\text{LIGAND}])/([\text{LIGAND}] + (1/K_D)) \qquad (10)$$

When plotted on a semilogrithmic scale the rectangular hyperbolic function takes on the form of a sigmoidal curve. Consequently, a plot of the fraction of functional response ($A_{fraction}$) vs the logarithmic concentration of drug (log[LIGAND]) can be fitted with Boltzman's equation describing sigmoidal functions (Fig. 4). The maximal function response or efficacy for a given ligand is the point in which the functional response reaches a plateau at higher concentrations of ligand (Fig. 4), although the concentration of ligand that produces half of the maximal response ($A_{fraction}/A_{max} = 0.5 = EC_{50}$) is defined as the potency. Both potency and efficacy are relative measures whose values rely in part on receptor density. Examples of the receptor mechanisms underlying the expected functional responses produced by ligands with different functional activities are depicted in Fig. 4.

The functional response term EC_{50} and the competitive ligand binding property IC_{50} bear some relation to one another, and although it is tempting to try to draw an analogy between them, there are some important distinctions. Both the EC_{50} and the IC_{50} are terms that correspond to concentrations of ligand that produce a half maximal measurement (i.e., activity or inhibition of binding). However, the IC_{50} is

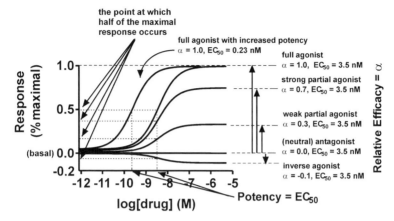

Fig. 4. Examples of responses for ligands with agonist, partial agonist, inverse agonist and (neutral) antagonist functional properties. The EC_{50} is the concentration of ligand that produces a half maximal effect, while the efficacy corresponds to the relative level of maximal effect, which can be denoted as intrinsic activity (α). (Copyright John A. Schetz, 2003.)

a measure of the ability of a competing ligand to inhibit the binding of a radioligand to its receptor that is both independent of receptor density and directly proportional to receptor occupancy. The EC_{50} is a measure of functional effect that is dependent on receptor density and not necessarily directly proportional to receptor occupancy. The reason that the functional response is not always directly proportional to receptor occupancy by ligand is that the strength of coupling between binding and response must be considered. This is not the case for a ligand–receptor-binding interaction because there is no additional coupling component to consider. This difference between binding interactions and functional responses is the molecular explanation regarding why, depending on the ligand's intrinsic activity and the conditions under which it is tested, a ligand's affinity value for its receptor may be different from its potency value.

5. PHARMACOKINETICS OF PHARMACOTHERAPIES

The clinical evaluation of a drug in vivo concerns dose–effect relationships, but the pharmacodynamic measures of the concentration–effect of drugs, described above, provide only part of the information. Relating dose to effect requires one to consider the dose–concentration relationships of a drug and then associate this with its concentration–effect relationships. A knowledge of pharmacokinetics, which is what the body does to or with a drug once it is administered, is key to understanding the relationship between drug dose and attaining a concentration of drug at the desired target site for an appropriate period of time to produce the intended therapeutic effect.

Because the drug targets for neuropsychiatric disorders are embedded in brain structures that are not readily accessible, drugs cannot be easily applied directly to the target tissues. Rather neuropsychiatric drugs must be introduced into the body at some distal site and then travel to their target sites in the brain. Of great importance to dosing is what happens to a drug once it is administered and en route to its target site. Although some drugs are applied intravenously in clinical trails, once their effectiveness is established most drugs are formulated for oral dosing. The oral administration of drugs is the preferred route of administration for clinical applications, because it eliminates safety concerns associated with the use of needles and it facilitates outpatient treatment. Following oral administration and on its way to its target site, a drug will encounter various biological barriers, metabolic tissues, and nontarget tissue deposition sites. The collective effect of these factors largely determines the amount of intact drug that is free to interact with the intended receptor target within a given time frame after dosing. Some critical pharmacokinetic parameters to consider for a drug are the time and concentration of its maximal blood levels, its apparent volume of distribution, its rate of clearance and its half-life. These parameters depend on the processes of drug absorption, distribution, metabolism, and excretion.

5.1. Absorption of Orally Administered Drugs and the Time and Amount of Maximal Drug Levels in Blood

For orally administered drugs, absorption begins with the transport of a drug from the gut to portal blood, continues as the drug passes through the liver, and ends when the drug reaches systemic circulation. If the drug is metabolized by the liver or its passage across the gastrointestinal barrier is incomplete, then the drug has reduced bioavailability. Bioavailability is defined as the fraction of intact drug that reaches the systemic circulation relative to the administered dose. With the exception of replacement strategies, such as L-DOPA treatment for Parkinson's disease, most drugs cannot utilize existing active transport mechanisms utilized by endogenous agents, and consequently, their transport properties are largely determined by passive diffusion across biological barriers. The rate and extent of oral drug absorption depends strongly on the physiochemical characteristics of the drug, the formulation state of the drug, and the gastric composition. Because the gut–blood barrier is comprised of cells with lipid membranes and aqueous interiors, the passive transport properties of a drug correlates well with partition coefficient measures of its preference for octanol (a lipophilic environment) over water (a polar environment). Consequently, octanol–water partition coefficients expressed as logarithmic values are frequently used to estimate a drug's absorption. Although it is true that lipophilic drugs are readily transported across lipid barriers, extreme lipophilicity is detrimental to transport. The reason for this parabolic nature of drug transport is that drugs with low lipophilicity will have a low probability of entering the lipid barrier, and those that are very lipophilic have a high probability of entering the lipid barrier but a low probability of leaving it. If a drug has an ionizable group, then the pH of the gastric contents can alter lipophilicity by changing the overall charge character of the drug resulting in altered absorption from the gut.

The drug formulation is another factor that can affect absorption of a drug. For example, oral formulations for the antiparkinsonian drug Sinemet® (L-DOPA plus carbidopa) can range from a rapidly absorbed liquid to a slowly absorbed capsule and even more slowly absorbed controlled release tablet. For many therapeutic applications it is desirable to gradually increase and then maintain steady blood levels, as rapid rises in blood levels of drugs can desensitize receptor responses or produce significant adverse side effects (e.g., nausea in the case of DA receptor agonists), and large changes in blood levels can result in fluctuating therapeutic responses. The blood adsorption characteristics of a drug that are usually of most interest are its maximal blood concentration and the time at which this maximum is achieved.

5.2. Distribution of Absorbed Drugs and Apparent Volume of Distribution

Distribution is a process involving the exchange of drug in systemic blood with tissues that it comes in contact with as it travels throughout the body. Circulating drugs can either remain soluble in the aqueous blood phase or they can be carried by blood components. Usually the carrier components in blood are proteins, but in rare instances, such as for the mood stabilizer sodium valproate, lipids can be the carrier. In many cases, the drug is not very tightly bound to blood components and it will prefer to associate with a tissue with which it comes in contact. Once the drug has transferred from blood to a tissue it is said to have been distributed or deposited. In certain cases, a drug may bind so tightly to carrier proteins that it cannot readily dissociate and interact with other tissues, and the blood proteins then act as a nontarget tissue deposition sites. Such tightly protein-bound drugs are usually therapeutically inactive in vivo.

Distribution can be a complex process requiring passage across more than one barrier that separates biological compartments. For example, neuropsychiatric drugs must cross the bloodbrain barrier (central nervous system compartment) before they can cross the cellular membrane barriers (cellular compartment) surrounding their target tissues in the brain. Some drugs can redistribute themselves to the periphery once deposited in the brain, but this effect is rarely significant for neuropsychiatric drugs. More relevant to the pharmacokinetics of neuropsychiatric drugs is the distribution of antipsychotic and antidepressant drugs into lipophilic stores such as fat. The reason for this is that antipsychotic and antidepressant drugs tend to be very lipophilic owing to having a number of aromatic rings. Such antipsychotic or antidepressant drugs can remain intact when stored in fatty tissues, and they can be slowly released over time, which can account for their sometimes long washout period. On the other hand, the antimania drug lithium is a very water-soluble elemental ion that distributes in a manner similar to bulk water. Lithium is also unique among neuropsychiatric agents in that it is not protein bound, and it is primarily transported into cells via passage through voltage-dependent sodium channels. Once inside cells, lithium is only slowly released, because it does not substitute for sodium for active transport through the sodium-potassium pump.

A useful parameter for describing drug distribution is the volume of distribution (V_d), which is an apparent measure of the accessible space in the body that is available to contain a drug. It can be defined as the ratio of the amount of drug in the body to the concentration present in the aqueous portion of blood (blood water) as shown in Eq. 11.

$$V_d = \text{amount of drug/concentration of drug in blood water} \tag{11}$$

V_d is only an apparent value, because it often does not relate to the real volume of the body. Instead, V_d is an operational definition that relates to a volume that would be required to homogeneously contain drug at the concentration found in blood. Large volumes of distribution indicate that the amount of drug measured in the blood is low as a result of distribution of the remaining drug into various tissues. Drugs that are not highly bound to blood constituents and that readily distribute into body tissues will have larger volumes of distribution. Note that the V_d values apply to intravenously administered drugs, unless an orally administered drug is completely or almost completely bioavailable, otherwise V_d values for an orally administered drug must be estimated by multiplying V_d by drug bioavailability.

5.3. Termination of Drug Responses

A drug response is terminated by excreting the drug from the body or by metabolically inactivating it. The excretion of a drug from the body depends on its clearance. Systemic clearance is a process by which the portion of drug that it is not metabolized and not protein-bound is removed from systemic circulation by hepatic excretion into the bile and/or by renal excretion into the urine. Renal excretion is common for small or polar drugs. For the majority of neuropsychiatric drugs at the doses utilized in clinical settings, the clearance is assumed to be a first-order process and is constant.

Another parameter that describes the elimination of drug is the elimination rate constant (K_e). The constant K_e is the fraction of drug excreted at any instant in time, and it is a function of clearance and volume of distribution as shown in Eq. 12.

$$K_e = \text{systemic clearance}/V_d \tag{12}$$

The elimination half-life ($t_{1/2}$) is the time needed to eliminate half of the drug from the body. The K_e, or its related clearance and V_d values, can be used to estimate the elimination half-life ($t_{1/2}$) of a drug as shown in Eq. 13.

$$\text{Elimination half-life} = t_{1/2} = ((\ln(2))(V_d))/\text{systemic clearance} = (\ln(2))/K_e \tag{13}$$

The value $\ln(2)$ in Eq. 13 is the proportionality constant for the first-order elimination of half of the drug. The elimination half-life value can be utilized to estimate drug-dosing regimens, the time needed to achieve steady-state levels, and the time needed to wash out the drug following the last dose. In general, the time needed to attain steady-state drug levels, or to approximate the drug wash out period is estimated to be greater than five elimination half-lives.

The dependence of the elimination half-life on V_d is as a result of the fact that only drugs that are in systemic circulation and in contact with organs of elimination (e.g., liver and kidney) can be cleared, although drugs distributed into other tissues cannot. The clearance of many drugs relies on the rate of blood flow to the organs of elimination. In these cases, the functional status of the heart, as a result of age, disease, or drugs that alter cardiac function, can significantly affect clearance, because blood flow rate is altered. The functional status of the major organs of elimination, owing to disease or age, for example, can also affect clearance rates, and consequently, the elimination half-life of drugs that are cleared by these organs. For example, impaired renal function, which is common in the elderly populations, can essentially double the elimination half-life of lithium as it is primarily cleared by the kidney *(13)*.

Although clearance is often the predominant factor in the termination of responses for drugs with low-molecular weights or significant polarity, most drugs used to treat neuropsychiatric disorders tend to be lipophilic and to have relatively large molecular volumes. Thus, the majority of such drugs must undergo bio-transformation to more polar metabolites before they can be effectively excreted. The production of more polar metabolites can occur by enzymatic reactions that either induce or unmasked polar functional groups (phase I reactions), or that con-jugate endogenous polar groups like sugars and polar amino acids (phase II reactions), or both. For example, desimipramine metabolism involves hydroxylation followed by glucuronidation.

Although many drug metabolites are biologically inactive, some retain activity or have modified activity. A variety of drugs used to treat neuropsychiatric disorders have active metabolites. For example, desimipramine is an active metabolite of the tricyclic antidepressant imipramine, and norfluoxetine is an active metabolite of the selective serotonin reuptake inhibitor fluoxetine; in both cases the metabolites have the same targets as the parent drug. In other cases, the activity profile of the metabolites is significantly different from the parent drug. For example, buproprion selectively blocks the DA transporter over the norepinephrine (NE) transporter, although one of its hydroxylated metabolites gains significant affinity for the NE transporter *(14,15)*. In another example, the antipsychotic drug loxapine is metabolized to the antidepressant amoxapine, which converts it from a D_2 DA receptor-blocking drug to a drug with significantly more norepinephrine transport blocking activity. Consequently, the metabolism of drugs can either terminate their actions, by forming inactive metabolites, or when active metabolites are formed, metabolism can be an underlying reason for their unique pharmacological effects.

6. RECEPTOR RESPONSIVENESS AND TIME OF ONSET OF THE THERAPEUTIC ACTIONS OF DRUGS

The relationship between drug concentration and functional effect described in the sections above is for a single challenge of drug at a naïve receptor. Following prolonged or repeated occupancy, most receptors undergo changes in responsiveness or density that protects them from excessive stimulation or blockade. Such adaptive responses to the repeated application of drugs can have significant consequences with respect to their actions. For example, attenuated responsiveness may limit the effective therapeutic use of a drug, it may result in tolerance to side effects, or it may be the underlying cause for their effectiveness.

Persistent activation as a result of persistent receptor occupancy by agonists leads to a reduction in receptor responsiveness. In the case of G protein-coupled receptors (GPCR), such as DA receptors, NE receptors, and most serotonin receptors, attenuated responsiveness is characterized by three types of temporally and mechanistically distinct adaptive processes *(16)*. Persistent receptor stimulation by acutely administered agonists results in GPCR desensitization followed by internalization. Receptor desensitization is the result of an uncoupling of the GPCRs from their G proteins. This uncoupling involves a phosphorylation-dependent (e.g., by kinases) blocking by cytoplasmic accessory proteins (e.g., arrestins) of intracellular portions of the GPCR that interact with G proteins (e.g., the intracellular loops and cytoplasmic tail). Desensitized receptors then undergo internalization whereby GPCRs are redistributed from plasma membranes to intracellular membranes via endocytosis. In some case, the internalized receptors are resensitized by dephosphorylation in clathrin-coated vesicles and recycled back to the plasma membrane. Under conditions of chronic stimulation, internalized GPCRs are not resensitized; rather, they are downregulated, which leads to a reduction in receptor density owing to proteolytic degradation. In some cases, chronic stimulation is additionally associated with a reduction in the amount of newly synthesized receptor. Although most GPCRs display attenuated responsiveness following persistent activation, the rate and extent of this effect can vary considerably depending on the receptor subtype and drug pharmacokinetics. In contrast to persistent activation, persistent blockade of GPCRs can lead to receptor supersensitivity or receptor upregulation. Neurotransmitter transporters and metabolic enzymes can also display changes in responsiveness as a result of persistent occupancy, but the details of the molecular mechanisms are distinct from those described for GPCRs *(17,18)*.

The general expectation is that the onset of drug action will be a function of how long it takes for a drug to reach its target tissue and then act on its receptor, which in most cases is rapid. For instance, intravenous bolus injection of the appropriate dose of phenobarbital into the tail vein of a rat produces sedation in less than 1 minute. However, the rate of onset of the therapeutic actions of drugs used to treat neuropsychiatric disorders can vary considerably. The anti-attention deficit hyperactivity disorder effect of psychostimulants, like D-amphetamine and methylphenidate, produce dramatic changes in behavior that closely parallels the expected dose–effect relationship. In contrast, the onset of action of chronically administered antipsychotic or antidepressant drugs can be much longer, requiring weeks for a full therapeutic effect to be achieved. In these cases, the large disparity between the expected and actual time course of the therapeutic effect implies that clinical efficacy is not as a result of acute effects on the target receptor; rather, it is because of chronic compensatory changes in the target receptor (e.g., up- or downregulation of receptor density) or some other receptor system whose function is linked to the target receptors. For instance, the therapeutic effect of chronic antidepressant treatment may be as a result of desensitization of presynaptic autoreceptors, such as somatodendritic serotonin 5-HT1A receptors *(19)* or terminal serotonin 5-HT1B receptors *(20)*, and/or downregulation of serotonin transporters *(21)*. The end result of each of these effects is an increase in the level of synaptic serotonin. A chronic elevation in synaptic serotonin could be signaling changes in the levels of nuclear transcription factors, which then regulate the expression of genes related to neurotransmission, and this might also account for the delay between the onset of drug treatments and their therapeutic effect.

7. THE MEANING OF DRUG SELECTIVITY

When the term "selectivity" is used to describe a drug it can take on a variety of contextual meanings. Selective effects of drugs can be as a result of differences in potency, efficacy, or pharmacokinetic accessibility. However, drug selectivity usually refers to the binding affinity for one receptor (or a subfamily of receptors) over others. The most important factors to consider are the relative frame of reference and the magnitude of the drug selectivity. Although it may be possible to accurately measure a fivefold difference in the affinity for one drug over another in isolated tissue fractions or when dealing with cloned receptor systems, for whole tissue in vitro or in vivo work, in which a large number of potential receptor sites are available, at least a 200-fold difference in affinity is usually required to elicit a truly selective response. A selectivity window of this size allows for dosing that will result in a maximal occupancy of the intended receptor target with little or no occupancy at nontarget receptors. An important caveat with respect to drug selectivity is that the selectivity of any drug may be difficult to rigorously define, because it is not feasible to screen all known related receptor sites and a drug may bind to receptor sites that have yet to be discovered or pharmacologically characterized.

The term "frame of reference" refers to the number of competing targets for a particular drug. For instance, a compound like NGD 94-1 has an affinity that is over 500-fold higher for the D_4 subtype of DA receptor than for any of the other DA receptor subtypes (D_1, D_2, D_3, and D_5). It also has over a 500-fold higher affinity for the D_4 receptor than for other GPCRs (e.g., serotonin, sigma, and adrenergic receptors) for which it has been evaluated *(22)*. Thus, within the frame of reference of receptor sites that were tested, it can be said that NGD 94-1 is a DA D_4 receptor-selective drug. However, drugs this selective for a particular receptor subtype are not available for many key receptor systems. The antipsychotic haloperidol is a more prototypical example as it binds with high affinity to cloned D_2, D_3, and D_4 receptors (K_i = 1.2, 4.1, and 1.6 nM, respectively). Because haloperidol has less than a four-fold lower affinity for the D_3 subtype, its in vivo selectivity over the D_2 and D_4 subtypes is negligible. However, if the comparison is expanded to include the entire DA family of receptors, then it can be said that haloperidol is D_2-like selective, as it binds with higher affinity to all members of the D_2-like subfamily (i.e., D_2, D_3, D_4) than to the D_1-subfamily (D_1 and D_5, K_i = 63 and 124 nM, respectively). If our frame of reference is among serotonin 5-HT1A, 5-HT2A, and 5-HT2C receptors (K_i = 2425, 54, and 4475 nM, respectively), then haloperidol can be said to be 5-HT2A selective. If we extend our frame of reference to include both these serotonin receptor subtypes and the entire family of DA receptors, then haloperidol's selectivity can be said to be mixed and would thus more accurately be defined as being 5-HT2A/D_2-like receptor selective. For these reasons, quantitative in vitro tissue or in vivo studies often must be interpreted with caution, especially if one neglects to selectively block, with other selective drugs, known sites that are not of interest. For instance, low concentrations of the high-affinity serotonin receptor selective antagonist mianserin and the high-affinity D_1-like selective antagonist SCH23390 could be added to block 5-HT2A and D_1-like sites in brain tissue when using [^{3}H]haloperidol as a radioligand to detect D_2-like sites. By analogy, in vivo chemical lesioning with the neurotoxin 6-hydroxydopamine (6-OH) is usually performed in the present of a norepinephrine transporter inhibitor, like imipramine, to permit uptake (via catecholamine transporters) into dopaminergic, but not noradrenergic neurons.

8. TARGETED PHARMACOTHERAPEUTIC MANAGEMENT OF SELECTED SYMPTOM MODALITIES

Drugs that target dopaminergic and serotonergic, and to a lesser extent noradrenergic systems, are the ones most often encountered in the pharmaco-therapeutic management of the neurological and psychiatric disorders discussed throughout the following chapters. This may seem odd given the vast array of unique clinical symptoms observed for the different neuropsychiatric disorders, but sense can be made of this by realizing that the pharmacotherapies for neuropsychiatric disorders are largely palliative, and usually, they are designed to provide relief for only one of a range of symptom modalities encountered for each disorder. For example, antipsychotic drugs are prescribed for the treatment of disorders as divergent as autism, Tourette's syndrome, and schizophrenia, but their application is designed to alleviate different symptoms associated with each: aggression and self-injurious behavior for autism, repetitive motor behaviors for Tourette's, and psychosis for schizophrenia. Utilization of similar treatments for different neuropsychiatric symptom modalities is thus possible because of the key roles that the various dopaminergic pathways play in the modulation of a range of cognitive and motor functions.

ACKNOWLEDGMENTS

The author thanks Drs. Michael Oglesby, Robert Luedtke, and Anna Ratka for insightful discussions and helpful comments. This work was supported in part by grant R01 MH063162-01 awarded to J.A.S.

REFERENCES

1. Jones BJ, Blackburn TP. The medical benefit of 5-HT research. Pharmacol Biochem Behav. 2002;71:555–568.
2. Xu Y, Ito A, Arai R. Immunohistochemical localization of monoamine oxidase type B in the taste bud of the rat. Neurotoxicology. 2004;25:149–154.
3. Mannisto PT, Kaakkola S. Catechol-*O*-methyltransferase (COMT): biochemistry, molecular biology, pharmacology, and clinical efficacy of the new selective COMT inhibitors. Pharmacol Rev. 1999;51:593–628.
4. Hall DA, Strange PG. Evidence that antipsychotic drugs are inverse agonists at D_2 dopamine receptors. Br J Pharmacol. 1997;121:731–736.
5. Wilson J, Lin H, Fu D, Javitch JA, Strange PG. Mechanisms of inverse agonism of antipsychotic drugs at the $D_{(2)}$ dopamine receptor: use of a mutant $D_{(2)}$ dopamine receptor that adopts the activated conformation. J Neurochem. 2001;77:493–504.
6. Weiner DM, Burstein ES, Nash N, et al. 5-hydroxytryptamine2A receptor inverse agonists as antipsychotics. J Pharmacol Exp Ther 2001;299:268–276.
7. Schetz JA. Allosteric modulation of dopamine receptors. Mini-review. Med Chem. 2004; in press.
8. Limbird LL. Identification of receptors using direct radioligand binding techniques. In: Cell Surface Receptors: A short course on Theory and Methods. Martinus Nijhoff Publishing, 1986:51–96.
9. Cheng Y-C, Prusoff WH. Relationship between the inhibition constant (K_i) and the concentration of inhibitor which causes 50 percent inhibition (IC_{50}) of an enzymatic reaction. Biochem Pharmacol. 1973;22:3099–3108.
10. Ehlert FJ. Estimation of the affinities of allosteric ligands using radioligand binding and pharmacological null methods. Mole Pharmacol. 1988;33:187–194.
11. Christopoulos A, Kenakin T. G protein-coupled receptor allosterism and complexing. Pharmacol Rev. 2002;54:323–374.
12. Ariens EJ. Affinity and intrinsic activity in the theory of competitive inhibition. Arch Int Pharmacodyn Ther. 1954;99:32–49.
13. Ritschel WA. Pharmacokinetics in the aged. In: Pagliaro LA and Pagliaro AM, eds. Pharmacologic aspects of aging. Mosby, 1983.
14. Ascher JA, Cole JO, Colin, J-N, et al. Bupropion: a review of its mechanism of antidepressant activity. J Clin Psychiatry. 1995;56:395–401
15. Bondarev ML, Bondareva TS, Young R, Glennon RA. Behavioral and biochemical investigations of bupropion metabolites. Eur J Pharmacol. 2003;474:85–93.
16. Tsao P, Cao T, von Zastrow M. Role of endocytosis in mediating downregulation of G-protein-coupled receptors. Trends Pharmacol Sci. 2001;22:91–96.
17. Torres GE, Gainetdinov RR, Caron MG. Plasma membrane monoamine transporters: structure, regulation and function. Nat Rev Neurosci. 2003;4:13–25.
18. Kumer SC, Vrana KE. Intricate regulation of tyrosine hydroxylase activity and gene expression. J. Neurochem. 1996;67:443–462.
19. Hensler JG. Regulation of 5-HT1A receptor function in brain following agonist or antidepressant administration. Life Sci. 2003;72:1665–1682.
20. Blier P. Pharmacology of rapid-onset antidepressant treatment strategies. J Clin Psychiatry. 2001;62 Suppl 15:12–17.
21. Benmansour S, Owens WA, Cecchi M, Morilak DA, Frazer A. Serotonin clearance in vivo is altered to a greater extent by antidepressant-induced downregulation of the serotonin transporter than by acute blockade of this transporter. J Neurosci. 2002;22:6766–6772.
22. Tallman JF, Primus RJ, Brodbeck R, et al. NGD 94-1: identification of a novel, high-affinity antagonist at the human dopamine D4 receptor. J Pharmacol Exp Ther. 1997;282:1011–1019.

II Neurological Disorders

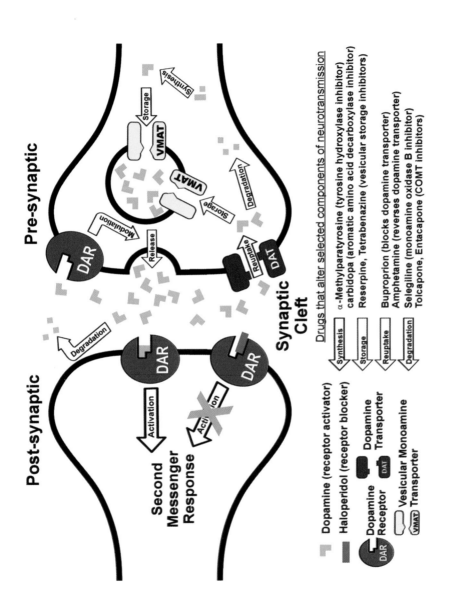

Color Plate 1, Fig. 1 (*see* full caption and discussion in Ch. 2, p. 30). Schematic of a chemical synapse.

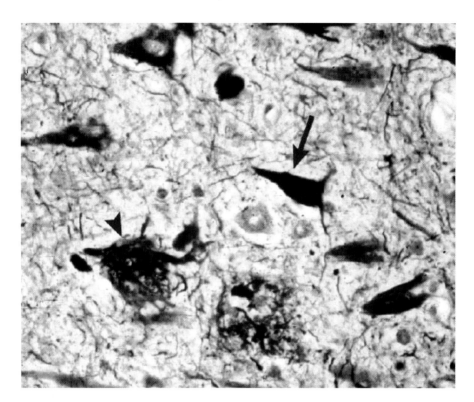

Color Plate 2, Fig. 1 (*see* full caption and discussion in Ch. 3, p. 52). Histopathological abnormalities in Alzheimer's disease (AD).

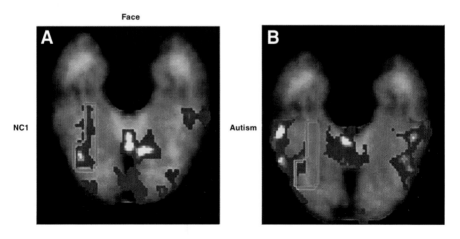

Color Plate 3, Fig. 1 (*see* full caption and disscusion in Ch. 7, p. 133). Composite activation maps superimposed on averaged anatomic images.

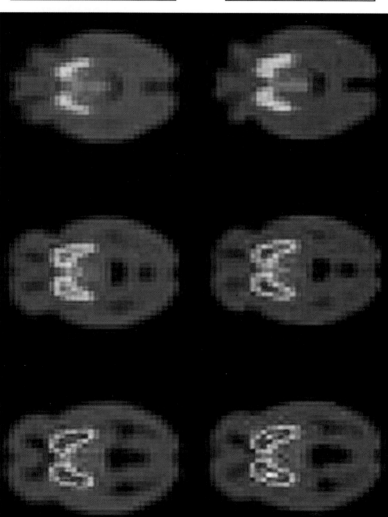

Group
means of 27
control
subject
adults

Group
means of 19
TS adults

Color Plate 4, Fig. 1 (*see* full caption and discussion in Ch. 8, p. 156). This figure depicts a false-color signal proportional to dopaminergic terminal innervation in axial views.

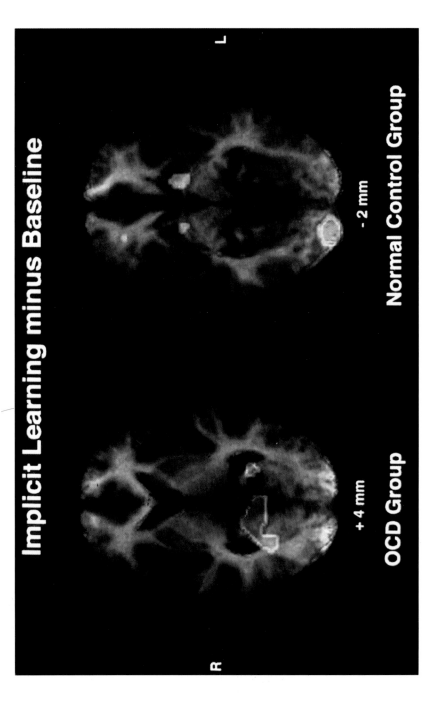

Color Plate 5, Fig. 1 (*see* full caption and discussion in Ch. 9, p. 173). Positron emission tomography demonstrates bilateral activation of the hippocampal/parahippocampal region of the brain in patients with obsessive-compulsive disorder.

3

Alzheimer's Disease

Mark P. Mattson

Summary

Cognitive impairment and psychiatric disturbances in Alzheimer's disease (AD) result from the dysfunction and degeneration of synapses, and consequent death of neurons, in the limbic system and associated regions of the cerebral cortex. A major molecular alteration in AD is increased amyloidogenic processing of the amyloid precursor protein (APP) resulting in increased production and accumulation of amyloid β-peptide (Aβ) in the brain. Aβ may promote synaptic dysfunction and can render neurons vulnerable to excitotoxicity and apoptosis by a mechanism involving oxidative stress and disruption of cellular calcium homeostasis. Some cases of inherited AD are caused by mutations in presenilins (PS)1 and PS2, which perturb cellular calcium homeostasis. Abnormalities in astrocytes, oligodendrocytes, and microglia have also been documented in studies of experimental models of AD, suggesting contributions of these alterations to neuronal dysfunction and cell death.

Key Words: Amyloid; apolipoprotein E; apoptosis; astrocytes; microglia; oligodendrocytes; presenilin.

1. BRAIN PATHWAYS

Alzheimer's disease (AD) is a devastating, and always fatal, neurodegenerative disorder characterized by progressive impairment of cognitive function and emotional disturbances *(1)*. AD is most commonly associated with cognitive impairment that results from degeneration of neurons in brain regions involved in learning and memory including the hippocampus, entorhinal cortex, and basal forebrain. Within each of the latter brain regions, subpopulations of neurons are selectively vulnerable including CA1 pyramidal neurons in the hippocampus, layer 2 neurons in the entorhinal cortex, and cholinergic neurons in the basal forebrain. However, degeneration of neurons in limbic structures including the amygdala and frontal cortex, and in serotonergic and noradrenergic pathways also occur in AD *(2,3)*. Degeneration of the latter pathways may play a major role in the depression, anxiety, and anger of AD patients *(4,5)*. Brain-imaging analyses of AD patients have revealed significant atrophy of brain structures that control affective behaviors including the amygdala, hippocampus, and septal area *(6)*.

From: *Current Clinical Neurology: Neurological and Psychiatric Disorders:
From Bench to Bedside*
Edited by: F. I. Tarazi and J. A. Schetz © Humana Press Inc., Totowa, NJ

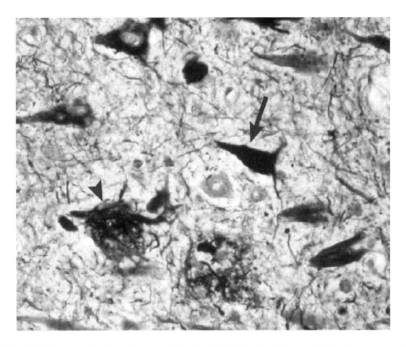

Fig. 1. Histopathological abnormalities in Alzheimer's disease (AD). A tissue section from the hippocampus of an AD patient shows the two cardinal features of AD, amyloid plaques with associated dystrophic neurites (arrowhead) and neurofibrillary tangles (arrow). *See* color insert preceding p. 51.

2. MOLECULAR MECHANISMS AND TARGETS

Two major histopathological alterations in AD (Fig. 1) are the accumulation of insoluble aggregates of the amyloid β-protein (Aβ) that form plaques, and the degeneration and death of neurons containing "neurofibrillary tangles," which are fibrillar aggregates of the microtuble-associated protein τ *(7)* (Fig. 1). Most cases of AD are sporadic with no clear genetic basis. However, some cases are caused by mutations in the amyloid precursor protein (APP), or presenilins (PS1 and PS2) *(8)*. The genetic mutations, and age-related increases in oxidative stress and metabolic impairment alter the proteolytic processing of APP such that increased amounts of a long 42-amino acid form of Aβ are produced. Aβ may promote neuronal dysfunction and death in AD by inducing oxidative stress and disrupting cellular calcium homeostasis *(8)*. Because of their high-energy demands and their subjection to heavy loads of ion fluxes and oxyradical production, synapses are particularly sensitive to the adverse effects of Aβ *(9,10)*. Aβ can activate apoptotic biochemical cascades in synapses that may be pivotal for the dysfunction and death of neurons that occurs in AD *(11,12)*. Several risk factors for AD have been identified, including apolipoprotein E (ApoE) genotype *(13)*, a high calorie intake *(14)*, elevated homocysteine levels and folate deficiency *(15)*, and reduced levels of intellectual and physical activities in midlife *(16)*.

Mutations in PS1 and PS2 are believed to cause AD, in part, by increasing production of the neurotoxic forms of Aβ *(17)*. However, studies of the pathogenic mechanism of PS1 mutations have revealed a role for perturbed cellular calcium homeostasis. When AD-linked mutant forms of PS1 are overexpressed in cultured neural cells or transgenic mice, the cells exhibit increased elevations of cytoplasmic calcium levels when stimulated with agonists, such as carbachol and glutamate, that induce calcium release from the endoplasmic reticulum (ER) *(18–20)*. The PS1 mutations increase the pool of ER calcium and may thereby render cells vulnerable to death induced by a variety of stimuli including trophic factor withdrawal and exposure to oxidative, ischemic, and metabolic insults *(19,21,22)*.

Inflammation-like processes occur in association with amyloid plaques and degenerating neurons in the brains of AD patients *(23)*. These inflammatory processes may be a response to neuronal degeneration, but may also be key events in the propagation of the disease process. Aβ may trigger activation of microglia and cytokine cascades involving tumor necrosis factor (TNF)-α and interleukin (IL)-1β *(24)*. Microglia express PS1 and PS1 mutant knock-in mice exhibit abnormal calcium homeostasis and an enhanced inflammatory cytokine response to immune challenge with bacterial lipopolysaccharide (LPS) *(25)*. The latter study showed that levels of TNF-α, IL-1α, IL-1β, IL-1 receptor antagonist, and IL-6 were induced by LPS to significantly greater amounts in the hippocampus and cerebral cortex of PS1 mutant mice as compared to wild-type mice. LPS also induced a greater increase in levels of inducible nitric oxide synthase and activation of mitogen-activated protein kinase in cultured microglia from PS1 mutant mice compared to microglia from control mice *(25)*. Oligodendrocytes, the myelinating cells in the central nervous system, may also be adversely affected in AD. As evidence, the vulnerability of oligodendrocytes to damage and death induced by demyelinating agents and glutamate is increased by AD-linked PS1 mutations *(22)*. Experiments in which cultured astrocytes were exposed to Aβ and related insults have suggested roles for perturbed calcium homeostasis *(26)* and impaired glutamate transport *(27)* in the pathogenesis of AD. Collectively, the available data suggest that abnormalities in glial cell function caused by Aβ, oxidative stress, and perturbed calcium regulation, contribute to neuronal dysfunction and death in AD.

It has recently become clear that adult mammals, including humans, contain populations of neural stem cells in their brains that are capable of proliferating and of differentiating into neurons—some of these newly generated neurons may integrate into circuits and become functional *(28)*. Such adult neurogenesis may even play an important role in learning and memory processes *(29)*. Although it is not known if neurogenesis is adversely affected in AD patients, recent studies of mouse models of AD suggest such a possibility. Hippocampal neurogenesis is impaired in APP mutant mice with Aβ deposits *(30)*. The latter studies further showed that subtoxic amounts of Aβ can impair neurogenesis in human neurosphere cultures. In other studies, it was shown that infusion of Aβ into the lateral ventricles of mice impairs neurogenesis in the subventribular zone *(31)*. There may be ways in which neurogenesis can be enhanced so as to prevent the onset or slow the progression of AD. Animal studies have identified three manipulations that can stimulate hippocampal neurogenesis—dietary restriction *(32)*, environmental enrichment *(33)*, and physical exercise *(34)*. These different environmental factors appear to act through a common pathway involving upregulation of brain-derived neurotrophic factor signaling *(14,35)*. Thus, it may be possible to reduce the risk of AD, and perhaps to the slow the progression of the disease, by environmental manipulations.

3. GENETICS

In rare inherited cases of AD, the alteration in APP processing results from mutations in APP itself or in PS1 or PS2 *(36)*. In contrast to sporadic forms of AD in which the age of disease onset is 70 years or older, the age of onset in familial AD cases caused by APP or PS mutations is typically in the age range of 35 to 50 years. The histopathological and clinical features of familial AD are indistinguishable from those of sporadic AD, although disease progression is typically much more rapid in familial AD cases. The APP mutations result in amino acid substitutions near or within the Aβ sequence, and each mutation increases the amount of Aβ, especially the 42 amino acid form of Aβ. Numerous missense mutations in PS1, and a few PS2 mutations are responsible for early onset autosomal dominant forms of AD. PS1 is an essential component of the γ-secretase activity that cleaves APP at the N-terminus of Aβ, and PS mutations may therefore increase production of Aβ. However, PS mutations may also perturb cellular calcium homeostasis in ways that render neurons vulnerable to synaptic dysfunction and cell death *(8,37)*.

In addition to disease-causing mutations in APP and PS, genetic factors may influence the risk of AD. One such genetic risk factor is the ApoE gene, which can encode one of three isoforms of ApoE (E2, E3, and E4). Individuals who inherit the E4 isoform of ApoE are at increased risk for AD, whereas those with one or both of the other two isoforms (E2 and E3) are at reduced risk *(38)*. Several hypotheses have been forwarded to explain how E4 increases the risk of AD. Three such possibilities include differential effects of the various ApoE isoforms on APP processing *(38)*, oxyradical metabolism *(39,40)*, and cellular calcium homeostasis *(41,42)*. Further studies will be required to better understand how ApoEs modulate neuronal plasticity and survival, and so influence risk of AD.

4. ANIMAL MODELS

Prior to the discovery of genes responsible for inherited forms of AD, animal models were based on the selective damage to neurons in brain regions in which neuronal degeneration occurs in humans with AD. For example, administration of the excitotoxin kainic acid to rats results in selective destruction of hippocampal pyramidal neurons and impairment of spatial learning and memory *(43)*. Injection of ibotenic acid or *N*-methyl-D-aspartate into the basal forebrain damages cholinergic neurons and impairs learning and memory in rats *(44)*. Once the amino acid sequence of Aβ was determined, synthetic Aβ was shown to be neurotoxic in cell culture and in vivo *(45,46)*. When administered into the lateral ventricles or basal forebrain of rats, Aβ can impair learning and memory *(47)*. Excitotoxins can induce some changes in τ and the cytoskeleton of hippocampal neurons similar to those seen in the neurofibrillary tangles *(48)*, suggesting a role for excitotoxicity in the pathogenesis of AD. Although informative, the lack of Aβ deposition in the toxin-based models, clearly made these animal models inadequate replicates of the human disease.

Once mutations in APP and PS were identified as being responsible for early onset autosomal dominant AD, transgenic mouse models were developed in which progressive plaque-like deposits of Aβ occur. Transgenic mice overexpressing the APP Swedish mutation exhibited Aβ deposits in the hippocampus and cerebral cortex and impaired performance in spatial learning tasks *(49,50)*. Interestingly, learning and memory impairment occurs very early in these mice, prior to the appearance of visible deposits of Aβ, suggesting that soluble oligomeric forms of Aβ may be neurotoxic. Mice expressing AD mutations in both APP and PS1 exhibit more rapid Aβ deposition and more severe deficits in spatial learning, as well as an increase in open field activity and motor dysfunction *(51)*. Transgenic and knock-in mice expressing disease-causing PS1 mutations exhibit no overt abnormalities, but neurons in their brains are more vulnerable to oxidative, excitotoxic, and apoptotic insults *(19,37)*. PS1 mutant transgenic mice exhibit enhanced hippocampal synaptic potentiation, which can be normalized by treatment with a γ-aminobutyric acid receptor agonist *(52,53)*.

Although τ mutations have not been linked to familial AD, they have been identified in families with the inherited disorder frontotemporal dementia and Parkinsonism linked to chromosome 17 (FTDP-17), a disorder characterized by extensive degeneration of neurons that accumulate neurofibrillary tangles indistinguishable from those in AD. τ deficient mice exhibit hyperactivity in a novel environment and an impairment in contextual fear conditioning *(54)*, suggesting a role for τ in regulating behavior. Most recently, a triple-mutant mouse model of AD ($3 \times$ TgAD mice) was produced, which express APP, PS1, and τ mutations *(53)*. In these mice, Aβ first accumulates intracellularly in CA1 hippocampal pyramidal neurons and neurons in layer IV of the neocortex. Subsequently, plaque-like Aβ deposits accumulate in the hippocampus and cortex and activated microglia are associated with these Aβ deposits. The $3 \times$ TgAD mice also develop progressive neurofibrillary tangle-like τ pathology in the hippocampus and cerebral cortex. Severe impairment of hippocampal synaptic plasticity occurs relatively early in the $3 \times$ TgAD mice, during a time period when intracellular Aβ begins to accumulate *(53)*. The abnormalities of CA1 and cortical layer IV neurons in the $3 \times$ TgAD mice is of interest from the perspective of the role of neuroendocrine stress in the pathogenesis of AD, because these two populations of neurons contain very high amounts of glucocorticoid receptors. Studies of other animal models of AD suggest a role for abnormal neuroendocrine stress responses in disease pathogenesis. For example, prolonged uncontrollable stress can promote neuronal degeneration and may contribute to neuronal degeneration in AD *(48)*. Additionally, recent studies have documented abnormal stress responses in APP mutant mice characterized by an enhanced glucocorticoid response and hypoglycemia following immobilization stress *(55)*.

Many of the features of AD in humans are reproduced in the $3 \times$ TgAD mice *(53)* including Aβ deposition, neurofibrillary pathology, synaptic dysfunction, and memory impairment. However, overt death of neurons has not yet been clearly established in this or any other transgenic model of AD. The reasons for the lack of neuronal death are unclear and it will be important to elucidate the cellular and molecular basis of this relative resistance of neurons to death in the mouse models.

5. DISEASE PREVALENCE

Obtaining accurate estimates of the prevalence rates for AD among populations throughout the world is difficult because there is no definitive premortem diagnostic test and symptoms similar to those in AD occur in other disorders. The available epidemiological data suggest that there are no major differences in the prevalence of AD among countries or ethnic groups. However, women have a greater risk of AD than do men. The prevalance of AD in the United States has been estimated in several studies *(56)* with the resulting numbers of AD cases ranging from 2 to 5 million in the year 2000. Taking into account the increasing number of individuals that live to more advanced ages in which their likelihood of developing AD increases, it is estimated that there will be 8 to 13 million Americans living with AD in the year 2050. The estimated health care cost for patients with AD is $38,000 per patient per year. The dire projections for large increases in the number of individuals with AD in the coming decades are, of course, based on the assumption that no effective means of preventing the disease are identified. In this regard, there is room for optimism based on recent research findings in several areas of investigation. One example comes from studies showing that dietary restriction is effective in protecting neurons from degeneration in mouse models relevant to AD *(57)* and that individuals with high-calorie intakes may be at increased risk of AD *(58)*.

6. SIGNS AND SYMPTOMS

Impairment of short-term memory is considered the behavioral hallmark of AD *(1)*. The memory deficits arise insidiously and progressively worsen over periods of years. Most patients die within 5 to 10 years of diagnosis, but some may live for several decades. In addition to memory impairment, anxiety, aggression, depression, perturbed sleep–wake cycles, and other behavioral abnormalities are prominent symptoms of patients with AD *(59,60)*. Severe behavioral problems are often the reason that AD patients are placed in a nursing home. AD patients are typically prescribed a variety of drugs to alleviate their psychiatric symptoms including antipsychotics, sedatives, and antidepressants *(61)*. Patients with AD often suffer from depression and aggression and agitation and these disturbances may occur very early in the course of the disease *(62)*.

Damage to serotonergic pathways is a likely explanation for the anxiety and aggressive behaviors of patients with AD. Genetic factors related to serotonin signaling may influence psychiatric symptoms in patients with AD as is suggested by a study showing that patients with AD homozygous for the long variant of a biallelic polymorphism of the serotonin transporter promoter region have an increased risk of aggressive behavior *(63)*. Links between psychiatric disturbances and polymorphisms in dopamine receptor genes have also been reported *(64)*.

7. PREVENTION AND TREATMENT

Advances are being made in identifying ways to prevent AD and to treat symptomatic patients. On the prevention front there are several promising approaches. Data from epidemiological and animal studies suggest that individuals with high-calorie intakes and elevated homocysteine levels are at increased risk of AD *(65,66)*. Dietary restriction or dietary supplementation with folic acid (which lowers homocysteine levels) can protect neurons against neuronal dysfunction and degeneration. By keeping homocysteine levels low, folic acid may prevent DNA damage and protect neurons against age-related oxidative and metabolic stress. In rodents, dietary restriction can enhance learning and memory during aging *(67)* and can protect synapses against insults relevant to AD pathogenesis *(68)*. Moreover, neurogenesis in the hippocampus is stimulated by dietary restriction in mice *(32,35)*, suggesting another way in which dietary restriction might protect against AD. Oxidative stress is thought to play an important role in various steps of the neurodegenerative process in AD, with production of superoxide anion radical, hydroxyl radical, peroxynitrite, and lipid peroxidation being increased in cell culture and animal models of AD, as well as in vulnerable brain regions of AD patients *(69,70)*. Dietary supplementation with antioxidants such as vitamin E, lipoic acid, and polyphenols might be expected to reduce the risk of AD, although this remains to be established. Because there is evidence that iron plays a role in the neurodegenerative process in AD, studies should be conducted to determine if dietary iron is a risk factor for AD.

Another promising approach for the prevention of AD is the use of a vaccine. When APP mutant mice with extensive amyloid deposits in their brains were immunized with aggregated forms of human Aβ1-42 much of the amyloid deposits were cleared from their brains *(71,72)*. Passive immunization with Aβ antibodies also resulted in a reduction in the amyloid burden in mouse models of AD *(73)*. Some data suggest that behavioral deficits of APP mutant mice can be improved by Aβ immunization *(74)*. However, the initial results of a clinical trial of an Aβ vaccine in patients with AD suggest that there are potential side effects of Aβ immunization including an encephalitis-like condition *(75)*. It has been suggested that, depending on the specific Aβ antibodies that the patient's immune system produces, the antibodies may either promote Aβ clearance and reduce neurotoxicity, or they may enhance the toxicity of Aβ *(76)*.

There are currently no treatments that can slow the progression of the neurodegenerative process in AD. However, some patients show improved memory when treated with acetylcholinesterase inhibitors *(77)*, and psychiatric/behavioral abnormalities can be relieved by drugs used to treat anxiety disorders and depression *(78)*. Acetylcholinesterase inhibitors are particularly beneficial in the early stages of the disease, presumably during a time period when cholinergic synapses are still present, but dysfunctional. There have been clinical trials of several promising approaches for slowing the neurodegenerative process including antioxidants such as vitamin E *(79)*, anti-inflammatory agents *(80)*, and estrogens *(81)*. However, no evidence of a clear slowing of the course of the disease was obtained in these studies. The vaccine—or passive immunization—approaches hold promise and the results of further clinical studies are eagerly awaited. Another approach that initial results suggest may prove effective in treating patients with AD involves administration of a copper-chelating drug called clioquinol, which was effective in removing amyloid from the brains of APP mutant mice, and is currently being evaluated in clinical trials in AD patients *(82)*. Finally, glutamate receptor-modulating drugs have proven beneficial in the treatment of AD patients *(83)*.

One continuing impediment to developing effective treatments for AD is the inability to identify patients in presymptomatic stages of the disease. Additionally, it would be of great value to identify healthy individuals with increased risk of AD. Early diagnosis will likely result in treatments that delay the onset of the disease.

GLOSSARY OF MEDICAL TERMINOLOGY

Alzheimer's disease (AD): A neurodegenerative disorder in which neurons in brain regions involved in learning and memory processes become dysfunction and die, and characterized by amyloid deposits and neurofibrillary tangles.

Amyloid β-peptide (Aβ): A 40- to 42-amino acid peptide generated by proteolytic processing of the amyloid precursor; Aβ is the major component of amyloid deposits in the brains of AD patients.

Amyloid precursor protein (APP): A transmembrane protein that is the source of Aβ; APP may normally function in the regulation of synaptic plasticity and cell survival.

Dementia: An impairment of cognitive function that is a major symptom of AD, but may also occur in other disorders including cerebrovascular disease.

Dietary restriction (DR): A reduction in the size and/or frequency of meals with maintenance of nutritional requirements; DR can increase life span and may reduce the risk of AD.

Hippocampus: A brain region that plays a central role in learning and memory processes, and a site of pathology in AD.

Homocysteine: An amino acid derivative of methionine that can promote damage to cells; individuals with elevated homocysteine levels are at increased risk of AD.

Membrane lipid peroxidation: An autocatalytic process in which free radicals attack double bonds in unsaturated membrane fatty acids resulting in the production of neurotoxic peroxidation products such as 4-hydroxynonenal.

Neurofibrillary tangles: Abnormal intracellular accumulations of fibrillar deposits of the microtubule-associated protein τ in neurons.

Neurogenesis: The process in which neurons are produced from neural stem cells; neurogenesis occurs in some regions of the adult brain and may be impaired in AD.

Oxidative stress: A circumstance in which levels of reactive oxygen species (e.g., superoxide anion radical, hydrogen peroxide, hydroxyl radical, and peroxynitrite) are such that oxidative damage to proteins, lipids, and DNA occurs to such an extent that it disrupts cellular functions.

Presenilins: Integral membrane proteins localized primarily in the endoplasmic reticulum; mutations in presenilins are responsible for many cases of inherited forms of early onset AD.

Synaptic plasticity: Changes in synaptic structure and function that occur in response to environmental demands including learning and memory

REFERENCES

1. DeKosky ST, Orgogozo JM. Alzheimer disease: diagnosis, costs, and dimensions of treatment. Alzheimer Dis Assoc Disord 2001;15:S3–7.
2. Engelborghs S, De Deyn PP. The neurochemistry of Alzheimer's disease. Acta Neurol Belg 1997;97:67–84
3. Buhot MC, Martin S, Segu L. Role of serotonin in memory impairment. Ann Med 2000;32: 210–221.
4. Braak H, Braak E, Yilmazer D, de Vos RA, Jansen EN, Bohl J. Pattern of brain destruction in Parkinson's and Alzheimer's diseases. J. Neural. Transm. 1996;103:455–490.
5. Kromer Vogt LJ, Hyman BT, Van Hoesen GW, Damasio AR. Pathological alterations in the amygdala in Alzheimer's disease. Neuroscience 1990;37:377–385.
6. Callen DJ, Black SE, Gao F, Caldwell CB, Szalai JP. Beyond the hippocampus: MRI volumetry confirms widespread limbic atrophy in AD. Neurology 2001;57:1669–1674.
7. Yankner BA. Mechanisms of neuronal degeneration in Alzheimer's disease. Neuron 1996;16: 921–932.
8. Mattson MP. Cellular actions of beta-amyloid precursor protein and its soluble and fibrillogenic derivatives. Physiol Rev 1997;77:1081–1132.
9. Mark RJ, Hensley K, Butterfield DA, Mattson MP. Amyloid beta-peptide impairs ion-motive ATPase activities: evidence for a role in loss of neuronal calcium homeostasis and cell death. J Neurosci 1995;15:6239–6249.
10. Keller JN, Pang Z, Geddes JW, et al. Impairment of glucose and glutamate transport and induction of mitochondrial oxidative stress and dysfunction in synaptosomes by amyloid beta-peptide: role of the lipid peroxidation product 4-hydroxynonenal. J Neurochem 1997;69:273–284.
11. Mattson MP, Partin J, Begley JG. Amyloid beta-peptide induces apoptosis-related events in synapses and dendrites. Brain Res 1998;807:167–176.
12. Mattson MP. Apoptotic and anti-apoptotic synaptic signaling mechanisms. Brain Pathol 2000; 10:300–312.
13. Smith JD. Apolipoproteins and aging: emerging mechanisms. Ageing Res Rev 2002;1:345–365.
14. Mattson MP, Chan SL, Duan W. Modification of brain aging and neurodegenerative disorders by genes, diet, and behavior. Physiol Rev 2002;82:637–672.
15. Mattson MP, Shea TB. Folate and homocysteine metabolism in neural plasticity and neurodegenerative disorders. Trends Neurosci 2003;26:137–146.
16. Friedland RP, Fritsch T, Smyth KA, et al. Patients with Alzheimer's disease have reduced activities in midlife compared with healthy control-group members. Proc Natl Acad Sci USA. 2001;98:3440–3445.
17. Esler WP, Wolfe MS. A portrait of Alzheimer secretases—new features and familiar faces. Science 2001;293:1449–1454.
18. Guo Q, Sopher BL, Furukawa K, et al. Alzheimer's presenilin mutation sensitizes neural cells to apoptosis induced by trophic factor withdrawal and amyloid beta-peptide: involvement of calcium and oxyradicals. J Neurosci 1997;17:4212–4222.
19. Guo Q, Fu W, Sopher BL, et al. Increased vulnerability of hippocampal neurons to excitotoxic necrosis in PS-1 mutant knock-in mice. Nat Med. 1999;5:101–106.
20. Chan SL, Culmsee C, Haughey N, Klapper W, Mattson MP. PS-1 mutations sensitize neurons to DNA damage-induced death by a mechanism involving perturbed calcium homeostasis and activation of calpains and caspase-12. Neurobiol Dis 2002;11:2–19.

21. Mattson MP, Zhu H, Yu J, Kindy MS. PS-1 mutation increases neuronal vulnerability to focal ischemia in vivo and to hypoxia and glucose deprivation in cell culture: involvement of perturbed calcium homeostasis. J Neurosci 2000;20:1358–1364.

22. Pak K, Chan SL, Mattson MP. PS-1 mutation sensitizes oligodendrocytes to glutamate and amyloid toxicities, and exacerbates white matter damage and memory impairment in mice. Neuromolecular Med 2003;3:53–64.

23. McGeer PL, McGeer EG. Anti-inflammatory drugs in the fight against Alzheimer's disease. Ann NY Acad Sci 1996;777:213–220.

24. Benveniste EN, Nguyen VT, O'Keefe GM. Immunological aspects of microglia: relevance to Alzheimer's disease. Neurochem Int 2001;39:381–391.

25. Lee J, Chan SL, Mattson MP. Adverse effect of a PS-1 mutation in microglia results in enhanced nitric oxide and inflammatory cytokine responses to immune challenge in the brain Neuromolecular Med. 2002;2:29–45.

26. Haughey NJ, Mattson MP. Alzheimer's amyloid beta-peptide enhances ATP/gap junction-mediated calcium-wave propagation in astrocytes. Neuromolecular Med. 2003;3:173–180.

27. Blanc EM, Keller JN, Fernandez S, Mattson MP. 4-hydroxynonenal, a lipid peroxidation product, impairs glutamate transport in cortical astrocytes. Glia. 1998;22:149–160.

28. Van Praag H, Schinder AF, Christie BR, Toni N, Palmer TD, Gage FH. Functional neurogenesis in the adult hippocampus. Nature 2002;415:1030–1034.

29. Feng R, Rampon C, Tang YP, et al. Deficient neurogenesis in forebrain-specific PS-1 knockout mice is associated with reduced clearance of hippocampal memory traces. Neuron. 2001;32: 911–926.

30. Haughey NJ, Nath A, Chan SL, Borchard AC, Rao MS, Mattson MP. Disruption of neurogenesis by amyloid beta-peptide, and perturbed neural progenitor cell homeostasis, in models of Alzheimer's disease. J. Neurochem. 2002;83:1509–1524.

31. Haughey NJ, Liu D, Nath A, Borchard AC, Mattson MP. Disruption of neurogenesis in the subventricular zone of adult mice, and in human cortical neuronal precursor cells in culture, by amyloid beta-peptide: implications for the pathogenesis of Alzheimer's disease. Neuromolecular Med. 2002;1:125–135.

32. Lee J, Seroogy KB, Mattson MP. Dietary restriction enhances neurotrophin expression and neurogenesis in the hippocampus of adult mice. J. Neurochem. 2002;80:539–547.

33. Kempermann G, Gast D, Gage FH. Neuroplasticity in old age: sustained fivefold induction of hippocampal neurogenesis by long-term environmental enrichment. Ann. Neurol. 2002;52: 135–143.

34. Cotman CW, Berchtold NC. Exercise: a behavioral intervention to enhance brain health and plasticity. Trends Neurosci. 2002;25:295–301.

35. Lee J, Duan W, Mattson MP. Evidence that brain-derived neurotrophic factor is required for basal neurogenesis and mediates, in part, the enhancement of neurogenesis by dietary restriction in the hippocampus of adult mice. J. Neurochem. 2002;82:1367–1375.

36. Hardy J. Amyloid, the presenilins and Alzheimer's disease. Trends Neurosci 1997;20:154–159.

37. Mattson MP, Chan SL, Camandola S. Presenilin mutations and calcium signaling defects in the nervous and immune systems. Bioessays 2001;23:733–744.

38. Cedazo-Minguez A, Cowburn RF. Apolipoprotein E: a major piece in the Alzheimer's disease puzzle. J. Cell. Mol. Med. 2001;5:254–266.

39. Miyata M, Smith JD. Apolipoprotein E allele-specific antioxidant activity and effects on cytotoxicity by oxidative insults and beta-amyloid peptides. Nat. Genet. 1996;14:55–61.

40. Pedersen WA, Chan SL, Mattson MP. A mechanism for the neuroprotective effect of apolipoprotein E: isoform-specific modification by the lipid peroxidation product 4-hydroxynonenal. J. Neurochem. 2000;74:1426–1433.

41. Hartmann H, Eckert A, Muller WE. Apolipoprotein E and cholesterol affect neuronal calcium signalling: the possible relationship to beta-amyloid neurotoxicity. Biochem. Biophys. Res. Commun. 1994;200:1185–1192.

42. Tolar M, Keller JN, Chan SL, Mattson MP, Marques MA, Crutcher KA. Truncated apolipoprotein E (ApoE) causes increased intracellular calcium and may mediate ApoE neurotoxicity. J. Neurosci. 1999;19:7100–7110.

43. Bruce-Keller AJ, Umberger G, McFall R, Mattson MP. Food restriction reduces brain damage and improves behavioral outcome following excitotoxic and metabolic insults. Ann. Neurol. 1999;45:8–15.

44. Boegman RJ, Cockhill J, Jhamandas K, Beninger RJ. Excitotoxic lesions of rat basal forebrain: differential effects on choline acetyltransferase in the cortex and amygdala. Neuroscience 1992;51:129–135.

45. Yankner BA, Duffy LK, Kirschner DA. Neurotrophic and neurotoxic effects of amyloid beta protein: reversal by tachykinin neuropeptides. Science. 1990;250:279–282.

46. Geula C, Wu CK, Saroff D, Lorenzo A, Yuan M, Yankner BA. Aging renders the brain vulnerable to amyloid beta-protein neurotoxicity. Nat. Med. 1998;4:827–831.

47. Tran MH, Yamada K, Nabeshima T. Amyloid beta-peptide induces cholinergic dysfunction and cognitive deficits: a minireview. Peptides 2002;23:1271–1283.

48. Stein-Behrens B, Mattson MP, Chang I, Yeh M, Sapolsky RM. Stress exacerbates neuron loss and cytoskeletal pathology in the hippocampus. J. Neurosci. 1994;14:5373–5380.

49. Hsiao K, Chapman P, Nilsen S, et al. Correlative memory deficits, Abeta elevation, and amyloid plaques in transgenic mice. Science 1996;274:99–102.

50. Chapman PF, White GL, Jones MW, et al. Impaired synaptic plasticity and learning in aged amyloid precursor protein transgenic mice. Nat. Neurosci. 1999;2:271–276.

51. Arendash GW, King DL, Gordon MN, et al. Progressive, age-related behavioral impairments in transgenic mice carrying both mutant amyloid precursor protein and PS-1 transgenes. Brain Res 2001;891:42–53.

52. Zaman SH, Parent A, Laskey A, et al. Enhanced synaptic potentiation in transgenic mice expressing presenilin 1 familial Alzheimer's disease mutation is normalized with a benzodiazepine. Neurobiol. Dis. 2000;7:54–63.

53. Oddo S, Caccamo A, Shepherd JD, et al. Triple-transgenic model of Alzheimer's disease with plaques and tangles: intracellular Abeta and synaptic dysfunction. Neuron. 2003;39:409–421.

54. Ikegami S, Harada A, Hirokawa N. Muscle weakness, hyperactivity, and impairment in fear conditioning in tau-deficient mice. Neurosci. Lett. 2000;279:129–132.

55. Pedersen WA, Culmsee C, Ziegler D, Herman JP, Mattson MP. Aberrant stress response associated with severe hypoglycemia in a transgenic mouse model of Alzheimer's disease. J. Mol. Neurosci. 1999;13:159–165.

56. Sloane PD, Zimmerman S, Suchindran C, et al. The public health impact of Alzheimer's disease, 2000–2050. Annu. Rev. Public Health 2002;23:213–231.

57. Zhu H, Guo Q, Mattson MP. Dietary restriction protects hippocampal neurons against the death-promoting action of a PS-1 mutation. Brain Res 1999;842:224–229.

58. Luchsinger JA, Tang MX, Shea S, Mayeux R. Caloric intake and the risk of Alzheimer disease. Arch. Neurol. 2002;59:1258–1263.

59. Aarsland D, Cummings JL, Yenner G, Miller B. Relationship of aggressive behavior to other neuropsychiatric symptoms in patients with Alzheimer's disease. Am. J. Psychiatry 1996;153:243–247.

60. Devanand DP, Jacobs DM, Tang MX, et al. The course of psychopathologic features in mild to moderate Alzheimer disease. Arch. Gen. Psychiatry 1997;54:257–263.

61. Stoppe G, Brandt CA, Staedt JH. Behavioural problems associated with dementia: the role of newer antipsychotics. Drugs Aging 1999;14:41–54.

62. Lyketsos CG, Steinberg M, Tschanz JT, Norton MC, Steffens DC, Breitner JC. Mental and behavioral disturbances in dementia: findings from the Cache County Study on Memory in Aging. Am. J. Psychiatry 2000;157:708–714.

63. Sukonick DL, Pollock BG, Sweet RA, et al. The 5-HTTPR*S/*L polymorphism and aggressive behavior in Alzheimer disease. Arch. Neurol. 2001;58:1425–1428.

64. Holmes C, Smith H, Ganderton R, et al. Psychosis and aggression in Alzheimer's disease: the effect of dopamine receptor gene variation. J. Neurol. Neurosurg. Psychiatry 2001;71:777–779.
65. Mattson MP. Gene–diet interactions in brain aging and neurodegenerative disorders. Ann Intern Med. 2003;139:441–444.
66. Mattson MP. Will caloric restriction and folate protect against AD and PD? Neurology. 2003;60:690–695.
67. Ingram DK, Weindruch R, Spangler EL, Freeman JR, Walford RL. Dietary restriction benefits learning and motor performance of aged mice. J. Gerontol. 1987;42:78–81.
68. Guo Z, Ersoz A, Butterfield DA, Mattson MP. Beneficial effects of dietary restriction on cerebral cortical synaptic terminals: preservation of glucose transport and mitochondrial function after exposure to amyloid beta-peptide and oxidative and metabolic insults. J. Neurochem. 2000;75: 314–320.
69. Mattson MP. Modification of ion homeostasis by lipid peroxidation: roles in neuronal degeneration and adaptive plasticity. Trends Neurosci. 1998;21:53–57.
70. Butterfield DA, Drake J, Pocernich C, Castegna A. Evidence of oxidative damage in Alzheimer's disease brain: central role for amyloid beta-peptide. Trends Mol. Med. 2001;7:548–554.
71. Selkoe DJ, Schenk D. Alzheimer's disease: molecular understanding predicts amyloid-based therapeutics. Annu. Rev. Pharmacol. Toxicol. 2003;43:545–584.
72. et al. A beta peptide immunization reduces behavioural impairment and plaques in a model of Alzheimer's disease. Nature. 2000; 408:979-982.
73. Mohajeri MH, Saini K, Schultz JG, Wollmer MA, Hock C, Nitsch RM. Passive immunization against beta-amyloid peptide protects central nervous system (CNS) neurons from increased vulnerability associated with an Alzheimer's disease-causing mutation. J. Biol. Chem. 2002;277: 33012–33017.
74. Morgan D, Diamond DM, Gottschall PE, et al. A beta peptide vaccination prevents memory loss in an animal model of Alzheimer's disease. Nature 2000;408:982–985.
75. Hock C, Konietzko U, Streffer JR, et al. Antibodies against beta-amyloid slow cognitive decline in Alzheimer's disease. Neuron 2003;38:547–554.
76. Mattson MP, Chan SL. Good and bad amyloid antibodies. Science, in press.
77. Lanctot KL, Herrmann N, LouLou MM. Correlates of response to acetylcholinesterase inhibitor therapy in Alzheimer's disease. J. Psychiatry Neurosci. 2003;28:13–26.
78. Tariot PN, Loy R, Ryan JM, Porsteinsson A, Ismail S. Mood stabilizers in Alzheimer's disease: symptomatic and neuroprotective rationales. Adv. Drug Deliv. Rev. 2002;54:1567–1577.
79. Rutten BP, Steinbusch HW, Korr H, Schmitz C. Antioxidants and Alzheimer's disease: from bench to bedside (and back again). Curr. Opin. Clin. Nutr. Metab. Care 2002;5:645–651.
80. Aisen PS. The potential of anti-inflammatory drugs for the treatment of Alzheimer's disease. Lancet Neurol. 2002;1:279–284.
81. Cholerton B, Gleason CE, Baker LD, Asthana S. Estrogen and Alzheimer's disease: the story so far. Drugs Aging 2002;19:405–427.
82. Bush AI. The metallobiology of Alzheimer's disease. Trends Neurosci. 2003;26:207–214.
83. Ferris SH. Evaluation of nemantine for the treatment of Alzheimer's disease. Expert Opin Pharmacother 2003;4:2305–2313.

4

Huntington's Disease

Susan E. Browne

Summary

Huntington's disease (HD) is an autosomal dominantly inherited, fatal neurodegenerative disorder, named for George Huntington, the author of the first definitive report of the condition in 1872. It is characterized by the progressive development of involuntary choreiform movements, although neuropsychiatric symptoms are sometimes the earliest and often the most devastating features of HD. These include detrimental emotional disturbances, behavioral and personality changes, and cognitive impairment. Gross pathological changes are restricted to the brain. Degeneration of specific basal ganglia neurons is a hallmark of HD, but dysfunction in multiple central nervous system pathways contributes to the motor and neuropsychiatric phenotype. HD is caused by an abnormal expansion of a trinucleotide repeat in the huntingtin gene. It is a relatively rare disease with highest prevalence rates of 5 to 10 per 100,000 found in Europe and the United States, whereas incidence is extremely low in Japan and Africa. The typical duration of disease before premature death is 15 to 20 years. Age of onset is associated with the size of the trinucleotide expansion and is generally in adulthood, although approx 10% of cases have juvenile onset. There are currently no effective treatments for the disease.

Key Words: Huntington's disease; trinucleotide; polyglutamine; neurodegeneration; striatum; movement disorder.

1. BRAIN PATHWAYS AFFECTED IN HUNTINGTON'S DISEASE

The motor and behavioral disturbances in Huntington's disease (HD) result from alterations in specific neurotransmitter systems and degeneration of selective neuronal subpopulations in the brain. The principal neuropathological feature of HD is progressive caudal to rostral degeneration of the neostriatum (caudate and putamen) *(1)*. A postmortem grading system classifies patients according to the extent of neuropathological severity at death, grades ranging from 0 to 4 with increasing severity and extent of striatal involvement. Grade 0 brains show 30 to 40% neuronal loss in the head of the caudate, with no visible gliosis. In grade 4 brains, the striatum is severely atrophic with neuronal depletion exceeding 95%, gliosis is

From: *Current Clinical Neurology: Neurological and Psychiatric Disorders: From Bench to Bedside*
Edited by: F. I. Tarazi and J. A. Schetz © Humana Press Inc., Totowa, NJ

extensive, and 50% of cases show cell loss in the nucleus accumbens. Most patients with HD reach grade 3 or 4 by the time of death, in which neuronal degeneration is evident in several nonstriatal regions including the globus pallidus (GP) and cerebral cortex, and to a lesser extent in thalamus, subthalamic nucleus, substantia nigra, white matter, and cerebellum. Cerebellar atrophy is particularly prevalent in juvenile-onset HD.

Striatal medium spiny projection neurons are most vulnerable to degeneration in HD. Positron emission tomography (PET) has demonstrated that the first clinical symptoms of the disease correlate with loss of 30 to 40% of striatal dopamine (DA) D_1 and D_2 receptors, which are localized on the medium spiny neurons *(2)*. These constitute 80% of all striatal neurons and are the principal input and output neurons of the striatum. They utilize the inhibitory neurotransmitter γ-aminobutyric acid (GABA), and subsets additionally contain either enkephalin (ENK), substance-P (SP), dynorphin, or calbindin. Aspiny interneurons containing nicotinamide adenine dinucleotide phosphate diaphorase (NADPH-d), neuropeptide-Y (NPY), somatostatin (SS), and nitric oxide synthase (NOS) are relatively spared in HD, but are eventually affected by the disease process. Striatal spiny projection neurons containing SP or ENK degenerate earliest in the disease, ENK-positive neurons projecting to the external segment of the globus pallidus (GPe) degenerating prior to SP-containing neurons that project to the internal segment (GPi). Neuronal degeneration eventually affects other brain regions and dysfunction within the cerebral cortex and limbic subcortical circuitry is thought to underlie the mood and personality changes prevalent in many HD patients *(3)*.

1.1. Neuropathologic Basis of Motor Dysfunction

The uncontrolled, hyperkinetic choreic movements typical of HD result from the disruption of basal ganglia–thalamocortical pathways that regulate movements *(4)*. Signals to stimulate initiation and execution of movements originate in the cerebral cortex in response to sensory afferent input. Excitatory glutamatergic efferents from the cortex innervate the neostriatum, which sends projections to other basal ganglia nuclei where signals are processed. Basal ganglia output nuclei (GPi, GPe, the substantia nigra pars reticulata [SNr], and ventral pallidum) then transmit "sorted" impulses to appropriate thalamic nuclei. From the thalamus, excitatory projections are sent back to topographically organized motor output areas of the frontal cortex to initiate execution of the appropriate motor response. The type of movement initiated thus depends on the combination of neostriatal neuron pathways activated, their downstream routing to the thalamus, and the resultant cortical activation (as discussed in Chapter 1). An imbalance in the relative contributions of the two regulatory basal ganglia pathways ("direct" mediated by GABA and SP, "indirect" mediated by GABA and ENK) triggers the motor dysfunction in HD and dictates its phenotype. In HD, there is preferential loss of the GABA/ENK neurons comprising the indirect pathway. Disinhibition of the thalamus and increased excitation of cortical motor output regions result (Fig. 1), manifest in HD patients by

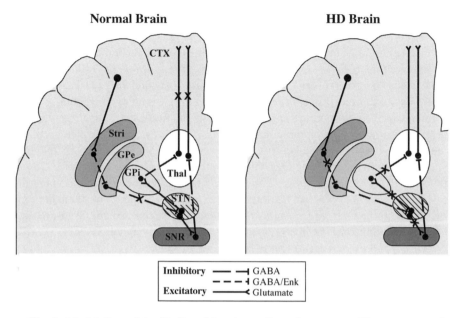

Fig. 1. Modulation of the "indirect" basal ganglia pathway controlling movement in Huntington's disease (HD). A representative diagram showing the major neurotransmitter systems involved in the indirect basal ganglia output pathways. Under normal circumstances (left), activation of the indirect pathway increases the inhibitory input to thalamic nuclei, resulting in reduced excitatory output to the cortex. Choreic movements in HD are thought to result from decreased activity of the indirect pathway as a result of loss of GABA/Enk neurons projecting from the striatum to GPe, reducing the tonic inhibition of the thalamo-cortical projection *(4)*. HD, Huntington's disease; CTX, cerebral cortex; GPe, Globus pallidus, external segment; GPi, Globus pallidus, internal segment; Thal, Thalamus; SNR, substantia nigra *pars reticulata*; STN, Subthalamic nucleus; Stri, Striatum. "X" represents pathways inhibited by presynaptic inhibitory input, or in the case of GABA/ENK Stri-GPe projection in HD, by neuronal loss.

the development of involuntary, unregulated choreic movements. The late onset of rigidity and akinesia in some HD patients is thought to be owing to disruption of the direct motor pathway following additional loss of striatal GABA/SP neurons. The predominance of bradykinesia in juvenile-onset HD results from simultaneous loss of SP and ENK neurons.

1.2. Neuropathological Basis of Psychiatric Symptoms

A number of psychiatric disorders are prevalent in HD, often occurring before motor symptoms. Although neuropathological pathways underlying these traits specifically in the context of HD are not well documented, these syndromes generally involve anatomical and neurotransmitter pathways that are disrupted by HD pathology. Common psychiatric syndromes including depression, apathy, mania, and cognition changes in HD generally involve dysfunction in the cerebral cortex and the subcortical limbic system.

Loss of cerebral cortex neurons is well documented in HD brain. At disease end-stage more than half the neurons in layer VI of frontal cortex that project to thalamus, claustrum, and other cortical regions are lost, and in excess of 70% of cortico-striatal projection neurons in layer V *(1)*. PET studies of cerebral glucose metabolism in presymptomatic and at-risk patients indicate cortical dysfunction prior to disease manifestation in many patients *(3)*. In particular, reduced cerebral metabolism in the prefrontal cortex of symptomatic and presymptomatic patients, and at-risk individuals, correlates with depression and increased suicide risk. Apathy is also associated with frontal lobe dysfunction. Bipolar disorder and mania are associated with alterations in neurotransmitter systems affected by HD pathology, including glutamatergic transmission in the cerebral cortex and striatum, and GABAergic transmission in cortex and hippocampus. Dysfunction and damage to neurons in the cerebral cortex and striatum, and subsequent dysfunction within synaptic projections from these regions to limbic structures including cingulate cortex and hippocampus are therefore likely to contribute to several of the emotional disturbances identified in HD.

2. GENETIC BACKGROUND

2.1. The HD Gene Mutation

HD is caused by a mutation in a gene on chromosome 4p16.3 termed *"huntingtin"* *(HD*; formally *IT15*, "interesting transcript 15") *(5)*. The mutation is an expansion of an unstable CAG repeat region in exon 1 of *HD* that is manifest as an expanded polyglutamine (Q_n) stretch in the 348 kDa protein product "huntingtin" (Htt). The polyQ stretch is associated with a proline (P)-rich domain. Wild-type *HD* in unaffected individuals contains 11 to 34 CAGs. Repeat lengths of 35 to 39 CAGs in one allele are variably penetrant, conferring the possibility of developing HD late in life, while the disease shows complete penetrance when triplet repeats exceed 39.

HD, generally a monozygotic trait, is considered a true dominant disorder with full penetrance because carriers with greater than 39 CAG repeats will develop the disease during a normal life span *(6)*. Homozygosity does not alter either age of onset, duration, or severity. Another disease trait is anticipation, whereby age of onset in an individual precedes that in their affected parent. Trinucleotide repeats of 27 or more are polymorphic and undergo alterations during meiosis, fluctuating by ±1 to 5 repeats per transmission with a bias toward expansion. Instability in spermatogenesis typically yields the largest expansions, meaning that anticipation is more pronounced following paternal inheritance. This characteristic contributes to the appearance of "sporadic" HD cases estimated to constitute about 8% of HD patients. Nonpenetrant but unstable repeats (27–35 CAGs) may expand to penetrant length during transmission, or expand owing to novel mutations. Other factors contributing to apparent sporadic onset include lack of knowledge of a family history of HD, for example because of adoption, no parental contact, or presymptomatic death or misdiagnosis of the affected parent.

Several features of the HD phenotype are influenced by CAG repeat length. Age of onset is inversely correlated with CAG expansion size, and especially long repeats (>55) confer juvenile onset. The most common repeat lengths of 42 to 50 generally correspond to symptom onset in the fourth and fifth decades, although the large variances in onset ages mean that repeat sizes in this range are often not accurate predictors for the age of symptom appearance. Disease severity, extent of neuropathological degeneration, and degree of DNA damage are all positively correlated with triplet repeat length. In contrast, rates of functional decline do not correspond with mutation size. It therefore seems likely that aspects of the disease process are influenced by extrinsic factors such as stochastic, environmental, or genetic modifiers. Genomic studies in HD families have revealed a number of genetic loci that may influence disease course including genes encoding ubiquitination enzymes (such as *UCHL1*, which encodes ubiquitin carboxyl-terminal hydrolase L1), the glutamate GluR6 kainate receptor subunit, and apolipoprotein E *(6,7)*.

Polymerase chain reaction (PCR)-based assays to quantify CAG repeat lengths are now available for confirmatory diagnostic testing, predictive testing in at-risk individuals, and prenatal testing in known mutation carriers (for review *see* ref. *8*). Linkage-based exclusion testing is offered to pregnant at-risk women who choose not to know their own gene status (termination is only an option if gene linkage analysis implies the fetus shows the same 50% genetic risk as the mother). Preimplantation testing of in vitro fertilized embryos is also available. Genetic testing is an emotive subject and testing procedures are closely governed by international guidelines. Genetic counseling is a prerequisite for participants. Current testing approaches are not 100% reliable, but identify CAG repeat number to within one or two triplets. Potential problems include interpretation of disease risk when CAG repeat lengths in the mutable or at-risk lengths are detected, which provide no accurate determination of the probability of disease onset or the risk of transmission to a child.

2.2 Htt Protein

Huntingtin (htt) protein was unknown until identification of the HD gene mutation in 1993, and the endogenous functions of both wild-type and mutant huntingtin have still to be definitively elucidated *(6)*.

2.2.1. Wild-Type Huntingtin (Htt)

A role in developmental apoptosis is suggested by observations that (a) mice entirely lacking the murine *HD* homologue gene *Hdh* die *in utero,* but heterozygous knock-out mice show little or no pathology, and (b) abnormally low levels of huntingtin expression are associated with developmental abnormalities. Huntingtin protein is ubiquitously expressed throughout the body. At the subcellular level it is present in multiple compartments with a largely cytoplasmic distribution in perikarya, axons, dendrites and some nerve terminals. The protein contains a nuclear export signal domain and at any given time approx 5% of the protein is found in the nucleus, suggesting that huntingtin shuttles between the nucleus and the cytoplasm. Reports of colocalization with synaptic vesicles and microtubules infer an involvement in trafficking, and possibly RNA biogenesis or signaling (*see* Section 3) *(9,10)*.

Htt is a large protein that takes on multiple conformations within cells, putatively as a result of multiple HEAT domains throughout the protein (approx 40 amino acid sequence repeats, named for the first four disease-related proteins this motif was identified in: <u>h</u>tt, <u>e</u>longation factor 3, regulatory <u>A</u> subunit of protein phosphatase 2A, and <u>TOR</u>1). HEAT repeats form hydrophobic α helices that can generate elongated superhelices. Htt binding with other proteins is facilitated by several protein components, including the HEAT superhelices, htt amino terminal, and the polyglutamine/proline tract.

2.2.2. Mutant Htt

Mutant htt's toxicity is a result of the gain of a novel function, rather than loss of wild-type huntingtin function, because (a) mice homozygous for the mutant gene still develop normally, and (b) expression of a single allele of mutant huntingtin is sufficient to rescue *Hdh*-null mice from death *in utero (6)*. Mutant htt is also expressed ubiquitously throughout the body and its distribution shows no apparent selectivity for cerebral regions targeted by the disease process, suggesting that another property of neurons within these regions confers vulnerability to htt toxicity.

Htt contains multiple cleavage sites and proteolytic processing of htt appears to be a normal physiological event *(11,12)*. Studies suggest that polyQ-induced toxicity is exacerbated in protein fragments, and is inversely correlated with fragment length. Therefore cleavage of mutant htt to generate N-terminal htt fragments encompassing the expanded polyQ region may contribute to htt toxicity. Htt fragments are most abundant in cortical projection neurons, suggesting that accumulation of mutant htt fragments contributes to cortico-striatal dysfunction in HD pathogenesis.

N-terminal fragments of mutant htt eventually form ubiquitinated sodium dodecyl sulphate-resistant protein aggregates in neuronal nuclei (neuronal intranuclear inclusions [NII]) and in dystrophic neurites (cytoplasmic inclusions). Aggregates have been identified in HD brain and in the brains of transgenic mice expressing mutant htt, but are not restricted to central nervous system (CNS) cells. Aggregate deposition patterns differ between CNS and somatic cells. In skeletal muscle cells, for example, aggregates are found solely within nuclei, whereas in the brain the bulk of aggregates are neuritic. The mechanism of inclusion formation is not yet known, but CAG repeat length is critical for aggregate formation and mutant polyglutamine stretches lend themselves to the formation of β-pleated sheets held together by hydrogen bonds between amide groups.

3. CELLULAR AND MOLECULAR TARGETS OF THE DISEASE

How the HD gene defect leads to progressive, selective neurodegeneration remains a tantalizing question. In vivo imaging and analysis of postmortem human tissue, in vitro studies, and animal models expressing mutant htt, have identified a number of cellular components and pathways that involve wild-type htt interactions, or are altered during mutant htt-mediated toxicity, discussed below and summarized in Table 1. The htt-mediated event triggering toxicity remains elusive.

3.1. Abnormal Protein–Protein Interactions

One hypothesis of neurotoxicity in HD is that mutant htt influences cellular functions via interactions with proteins that are either novel, or modify the effects of wild-type htt binding (reviewed in ref. 9). Htt contains several binding sites for protein interactions:

1. *The polyglutamine/proline (Q/P)-rich domain* binds with proteins with Src homology region 3 (SH3) or tryptophan (WW) residues. These include protein kinase C and casein kinase substrate 1 (PACSIN1) and SH3GL3/endophilin3 involved in endocytosis, the transcription factor p53, and the synaptic scaffold protein PSD-95. Other interactors include the multifunctional enzyme glyceraldehyde 3-phosphate dehydrogenase (GAPDH), the calcium sensor protein calmodulin, and pro-apoptotic caspase-3.
2. *HEAT domains* bind with several proteins, including the transcription factor NFkB, and contribute to binding with htt-associated protein (HAP) 1, and htt-interacting proteins (HIP) 1 and 14 (HYP-H) involved in intraneuronal trafficking and endocytosis.
3. *The amino terminal region* (including the polyQ region) binds to molecules involved in endocytosis (e.g., α-adaptin C/HYP-J) and several transcription regulators including cAMP response element binding protein (CREB) binding protein (CBP), specificity protein 1 (Sp1), TATA-binding protein-associated factor (TAFII-130), and Sin3a. Other interactors include components of signal transduction pathways including Cdc42-interacting protein 4 (CIP4), Akt/PKB, and Ras GTPase-activating protein (RasGAP). The functional consequences of some of these interactions are reviewed next.

Findings of increased transglutaminase (TGase) activity in HD caudate and in transgenic mouse models imply that the gene mutation increases the extent of htt–protein interactions. TGases catalyze the covalent linkage of Q residues with lysine (K) and polyamines in other proteins. The concentration of glutamyl-lysine crosslinks is also elevated in HD brain and cerebrospinal fluid, and crosslinks are found in htt-positive aggregates. TGase-mediated htt–protein interactions appear to contribute to htt-mediated toxicity, because knocking out the TGase-2 gene delayed neuronal damage in HD transgenic mice *(13)*.

3.2. Endocytosis Pathways

Endocytosis is the process whereby the cell membrane invaginates to form membrane-bound vesicles containing substances previously bound at the cell surface. A number of proteins that interact with htt modulate steps in the endocytosis process, and thus mutant htt may deleteriously affect this pathway (reviewed in ref. 9). An early stage in vesicle generation is the formation of pits in the cell membrane that are lined with the structural protein clathrin, via clathrin's interaction with adaptor protein-2 (AP2), which binds to membrane phospholipids. A number of htt-interacting proteins may modify the formation of clathrin-coated pits and vesicles. HIP1 can interact with clathrin, and both HIP1 and htt directly interact with the AP2 α-adaptin subunit. HIP1 and HIP12 influence vesicle budding and

Table 1
Synopsis of Wild-Type and Mutant Htts' Interactions With Cellular and Molecular Targets

Process altered	Htt target	Effect
Protein–protein interactions	Multiple, described below, plus calmodulin, GAPDH	Potential to modify or abrogate activity of bound protein. Many covalent interactions are catalyzed by transglutaminases, forming glutamyl-lysine crosslinks.
Endocytosis	HIP-1, HIP-12, HIP-14, AP-2αadaptin, PACSIN1, SH3GL3	Htt modulates clathrin-mediated vesicle formation and endocytosis. Mutant htt may disrupt vesicle formation and transport.
Intracellular trafficking	HAP-1	PolyQ increases axonal blockages
Gene transcription	CBP, p53 Sp1, TAFII-130, N-CoR, Sin3A	Mutant htt affects transcription factors, transcriptional activators and co-activators, and transcription repressor activities.
Postsynaptic signaling	PSD-95, CIP4, FIP-2	Htt influences organization of the post-synaptic density, including glutamate receptor subtypes, and dendrite morphology.
Apoptosis	HIP1, Caspase-3	Htt binding to HIP1 prevents HIP-induced caspase-dependent cell death cascades. PolyQ expansion reduces htt's binding to HIP1.
Energy metabolism	Mitochondrial enzymes (TCA cycle and respiratory chain)	Mitochondrial damage, reduced energy production, increased risk of excitotoxicity.
Glutamatergic signaling	NMDA receptor-bearing neurons	Brain regions receiving glutamatergic innervation at risk of excitotoxic damage.
Oxidative damage	Mutant htt-mediated cascades induce free radical generation	Oxidative damage to proteins, DNA, and phospholipids.
Htt aggregation	Mutant-length polyQ expansions lead to htt self-aggregation.	Deposition of ubiquitinated htt-positive protein aggregates, that may sequester or bind other proteins, and may disrupt proteosomal processing.

actin-mediated transport. PACSIN1 has roles in actin polymerization and phosphoinositide turnover, and is thought to contribute to vesicle detachment. Another htt interactor, SH3GL3 (endophilin 3), appears to affect membrane curvature, invagination and vesicle scission. Htt also binds to HIP14 (HYP-H), which has sequence similarity with a yeast endocytotic protein, Ark1p. Because HIP14 localizes to the Golgi apparatus and cytoplasmic vesicles in cell lines, it has been proposed to act as a perinuclear endocytosis regulator. Thus, wild-type htt may serve regulatory roles in clathrin-mediated endocytosis, and mutations in htt could deleteriously modify clathrin binding to membranes, vesicle budding, and actin-mediated vesicle transport.

3.3. Intraneuronal Trafficking

Mutant htt-induced defects in axonal trafficking were first proposed on the basis that distribution of htt aggregates within neuropil seemed to correlate with neurodegeneration more closely than nuclear deposition, in HD patients and "knock-in" mouse models. Additionally, htt is enriched in membranous cell fractions and shows affinity for cytoskeletal and vesicular components. More compelling evidence for a role of wild-type htt in trafficking is provided by a recent study demonstrating that reduced expression of htt in *Drosophila* induces abnormal accumulations of cellular organelles in larval neurons, termed axonal blockages, and concomitant disruption of axonal transport. Another study demonstrated that mutant polyQ expansions in truncated htt and androgen receptor (AR) proteins impair intergraded and retrograde fast axonal transport in squid giant axons. Increased polyQ repeat length exacerbates this defect (reviewed in ref. *10*).

3.4. Transcriptional Regulation

Huntingtin protein can bind to and functionally alter the activity of several transcription factors, co-activators, and repressors *(14)*.

1. *Transcription factors:* Mutant htt exon 1 interacts with both p53 and CBP and represses transcription of the p53-regulated promoters $p21^{WAF/CIP1}$ and MDR1. CBP colocalizes with htt aggregates in HD mouse models, cell culture preparations, and in human HD postmortem brain tissue. PolyQ toxicity in vitro can be blocked by overexpression of CBP.
2. *Transcriptional activators:* Htt binds to the transcriptional activator Sp1 that recruits the transcription factor TAFIID to DNA. It also binds the co-activator TAFII-130. Because TAFII-130 interacts directly with Sp1, it has been proposed that htt may form a support to facilitate transcription activation.
3. *Transcriptional repression:* Htt also interacts with repressor machinery, including the complex containing N-CoR and Sin3A that represses transcription induced by some ligand-activated nuclear receptors (e.g., retinoic acid receptors). N-CoR links DNA-binding proteins to histone deacetylases, and interacts directly with transcription factors through TFIIB. Several genes regulated by NcoR-Sin3A-mediated transcription are altered in HD *(9,14)*. Furthermore, mSin3 also colocalizes with htt and CBP in protein aggregates.

The mechanism underlying mutant htt's effects on gene transcription is currently unclear. It was initially suggested that reduced transcriptional activity of some factors (e.g., CBP and TAFII-130) might result from sequestration into htt-containing aggregates. Sequestration now seems unlikely to be the primary step in HD pathogenesis because transcriptional changes precede aggregate formation in several experimental models. An alternative hypothesis is that a deficiency in cAMP underlies decreases in CRE-mediated gene transcription. Adenosine triphosphate (ATP)-dependent cAMP generation is reduced in HD CSF, cerebral cortex, and lymphoblastoid cell lines, whereas the adenylate cyclase stimulator forskolin attenuates mutant htt-induced toxicity in cell lines. Reduced cortical and striatal levels of cAMP also precede alterations in PKA/CREB signaling, nuclear aggregate formation, and neuronal death in a mouse model of HD *(15)*.

Changes in cAMP-mediated transcription will have downstream effects on many cell components. There is substantial evidence of defects in brain-derived neurotrophic factor (BDNF) function, a cell-survival protein regulated by CREB, in HD. BDNF protein and mRNA levels are markedly reduced in the frontoparietal cortex of symptomatic patients. Reduced BDNF gene transcription and protein levels are also evident in cerebral cortex and striatum of multiple mouse models expressing mutant htt *(15)*. In contrast, mice expressing human wild-type huntingtin show increased levels of BDNF. It has therefore been hypothesized that the selective vulnerability of striatal neurons may result from loss of neurotrophic support by BDNF, because the striatal pool of BDNF arises from cortical projection neurons.

3.5. Postsynaptic Signaling

Htt binds to postsynaptic density-95 (PSD-95), a member of the membrane-associated guanylate kinase (MAGUK) protein family that is involved in organization of the postsynaptic density. PSD-95 binds to kainite and *N*-methyl-D-aspartate (NMDA) glutamate receptor subtypes, as well as to cytoplasmic signaling molecules including SynGAP (synaptic GTPase-activating protein). SynGAP also modulates excitatory synapses via down-regulation of GTPase Ras. PSD-95 further influences dendritic spine morphology via effects on Rac1 signalling involved in actin cytoskeleton remodeling. Htt binding to CIP4 and FIP-2 may also affect dendritic spine morphology *(9)*.

3.6. Apoptotic Cascades

One putative function of wild-type htt is regulation of apoptosis during development, and it has been suggested that striatal htt protects neurons from pro-apoptotic pathways, possibly through inhibition of the cytochrome *C* (cyt C)-dependent procaspase-9 pathway. The htt interactor HIP1 induces caspase-3-dependent cell death, but co-expression of htt abrogates this toxicity in cell lines. Mutant expansion of the htt polyQ tract reduces the ability of htt to bind HIP1, suggesting a possible pathway for increased apoptotic damage in HD. Free HIP1 can associate with HIP1 protein interactor (Hippi) to induce procaspase-8 cleavage and apoptosis in vitro *(16)*. It has also been proposed that htt acts as a survival factor in the phosphoinositide 3-kinase (PI3K)-Akt pathway, as it is a substrate for Akt. This pathway stimulates the expression of survival genes including Bcl-xL and BDNF, and represses death genes including BAX and Bcl-2.

3.7. Mitochondria and Energy Metabolism Pathways

Energy metabolism is impaired in affected brain regions of HD patients *(17)*. Reduced ATP generation can be detrimental to cells in a number of ways, including direct reduction of functional activity within cells, increasing free radical generation, and increasing neuronal vulnerability to excitotoxic damage. Thus energetic defects are postulated to be important contributors to HD pathogenesis.

The most prominent metabolic alteration in HD patients is profound weight loss, even when caloric intake is maintained. In the CNS, impairments in energy metabolism have been found in brain regions targeted by the disease. Glucose uptake is reduced in the caudate, putamen, and cerebral cortex prior to the bulk of tissue loss in symptomatic patients, and presymptomatically in approx 50% of gene-positive mutation carriers. Cerebral levels of lactate are abnormally elevated in affected basal ganglia and cerebral cortex of HD patients. This abnormality can be ameliorated by treatment with the metabolic co-factor Coenzyme Q_{10} (CoQ_{10}) *(18)*. Biochemical studies in HD postmortem tissue have revealed selective dysfunction of components of the mitochondrial tricarboxylic acid (TCA) cycle and electron transport chain (ETC) in affected brain regions, in particular succinate dehydrogenase in complex II and the TCA cycle, complex IV, and aconitase. Further indirect evidence that energetic defects contribute to neurodegeneration in HD is provided by findings that creatine and CoQ_{10} are protective in animal models of HD, putatively via enhancing the efficiency of energy production and delivery in neurons.

Involvement of mitochondrial damage in HD is supported by observations of degenerating mitochondria in mutant mouse models of HD, in some cases concomitant with symptom onset. Htt staining in degenerated mitochondria in symptomatic mice suggests that mutant htt may interact directly with neuronal mitochondria *(19)*. Another HD mouse line (N171-82Q) shows evidence of apoptotic cell death in the striatum and cerebral cortex associated with mitochondrial cytochrome *C* release and caspase-9 activation in the striatum and cerebral cortex. In vitro studies show that mutant htt can alter mitochondrial function by influencing mitochondrial calcium handling *(17)*. Pathogenic polyglutamine constructs have also been shown to decrease mitochondrial membrane potential and to increase mitochondrial vulnerability to Ca^{2+}-induced depolarization.

3.8. Excitotoxic Processes

Mutant htt expression induces alterations in several components of the glutamate neurotransmitter system in affected brain regions that may render cells vulnerable to glutamate-mediated excitotoxic damage *(17)*. The considerable glutamatergic innervation of the neostriatum from the cerebral cortex is postulated to exacerbate the risk of excitotoxic damage to striatal neurons.

Studies of glutamate receptor subtypes in postmortem tissue from late-stage and presymptomatic HD patients show that NMDA receptors are selectively depleted in HD striatum. Findings suggest that NMDA receptor-bearing neurons are preferentially vulnerable to degeneration, and that excitotoxic stress may occur early in the disease course. In animal models, striatal lesions induced by excitotoxins (glutamate receptor agonists) in rodents and primates closely resemble those seen in HD brain. The NMDA receptor agonist quinolinic acid produces neuronal-specific lesions typical of HD, with relative sparing of NADPH-diaphorase and parvalbumin-positive neurons. NMDA receptor-mediated lesions in primates are associated with an apomorphine-inducible movement disorder resembling the choreic movements in HD. Some genetic models of HD (discussed further in Section 4) also show age-dependent declines in glutamate receptor densities in striatum and cerebral cortex, and increased vulnerability to excitotoxic damage.

Excitotoxic damage may also occur in circumstances when extracellular glutamate levels are normal but energy metabolism is impaired, by so-called "secondary excitotoxicity" *(20)*. Reduced ATP production disrupts energy-dependent processes within neurons, including the maintenance of pumps regulating ionic and voltage gradients across cell membranes. Impaired Na^+/K^+-ATPase activities at the cell membrane may cause prolonged or inappropriate opening of voltage-dependent ion channels leading to partial depolarization. If depolarization is severe enough, normally inert extracellular levels of glutamate can trigger NMDA receptor activation resulting in Ca^{2+} influx, nitric oxide synthase (NOS) activation and free radical production. Secondary excitotoxicity is responsive to blockade by NMDA receptor antagonists and glutamate release inhibitors.

3.9. Htt and Oxidative Damage

Mutant htt expression is linked with oxidative damage to multiple cellular components in HD, including proteins, DNA and phospholipids *(21)*. Studies in HD postmortem brain show increased levels of DNA strand breaks, DNA oxidative damage products such as 8-hydroxydeoxyguanosine (OH^8dG), 3-nitrotyrosine (a marker for peroxynitrite-mediated protein nitration), malondialdehyde (marker for oxidative damage to lipids), lipofuscin accumulation (a marker of lipid peroxidation), and heme oxygenase (formed during oxidative stress) in HD striatum and cortex. Findings that oxidative damage to DNA and lipids is increased after symptom onset in mouse models of HD suggest that it is a downstream consequence of htt-induced damage. Glutamate agonists, Ca^{2+} influx, and nitric oxide can stimulate free radical generation, and therefore oxidative damage in HD may result from excitotoxic damage or energy impairments.

3.10. Htt Aggregates in Pathogenesis

Intracellular htt-containing protein aggregates are a hallmark of HD. In some experimental models, including *Drosophila* photoreceptors, mutant htt's toxicity is associated with the presence of neuronal aggregates (NII). Thus, it has been proposed that htt-positive aggregates could be detrimental to cells by sequestering other critical cell proteins and macromolecules, by preventing htt from performing its normal function, or by disrupting vital processes such as proteosome pathways. However, this hypothesis is countered by observations that aggregates are found throughout the body of HD patients and deposition patterns do not mirror cell death in postmortem tissue. Additionally, several studies in cell lines have shown that human mutant htt can induce cell-selective neurodegeneration independent of the presence of NII, whereas suppression of NII formation can increase htt-mediated toxicity, suggesting that aggregate deposition may be part of a protective mechanism within cells *(17)*. Transgenic and knock-in mouse models (discussed in Section 4) further support the argument that NII are not a prerequisite for toxicity in HD models, because there is no direct link between the timing and distribution of NII deposition and cell damage or dysfunction in the majority of models. Aggregates may, therefore, be the result of an intrinsic mechanism to remove toxic htt from the cell milieu, or alternatively be an inert side effect of the propensity for htt to self-aggregate.

4. ANIMAL MODELS

The existing approaches for modeling Huntington's disease in animals utilize knowledge of the genetic basis of the disease and neurochemical facets of its etiology (largely the involvement of the glutamate neurotransmitter system and energetic defects). Three categories predominate: models recapitulating specific neurotransmitter pathway lesions using either (a) excitotoxic or (b) mitochondrial toxins in rodents and nonhuman primates, and (c) models expressing the HD gene defect.

4.1. Excitotoxins

Excitotoxic striatal lesions in rodents and primates closely resemble those seen in HD brain *(17)*. Intrastriatal injection of the NMDA agonist quinolinic acid induces striatal neurodegeneration of medium spiny projection neurons, but spares NADPH-diaphorase and parvalbumin-positive neurons. In primates, NMDA receptor-mediated striatal lesions result in an apomorphine inducible movement disorder resembling that seen in HD patients. This phenomenon appears to be NMDA receptor-specific, because degeneration induced by AMPA and kainate receptor agonists does not target the same neuronal populations.

Expression of the HD gene mutation also confers some susceptibility to excitotoxic damage, but reports to date suggest that the context in which the mutant gene is expressed influences vulnerability. For example, striatal NMDA receptor-mediated quinolinic acid lesions are exacerbated in a full-length htt mouse model (YAC-72Q mice), possibly associated with expression of the NMDA receptor NR2B subunit in this model. In contrast, another transgenic mouse model expressing an N-terminal fragment of mutant huntingtin (N171-82Q) showed no preferential susceptibility to quinolinic acid lesions, while expression of a shorter gene fragment with longer CAG repeats (in R6/2 and R6/1 mice) conferred resistance to quinolinic acid, malonate, NMDA and 3-NP toxicity. Hypotheses to explain the differences between models include reduced synaptic activity in resistant lines, or differential vulnerabilities of background mouse strains. In contrast, R6/2 striatal and cortical neurons show increased susceptibility to NMDA ex vivo. The fact that the glutamate release inhibitor riluzole prolongs survival in R6/2 mice reinforces suggestions of an excitotoxic component of pathogenesis in this model.

4.2. Mitochondrial Toxins: 3-Nitropropionic Acid (3-NP) and Malonate

Mitochondrial defects are implicated in HD by findings of reduced glucose metabolism and mitochondrial succinate dehydrogenase (SDH) activity in the caudate and putamen of symptomatic patients. SDH, located on the matrix surface of the inner mitochondrial membrane, catalyzes the oxidation of succinate to fumarate in both the TCA cycle and complex II of the electron transport chain (ETC). Impaired SDH activity therefore decreases substrate delivery from the TCA cycle to complex I of the ETC and impairs electron transfer, ultimately reducing ATP generation. Some of the clinical and pathological characteristics of HD are replicated by inhibiting striatal SDH activity with 3-nitropropionic acid (3-NP) and malonate *(17)*.

4.2.1. 3-Nitropropionic Acid

Systemic administration of 3-NP causes selective degeneration of striatal medium spiny neurons and motor abnormalities resembling HD. 3-NP's utility as a HD mimetic was discovered by chance, when a group of children in China developed motor disturbances and dystonia associated with discrete basal ganglia lesions after eating sugar cane contaminated with the fungus *Arthrinium.* The toxic moiety was found to be the 3-nitopropanol metabolite 3-NP *(22)*. 3-NP toxicity in humans induces gait abnormalities, multiple cognitive symptoms including acute encephalopathies and coma, and may be fatal. Systemic administration of 3-NP to both rats and primates produces age-dependent striatal lesions that are strikingly similar to those seen in HD. For example, striatal 3-NP lesions in nonhuman primates show sparing of NADPH-d neurons and proliferative changes in the dendrites of spiny neurons. Animals also develop both spontaneous and apomorphine-inducible movement disorders. The extent of basal ganglia lesions induced in animals are minutely dependent on the dosing regimen used, with chronic low dose paradigms inducing cerebral pathology most closely mimicking HD.

4.2.2. Malonate

Malonate is another selective inhibitor of SDH activity that induces motor impairments following intrastriatal administration in rodents. Because malonate does not cross the blood brain barrier systemic administration is ineffective, but it remains a useful tool for modeling the effects of complex II inhibition in vitro and in vivo.

4.2.3. Selective Toxicity of Mitochondrial Toxins

The striatum is discretely targeted by 3-NP toxicity despite uniform distribution of 3-NP throughout the brain and uniform depression of SDH activity following systemic administration. It has been suggested that this susceptibility of striatal neurons to metabolic stress might contribute to their selective vulnerability in HD, supported by findings that improving energy generation within neurons (by creatine or CoQ_{10} administration) protects against 3-NP toxicity. 3-NP administration also causes activation of NMDA receptors, and lesions can be prevented by prior removal of glutamatergic excitatory cortico-striatal inputs by decortication, by glutamate release inhibitors, and by glutamate receptor antagonists, suggesting that 3-NP toxicity is mediated by excitotoxic mechanisms secondary to metabolic defects *(23)*. NMDA receptor antagonists also abrogate malonate toxicity. 3-NP and malonate lesions induce oxidative damage, resulting in increased hydroxyl radical generation, DNA, and protein damage. Free radical scavengers and nitric oxide synthase inhibitors attenuate lesions *(21)*.

4.3. Genetic Models of HD

One of the major drawbacks of relying on human tissue to determine disease mechanism in progressive neurodegenerative disorders is the inability to adequately map early events in the disease process. The development of animal models expressing the HD gene mutation has been invaluable in circumventing many of these issues. A number of model organisms have been utilized, including *C. elegans* and *Drosophila*, which are particularly useful for rapid, high-throughput screening applications, and HD-mutant rodent models, which allow multisystem evaluation of potential disease pathways.

Mutant mouse lines are the most thoroughly characterized HD genetic models currently available (Table 2) *(17,24)*. Several different mutants have been generated that vary in the technique used to incorporate the gene mutation into the mouse genome. As a result, phenotypes vary between mouse lines depending on the nature of the mutation incorporated (full-length human *HD*, a fragment of human *HD*, or precise "knock-in" of a polyglutamine repeat into the murine *HD* homologue *Hdh*), CAG repeat length, copy number of the mutant gene, promoter-dependent cellular specificity of expression, expression levels, and background strains of the mice. The utilities of these different types of mouse models can be divided into three broad categories.

4.3.1. Mice Expressing N-Terminal Exon-1 Fragments of the Human Huntingtin Gene Containing CAG Expansions (Plus Both Alleles of Murine Wild-Type Huntingtin, Hdh)

Typical characteristics of "fragment" mouse models are short life spans, and relatively rapid onset of phenotype that includes reductions in body weight and brain weight, htt aggregate formation, and neuronal atrophy. R6/2 mice expressing about 150 CAGs were the first mutant HD mice developed, and are therefore the best characterized to date *(25)*. Mice have extremely short life spans (approx 13–17 weeks), and develop NII (approx 3–4 weeks); gait abnormalities, rotarod impairments, glucose intolerance, body weight loss, brain weight loss, diabetes, striatal atrophy and ventricular enlargement (6–10 weeks); and cerebral neurotrans-

Table 2
Animal Models of Huntington's Disease

Approach	Model	HD-like phenotypes	Atypical phenotypes
Excitotoxic lesions	Intrastriatal injections of NMDA receptor agonists (quinolinic acid, kynurenic acid) in non-human primates, rats, mice	Striatal neurodegeneration. Medium spiny neurons targeted. Apomorphine-inducible movement disorder in primates.	Rapidly progressing, acute phenotypes. Toxins are not region-specific, and intrastriatal placement is required.
Mitochondrial toxins	SDH / Complex II inhibition by systemic administration of 3-NP; intrastriatal injection of malonate. Primates, rats, mice	Striatal neurodegeneration. Medium spiny neurons targeted. Often fatal. 3-NP's effects are striatal-specific. Induce motor disturbances and dystonia. Disrupt energy metabolism and induce oxidative damage.	Rapidly progressing, acute phenotypes (but can be titered for more chronic effects).
Gene constructs Fragment, human htt.	**Mouse lines** R6/2 [144Q], R6/1 [115Q], N171-82Q [82Q], HD100 [100Q]	Weight loss, movement disorder, htt aggregates, atrophy of cortex and striatum, neurotransmitter receptor changes, transcriptional dysregulation, reduced life span.	Little or no overt striatal cell death. Diabetes or glucose intolerance. Disease onset very rapid. Peripheral toxicity.
Full-length, human htt.	YAC [72Q & 128Q] HD89 [89Q]	Weight loss, movement disorder, htt aggregates, transcriptional dysregulation, atrophy of cortex and striatum, some cell death. Symptoms develop slowly.	Normal life span.
Inducible, human htt.	Tet-off [94Q]	Movement disorder, htt aggregates, atrophy of cortex and striatum, neurotransmitter receptor changes. (Many symptoms reversible on gene turn-off).	Normal life span. Symptom-onset rapid after gene turn-on.
CAG insertion, murine htt.	HdhQ111 [111Q], Hdh-150Q [150Q], Hdh4/6 Knock-in [80Q], HD/Hdh Chimera [80Q]	Selective cell death and atrophy of cortex and striatum observed in some models, htt aggregates. Subtle behavioral changes. Symptoms develop slowly.	Normal life span. No overt movement disorder.

From ref. 17.

78

mitter receptor alterations including depletions of metabotropic glutamate and DA receptors (approx 12 weeks). N171-82Q mice express a longer fragment of human htt exon 1 with a shorter polyQ repeat (82Q). As a result, phenotype onset is later and progression slower than R6/2s, but mice develop a behavioral phenotype more closely reminiscent of HD. Weight loss, gait abnormalities, impaired motor performance, systemic glucose intolerance, and NII deposition are evident by 3 to 4 months of age, before premature death at 4 to 6 months *(26)*. There is little evidence of overt neuronal loss in R6/2 mice, but degeneration of organelles including mitochondria has been reported in symptomatic mice *(19)*. End-stage N171-82Q mice show evidence of apoptotic cell death in striatum and cortex.

Another genetic HD modeling strategy uses an inducible tetracycline-responsive gene system to turn on expression of an *HD* gene fragment postnatally *(27)*. Gene expression in this context induced a progressive phenotype of intranuclear and cytoplasmic inclusion formation, striatal atrophy and astrocytosis, hind-limb clasping and rotarod motor impairments, and receptor changes in the striatum. Some of these changes partially reverse or resolve following transgene turn-off, including aggregate load, receptor fluctuations, and motor performance. These observations suggest that appropriate HD treatments may still be beneficial when applied after symptom onset.

4.3.2. Mice Expressing the Full-Length Human HD Gene (and Murine Hdh)

"Full-length" mouse models show behavioral phenotypes and selective neuronal degeneration more closely resembling HD than fragment models, but onset and progression is slower. YAC128 mice express full length HD using the human promoter, with expression levels approx 75% of endogenous *(28)*. Mice show early hyperkinetic movements, followed by impaired motor function, reduced brain weight, cortical and striatal atrophy, neuronal atrophy and striatal cell loss (affecting primarily medium spiny neurons), and late deposition of htt aggregates. These full-length mutant mice live normal life spans.

4.3.3. Mice With Pathogenic CAG Repeats Inserted Into Murine Hdh

"Knock-in" mice generated by inserting mutant CAG expansions into the murine *HD* homologue *Hdh* represent the most accurate models for mutant htt expression. In general, these models develop pathologic phenotypes most closely resembling HD, but behavioral phenotypes are less severe and slower progressing than human full-length and fragment *HD* models. Mice have normal life spans. Several knock-in models have been generated of which the Hdh^{Q92} and Hdh^{Q111} mice are the best characterized *(29)*. Mice show nuclear localization of htt selectively in striatal medium spiny neurons, eventual htt aggregate formation, and striatal-specific cell loss around 24 months of age in Hdh^{Q111} mice. Increased CAG repeat length is associated with acceleration of NII formation and cell death. Other knock-in models show overt behavioral abnormalities including hypoactivity, hindlimb clasping, and gait abnormalities *(24)*.

In summary, although all mutant HD models exhibit some features of the human disorder, invariably involving htt aggregate formation, few develop the cardinal

signs of striatal neuronal degeneration. Neurodegeneration seems to depend ultimately on the context in which the HD mutation is expressed. Some generalities
can be drawn from a survey of existing mouse lines. First, mice require longer CAG
repeats than humans to elicit pathogenic events, putatively as a result of their relatively short life spans. Second, onset is accelerated when gene fragments are
expressed, and both age of onset and survival decrease with shorter fragments.
In contrast, expression of longer fragments or full-length huntingtin is associated
with neuronal death patterns more closely resembling human HD pathology. Age
of phenotype onset, aggregate formation, and cell death are all slower in full-length
models (including knock-in mice), compared with fragment models. Within each
of these subsets, longer CAG repeats accelerate all phenotypes.

5. CLINICAL PHENOTYPES

A diagnosis of HD is based largely on the development of the hallmark choreic
movement disorder, and is aided by a positive family history. Genetic testing to
detect the abnormal CAG repeat may now be used to confirm suspected HD.
Approximately one-third of HD cases initially present with emotional disturbances
and neuropsychiatric conditions, however, which can lead to misdiagnosis. In the
absence of a family history, a correct diagnosis in these cases may be difficult until
the movement disorder presents.

The clinical phenotype of HD includes a primary movement disorder, emotional
disturbances, and cognitive decline. The heterogeneous clinical presentations of HD
and treatment paradigms are extensively reviewed by Rosenblatt and colleagues *(30)*.

5.1. HD Movement Disorder

The earliest motor abnormalities in HD typically affect the eye. Initiation of eye
movement is delayed, the speed of saccades declines, patients show impaired ability to suppress blinks when saccades are initiated, and pursuit movements become
jerky. Choreic body movements gradually develop, and are the most noticeable
feature of HD. The earliest changes are subtle and are often suppressible at first.
These include clumsiness, variable stride length, a propensity to fidget, restlessness, and the appearance of fragmentary or exaggerated facial expressions or gestures. As the movement disorder becomes more profound and disabling patients
develop a choreic "dancing" or "drunken" gait. Patients are unable to suppress
involuntary movements involving many muscle groups, principally affecting the
limbs and trunk generating irregular jerking and writhing movements, and often
face, mouth, and tongue. As a result, HD patients show an increasing frequency of
falls and muscle movements controlling respiration may become irregular. Motor
impersistence develops, typified by incomplete chewing (increasing the risk of
choking and aspiration), inconsistent driving speed, and a tendency to drop objects.
Dystonia and bradykinesia become prominent later in the disease. Voluntary movements and postural reflexes slow, and patients lose facial expression. As a result,
dysphagia, dysarthria, aspiration, reduced dexterity and coordination, and balance
problems are common occurrences in HD.

5.2. Emotional Disturbances

Mood and behavioral disorders are often the most disruptive features of HD not only for patients, but also their families and other relationships. Emotional changes precede the appearance of overt motor symptoms in approximately one-third of patients, and an increased risk of suicide has been identified in presymptomatic HD patients. Although the appearance of emotional disturbances is quite variable between individuals, they may include depression (with concomitant social withdrawal and suicide risk), increased impulsivity, obsessive-compulsive behavior, increased anxiety and irritability, or psychosis. Overt changes in personality are also common, including the development of uncharacteristically rude behavior and impatience, violent outbursts, changes in sexual behavior, and errors in social judgment.

5.3. Cognitive Decline

As the disease progresses, symptoms of cognitive decline become prevalent. Patients become easily distractible and the speed of their intellectual maneuvers decreases. Visuospatial abilities become impaired, often manifest as a decreased awareness of their environment and the relationship of their body to objects, and a tendency to get lost. Executive function is impaired, affecting attention, decision-making, planning, and organization abilities, and initiation and sequencing of actions. Decline in short-term memory and learning skills are also prevalent. Cognitive changes in HD are considered "subcortical" in origin, because they generally lack cortical-associated symptoms such as aphasia, agnosia, and amnesia typical of Alzheimer's type dementia.

5.4. Juvenile- and Late-Onset HD

Consistent with the pathological differences between adult and juvenile-onset forms, juvenile HD shows phenotypic variations. Chorea is much less prominent, and bradykinesia is overt and occurs early (the so-called Westphal variant). Juvenile patients also typically show tremor, rigidity, and dystonia. Myoclonic jerks and seizures may occur. Behavioral problems are often manifest as attention deficit, poor impulse control, inappropriate behavior, and failure at school. Late-onset HD may present purely as chorea.

6. CURRENT AND PROTOTYPICAL TREATMENTS

6.1. Current Treatments

There are no therapeutic approaches to prevent the neuronal degeneration in HD available at present (agents in clinical trial are discussed later). Approaches currently used treat the symptoms rather than the disease. The multiple neurological and psychological components of HD mean that medications used to treat these symptoms often have side effects that compound other features of the disease. Wherever possible, therefore, nonpharmacological techniques are applied first, and if pharmacological agents are necessary the lowest effective doses are used. HD is associated with reduced energy metabolism, weight loss, and associated loss of strength. Therefore, nutrition is important and patients should be maintained on high-calorie diets, with supplements if necessary. Swallowing is often impaired and easy-to-swallow food should be chosen. An eating environment designed to reduce distractions and improve food access (e.g., using adapted utensils) is also beneficial. Pharmacological and nonpharmacological approaches are discussed in detail in "A Physician's Guide to the Management of Huntington's Disease" *(30)*.

6.1.1. Movement Disorder

Although the appearance of involuntary choreic movements is typically the most overt feature of HD, it is often the least troublesome symptom for patients and therefore often needs no treatment. If chorea is severe and distressful, standard antipsychotics such as the neuroleptics haloperidol or fluphenazine may be used to suppress movements. Possible side effects include sedation, parkinsonism, and dystonia, of which the latter two can be addressed by using less potent antipsychotics (e.g., clozapine or quetiapine *[31]*). Benzodiazepines including clonazepam and diazepam, or DA-depleting agents (e.g., reserpine and tetrabenazine) may have some beneficial effects. The impaired initiation and control of voluntary movements have greater impacts on functional ability in HD, but no effective pharmacological agents are available. Physical, occupational, speech, and swallowing therapies can delay decline of these functions. Bradykinesia, dystonia, and spasticity may develop late in the disease. Antiparkinsonism drugs such as levodopa/carbidopa and amantadine can be used to treat bradykinesia, but are associated with delirium and tolerance. Benzodiazepines may relieve stiffness, although increased bradykineisa is a potential side effect. Myoclonus may respond to clonazepam or divalproex sodium, although it is often not debilitating enough to warrant treatment. Divalproex sodium is also used to treat myoclonic epilepsy or seizures that occur in approx 30% of juvenile HD patients.

6.1.2. Emotional Changes

Many of the symptoms of mood disturbances and personality changes can be improved by conventional pharmacological approaches. Antidepressants are commonly used, and do not generally affect motor deficits. Selective serotonin reuptake inhibitors (SSRIs; including fluoxetine, sertraline, paroxetine, and fluvoxamine) are usually the class chosen because they have less severe side effects and less chance of overdose. Tricyclic antidepressants are avoided if possible, especially in impulsive or suicidal patients, as a result of their adverse cardiovascular effects and relatively high risk of toxicity in overdose, although they may be used for acute treatment if depression is unresponsive to SSRIs (e.g., Nortryptaline). Psychotherapy can be beneficial, and in refractory or severe cases electroconvulsive therapy has been used *(30)*. Concomitant presentation of hallucinations, delusions, or severe agitation can be treated with antipsychotic medications. Standard antipsychotics should be administered at low doses to avoid the detrimental side effects of parkinsonism, rigidity, or sedation. If chorea is not an overt problem in psychotic patients, newer agents that are less sedative and display low or no parkinsonian side effects (e.g., quetiapine or aripiprazole) may be beneficial *(31)*.

A small cohort of patients with HD develop mania, and some may develop bipolar disorder (alternating between depression, mania, and normal mood). Mood stabilizers such as lithium are useful in these cases. Impulsivity can also be treated with mood stabilizers (e.g., carbamazepine, gabapentin, divalproex sodium, and valproic acid). SSRIs or the tricyclic antidepressant clomipramine are typically used to treat obsessive-compulsive behavior. Commonly used anti-anxiety agents include SSRIs and benzodiazepines. Mood stabilizers, SSRIs, and antipsychotic agents are often useful to treat irritability. One prevalent behavioral affect of HD is a change in sexual behavior. If inappropriate sexual activity is a problem, agents that reduce libido as a side effect such as propranolol or fluoxetine may be useful.

6.1.3. Cognitive Changes

No pharmacological interventions are currently available. Nonpharmacological approaches include compensating for poor organizational skills by instigating daily routines, prompting patients to initiate activity, and behavioral approaches to deal with impulsivity and temper outbursts.

6.2. Prototypical Treatments

Mutant htt interactions and animal models of the disease have revealed several targets for pharmacological interventions aimed at preventing or arresting the progression of neurodegeneration in HD. A number of agents induced moderate beneficial effects in animal models, including agents that improve energy metabolism, modulate glutamate receptor activation, inhibit free radical-mediated oxidative damage, modulate DA and cannabinoid neurotransmission, and prevent caspase activation. The most promising agents identified to date are being assessed in clinical trials in the HD population.

CoQ_{10} and creatine improve aspects of HD phenotype putatively via enhancing cerebral energy metabolism *(17)*. Oral administration of CoQ_{10} ameliorated elevated lactate levels seen in the cortex of patients with HD, an effect that was reversible on withdrawal of the agent *(18)*. CoQ_{10} attenuated neurotoxicity induced by the mitochondrial toxins MPTP and malonate in animal models, and increased survival and delayed symptom onset in genetic mouse models of HD. These findings led to CoQ_{10} being tested in a 30-month clinical trial in early-stage HD patients, both alone and in combination with the weak NMDA-receptor antagonist remacemide *(32)*. Although this multiarm trial did not detect a significant ameliorative effect of CoQ_{10}, it did demonstrate a trend toward a protective effect with treatment slowing the decline in "total functional capacity" of patients with HD by 13%. Although findings were not immediately conclusive, results are encouraging and further studies of different doses are planned.

An alternative strategy to enhance cerebral energy metabolism is to increase brain energy stores of the high-energy compound phosphocreatine (PCr) via systemic creatine administration. Oral creatine treatment successfully attenuated neurotoxicity induced by 3-NP in rats, ameliorating increases in striatal lactate levels and decreases in energy metabolites including ATP induced by the toxin *(17)*. Furthermore, oral creatine administration delayed disease onset in HD mouse models, and protected against purkinje cell loss in a transgenic mouse model of another polyglutamine repeat disease, SCA1. As a result of these promising effects, creatine's efficacy in HD is currently being assessed in clinical trials.

Riluzole is a glutamate release inhibitor that has been shown to abrogate damage in models of excitotoxic damage, and of HD and other neurodegenerative disorders. The effects of riluzole on components of the Unified HD Rating Scale (UHDRS) were recently assessed in an 8-week two-dose study in 63 patients with HD *(33)*. The higher dose tested (200 mg/kg per day) significantly reduced the progression of chorea over this period, but had no effects on motor, cognitive, behavioral, or functional components of the UHDRS.

The modified tetracycline antibiotic minocycline is currently in initial clinical trials as an HD therapeutic. This agent has been shown to inhibit htt aggregation, caspase-3 activation, and calpain cleavage. It has been reported to be protective in some animal models of focal and global cerebral ischemia, mitochondrial toxicity, and neurodegenerative disorders including HD and amyotrophic lateral sclerosis. However, beneficial effects are not universal, and a number of recent studies report no effects or even detrimental effects of this agent, suggesting its reported beneficial effects may be associated with a small dosing window. The potential utility of this agent in HD therapy is controversial.

A number of other therapeutic approaches are being actively explored for HD, including stem-cell transplantation, viral vector delivery of neurotrophic hormones, gene-therapy approaches, and genetic technology designed to silence mutant HD gene expression. As a result, HD is currently at the forefront of therapeutic design in neurodegenerative disorders, and the current high volume of HD-related research implies that ameliorative treatments may be available in the near future.

GLOSSARY OF MEDICAL TERMINOLOGY

Anticipation: Age of disease onset decreases in successive generations, owing to mutation instability.

Atrophy: A wasting or decrease in size of a body organ, tissue, or part, owing to disease, injury, or lack of use.

Apoptosis: Programmed cell death (or "cell suicide") induced by intracellular signals in response to a variety of stimuli. Apoptosis may occur in development, or as a result of disease, or age. Cell death occurs in a controlled fashion, requires energy, and generally occurs without inflammatory responses.

Autosomal dominant: A dominant trait (expressed even if represented in only one of two alleles) in a nongender-determining chromosome.

Chorea: Irregular, sustained jerking or writhing movements involving multiple muscle groups.

Dysarthria: Difficulty with the physical production of speech.

Dysphagia: Difficulty swallowing.

Dystonia: A neurologic movement disorder characterized by sustained muscle contractions, usually producing twisting and repetitive movements or abnormal postures or positions.

Monozygotic: Trait resulting from expression of a gene carried on only one of a pair of chromosome alleles.

Mutation: A random change in a gene or chromosome resulting in a new trait or characteristic that can be inherited.

Myoclonus: Sudden brief jerking movements involving discrete groups of muscles.

Oxidative damage: Detrimental events in cells induced by altering the function or bioavailability of molecules by oxidization, for example by interaction with free radicals.

Polyglutamine (polyQ): Repetitive sequence of glutamine amino acid moieties.

Transcription: The first step in converting genetic instructions encoded in DNA. The genetic code in DNA is transferred to messenger RNA molecules that carry the code to protein-generating machinery.

REFERENCES

1. Vonsattel JPG, DiFiglia M. Huntington Disease. J Neuropathol Exp Neurol 1998;57:369–384.
2. Backman L, Farde L. Dopamine and cognitive functioning: brain imaging findings in Huntington's disease and normal aging. Scand J Psychol 2001;42:287–296.
3. Mayberg HS, Starkstein SE, Peyser CE, Brandt J, Dannals RF, Folstein SE. Paralimbic frontal lobe hypometabolism in depression associated with Huntington's disease. Neurology 1992;42: 1791–1797.
4. Albin RL, Young AB, Penney JB. The functional anatomy of basal ganglia disorders. Trends Neurosci 1989;12:366–375.
5. The Huntington's Disease Collaborative Research Group. A novel gene containing a trinucleotide repeat that is expanded and unstable on Huntington's disease chromosome. Cell 1993;72: 971–983.
6. MacDonald ME, Gines S, Gusella JF, Wheeler VC. Huntington's disease. Neuromolecular Med 2003;42:7–20.
7. Kehoe P, Krawczak M, Harper PS, Owen MJ, Jones AL. Age of onset in Huntington disease: sex specific influence of apolipoprotein E genotype and normal CAG repeat length. J Med Genet 1999;36:108–111.
8. Margolis RL, Ross CA. Diagnosis of Huntington disease. Clin Chem 2003;49:1726–1732.
9. Harjes P, Wanker EE. The hunt for huntingtin function: interaction partners tell many different stories. Trends Biochem Sci 2003;28:425–433.
10. Feany MB, La Spada AR. Polyglutamines stop traffic: axonal transport as a common target in neurodegenerative diseases. Neuron 2003;40:1,2.
11. DiFiglia M. Huntingtin fragments that aggregate go their separate ways. Mol Cell 2002;10: 224,225.
12. Wellington CL, Ellerby LM, Gutekunst CA, et al. Caspase cleavage of mutant huntingtin precedes neurodegeneration in Huntington's disease. J Neurosci 2003;22:7862–7872.
13. Mastroberardino PG, Iannicola C, Nardacci R, et al. "Tissue" transglutaminase ablation reduces neuronal death and prolongs survival in a mouse model of Huntington's disease. Cell Death Differ 2002;9:873–880.
14. Sugars KL, Rubinsztein DC. Transcriptional abnormalities in Huntington disease. Trends Genet 2003;19:233–238.
15. Gines S, Seong IS, Fossale E, et al. Specific progressive cAMP reduction implicates energy deficit in presymptomatic Huntington's disease knock-in mice. Hum Mol Genet 2003;12:497–508.
16. Gervais FG, Singaraja R, Xanthoudakis S, et al. Recruitment and activation of caspase-8 by the Huntingtin-interacting protein Hip-1 and a novel partner Hippi. Nat Cell Biol 2002;4:95–105.
17. Browne SE, Beal MF. The energetics of HD. Neurochem Res 2004;29:531–546.

18. Koroshetz WJ, Jenkins BG, Rosen BR, Beal MF. Energy metabolism defects in Huntington's disease and possible therapy with coenzyme Q_{10}. Ann. Neurol 1997;41:160–165.

19. Yu Z-X, Li S-H, Evans J, Pillarisetti A, Li H, Li X-J. Mutant huntingtin causes context-dependent neurodegeneration in mice with Huntington's Disease. J Neurosci 2003; 23:2193–2202.

20. Albin RL, Greenamyre JT. Alternative excitotoxic hypotheses. Neurology 1992; 42:733–738.

21. Browne SE, Ferrante RJ, Beal MF. Oxidative stress in Huntington's disease. Brain Pathol 1999;9:147–163.

22. Ludolph AC, He F, Spencer PS, Hammerstad J, Sabri M. 3-nitropropionic acid: exogenous animal neurotoxin and possible human striatal toxin. Can J Neurol Sci 1990;18:492-498.

23. Beal MF. Huntington's disease, energy, and excitotoxicity. Neurobiol Aging 1994;15:275,276.

24. Hickey MA, Chesselet MF. The use of transgenic and knock-in mice to study Huntington's disease. Cytogenet Genome Res. 2003;100:276–286.

25. Mangiarini L, Sathasivam K, Seller M, et al. Exon 1 of the HD gene with an expanded CAG repeat is sufficient to cause a progressive neurological phenotype in transgenic mice. Cell 1996;87:493–506.

26. Schilling G, Becher MW, Sharp AH, et al. Intranuclear inclusions and neuritic aggregates in transgenic mice expressing a mutant N-terminal fragment of huntingtin. Hum Mol Genet 1999;8:397–407.

27. Yamamoto A, Lucas JJ, Hen R. Reversal of neuropathology and motor dysfunction in a conditional model of Huntington's disease. Cell 2000;101:57–66.

28. Slow EJ, van Raamsdonk J, Rogers D, et al. Selective striatal neuronal loss in a YAC128 mouse model of Huntington disease. Hum Mol Genet 2003;12:1555–1567.

29. Wheeler VC, Gutekunst CA, Vrbanac V, et al. Early phenotypes that presage late-onset neurodegenerative disease allow testing of modifiers in Hdh CAG knock-in mice. Hum Mol Genet 2002;15;11:633–640.

30. Rosenblatt A, Ranen NG, Nance MA, Paulsen JS. A Physician's Guide to the Management of Huntington's Disease. Huntington's Disease Society of America, 1999.

31. Tarsy D, Baldessarini RJ, Tarazi FI. Effects of newer antipsychotics on extrapyramidal function. CNS Drugs 2002;16:23–45.

32. Huntington Study Group. A randomized, placebo-controlled trial of coenzyme Q10 and remacemide in Huntington's disease. Neurology 2001;57:375,376.

33. Huntington Study Group. Dosage effects of riluzole in Huntington's disease: a multicenter placebo-controlled study. Neurology 2003;61:1551–1556.

5

Parkinson's Disease

Thomas Wichmann

Summary

Parkinson's disease (PD) is the second most common neurodegenerative disorder, affecting millions of patients worldwide. Individuals with parkinsonism develop a slowly progressive and disabling disorder with motor, cognitive, and behavioral symptoms. It is well established that neurodegeneration in this disease affects mainly dopaminergic neurons in the basal ganglia, and recent progress in neuroscience research has begun to establish the pathophysiological links that lead from loss of dopaminergic transmission to the symptoms of parkinsonism. The newly gained knowledge in this area has already resulted in the development of a number of new therapeutic options for patients with PD. The process of neurodegeneration itself is also under very active investigation, primarily using genetic and molecular research. Results from these studies promise to help in the future development of neuroprotective treatments. This chapter outlines the scientific basis for established treatments as well as therapeutic options that are currently under development.

Key Words: MPTP; primate; pathophysiology; pallidum; subthalamic nucleus; substantia nigra.

1. CLINICAL ASPECTS

1.1. Incidence and Prevalence

The incidence of Parkinson's disease (PD) is reported to be between 5 and 24 per 100,000 persons worldwide; in the United States, this figure is 20.5 per 100,000. Estimates of the prevalence of the disease are similarly wide ranging, between 57 and 371 per 100,000 worldwide, and about 300 per 100,000 for the United States and Canada. At any given time, about 40% of cases are considered undiagnosed. With the increasing age of the population, there will be a large (up to fourfold) increase in the prevalence of PD over the next 20 years. The age of onset differs substantially between patients. Although the average age of onset is 62 years, 4 to 10% of cases occur before the age of 40. The younger cases are commonly suffering from familial forms of PD (*see* Subheading 2.2.). Males appear to be affected slightly more frequently than females.

From: *Current Clinical Neurology: Neurological and Psychiatric Disorders:*
From Bench to Bedside
Edited by: F. I. Tarazi and J. A. Schetz © Humana Press Inc., Totowa, NJ

1.2. Signs and Symptoms

In his seminal paper, written in 1817 *(1)*, James Parkinson described many of the salient behavioral abnormalities of the disease that later went on to carry his name. He recognized that the disease manifests itself in most patients with prominent abnormalities of movement, including a tremor at rest, typically occurring at 5 Hz, rigidity (velocity-independent muscle stiffness), bradykinesia (slowness of movement), and akinesia (a failure of movement initiation). Bradykinesia and akinesia are often early and insidious signs, most evident in problems such as slowed and illegible handwriting, reduced volume of speech, dysarthria, freezing episodes, reduced arm swing, or facial masking, and varying degrees of apraxia or dystonia. Many of these motor signs predominate unilaterally early in the disease, with a gradual progression to involve the opposite side in later stages. Other symptoms and signs develop in more advanced phases of the disease, such as autonomic insufficiency, ranging from mild constipation to autonomic failure with severe orthostatic hypotension, impotence, or postural abnormalities, such as stooping or retropulsion (often described by patients as the experience of being "pulled backward"). Prominent psychiatric and cognitive complications also develop. The cognitive disability often represents a continuum of problems, starting with a mild disruption of sleep, followed by the development of a propensity to have nightmares, rapid eye movement sleep (REM) behavioral problems, drug-induced daytime hallucinations, and cognitive decline. Dementia has been described in up to 60 to 70% of patients.

1.3. Differential Diagnosis

PD has to be separated from a variety of other conditions that can mimic the parkinsonian phenotype. Some of the more important conditions are listed in Table 1. Typical "red flags" that betray the presence of a parkinsonian syndrome different from idiopathic PD include bilaterally symmetric onset of the disorder, an abrupt onset of motor abnormalities, the absence of tremor, or the presence of unusual physical signs that are not part of typical PD, such as oculomotor abnormalities, prominent apraxia, cerebellar signs, upper motor neuron signs, and the early development of dementia, hallucinations, or autonomic failure. In any patient with parkinsonism, a particularly important differential diagnostic consideration is the possibility that symmetrically appearing parkinsonian signs may be induced by medications such as commonly used antipsychotic drugs, for instance, haloperidol, antiemetics drugs, such as metoclopramide, or antihypertensive drugs, such as reserpine. All of these medications may produce parkinsonism by interference with dopaminergic transmission (*see* Section 3). In addition, other neurodegenerative conditions may mimic PD. These disorders are often accompanied by physical signs that are not usually part of parkinsonism. The most common among these disorders is progressive supranuclear palsy, a condition in which patients develop a prominent supranuclear gaze palsy, stiff posture, a typical "staring" facial expression and early dementia and autonomic signs. Another neurodegenerative disorder to con-

Table 1
Differential Diagnosis of Parkinson's Disease

1. Neurodegenerative diseases
   a. Idiopathic Parkinson's disease
      i. Sporadic forms
      ii. Genetic forms (PARK1–PARK11)
   b. Progressive supranuclear palsy
   c. Cortico-basal ganglionic degeneration
   d. Multiple systems atrophy
      i. Striatonigral degeneration
      ii. Shy-Drager syndrome
   e. Hallervorden-Spatz syndrome
   f. Neuroacanthocytosis
   g. Segawa syndrome (Dopa-responsive dystonia)
   h. Spinocerebellar ataxias (Machado-Joseph disease [SCA 3])
   i. Olivopontocerebellar atrophy
   j. Dementias
      i. Diffuse Lewy body disease
      ii. Alzheimer's disease
2. Drug-induced parkinsonism
   a. Antipsychotics: haloperidol, chlorpromazine, perphenazine, olanzapine, others
   b. Antiemetics: metoclopramide, perphenazine, prochloperazine
   c. Dopamine depleting agents: methyldopa, reserpine, tetrabenazine
3. Metabolic causes of parkinsonism
   a. Often reversible
   b. Hypo- or hyperthyroidism
   c. Hypo- or hyperparathyroidism
   d. Liver failure
   e. Central pontine myelinolysis
4. Infectious causes of parkinsonism
   a. Postencephalitic
   b. Prion diseases
   c. Brain abscess
   d. HIV infection
5. Toxic
   a. Mitochondrial toxins: MPTP, rotenone (?)
   b. Carbon monoxide
   c. Manganese
   d. Cyanide
6. Vascular parkinsonism

sider is cortico-basal ganglionic degeneration. In this condition, patients typically present with an akinetic rigid syndrome, associated with cortical signs, such as limb apraxia, or corticospinal tract signs, dystonia, and myoclonus. Striatonigral degeneration and the Shy-Drager syndrome are also in the differential diagnosis. Both are accompanied by early and severe autonomic insufficiency. Finally, the olivopontocerebellar atrophies are worth considering when cerebellar signs are prominent. More recently, these conditions, as well as others that are part of the differential diagnosis of Parkinson's disease, such as Machado-Joseph disease, and dentato-rubro-cerebellar atrophy have been grouped with the inherited spinocerebellar ataxias (SCAs) rather than with PD. In all of these conditions, some aspects of parkinsonism, particularly akinesia and rigidity, are present to varying degrees, although other aspects, such as tremor at rest, are often missing. All of these parkinsonian conditions differ pathologically from true idiopathic PD (*see* Subheading 2.1.).

Although the characteristics mentioned here appear to clearly distinguish PD from its look-alikes, in clinical practice, this distinction is often difficult, particularly in more advanced stages of the diseases. In a study by Hughes et al., it was found that one-fourth of cases of PD, diagnosed by experienced movement disorder specialists, may, in fact, represent one of the Parkinson-plus syndromes, as judged by autopsy examination *(2)*. Commonly available laboratory tests rarely help in making distinctions between these conditions, but magnetic resonance imaging scans of the brain may show lesions suggestive of vascular parkinsonism or olivopontocerebellar atrophy. 18F-DOPA-poistron emission tomography scans may demonstrate the striatal dopamine (DA) deficit typical of PD (*see* Section 3), and genetic testing may help with identifying the SCAs or one of the genetic forms of parkinsonism.

2. PATHOLOGIC SUBSTRATE, GENETIC ASPECTS, AND MOLECULAR TARGETS

2.1. Pathology

Although recent studies have suggested that the earliest pathological changes in PD may occur in structures outside of the basal ganglia, such as the lower brainstem nuclei or the olfactory bulb *(3)*, it is well documented that the most salient pathological abnormality in later stages of the disease is the relatively selective degeneration of dopaminergic neurons in the substantia nigra pars compacta (SNc), which projects to the striatum, and, to a lesser extent, to other basal ganglia nuclei such as the external and internal pallidal segments (GPe, GPi, respectively), the subthalamic nucleus (STN), and the substantia nigra pars reticulata (SNr). DA loss in these nuclei is easily compensated for in early stages of the disease; identifiable symptoms occur only when more than 70% of striatal DA is lost. Degenerating dopaminergic cells leave characteristic eosinophilic inclusions in their wake, called Lewy neurites and Lewy bodies. Recent studies have also shown that low-level inflammatory responses may accompany the loss of dopaminergic cells, and may contribute to cell death *(4)*.

In early phases of PD, DA loss affects particularly the sensorimotor portion of the striatum, the posterior putamen, resulting in the appearance of motor disturbances. In later stages, more widespread DA loss, affects other regions of the basal ganglia (such as the caudate nucleus and the pallidum) and extra-basal ganglia areas, such as cortex, hypothalamus, and thalamus. Further spread of neuronal degeneration to nondopaminergic systems, such as the locus coeruleus and the raphe nuclei, may cause the development of the aforementioned nonmotor signs and symptoms of the disease, such as cognitive disabilities, sleep disorders, and mood disturbances *(5)*.

2.2. Etiology

The etiology of the disease is varied. Most cases of parkinsonism are multifactorial in origin, caused by genetic as well as environmental/toxic factors. Purely genetic forms of the disease probably account for less than 10% of cases, but even in sporadic parkinsonism, the risk of family members of an affected patient to develop PD is significantly increased. Studying familial forms of parkinsonism has significantly enhanced our understanding of the molecular mechanisms that underlie the neurodegenerative process in PD. Such familial forms of parkinsonism have been known at least since the early 1900s. In the last decade, a large number of specific genetic mechanisms have been described to underlie specific forms of PD. Several of these genetic defects appear to interfere with DA metabolism or release. An example of this is Segawa's disease, also known as DA-responsive dystonia. This disease is caused by a defect in the gene coding for GTP-cyclohydrolase *(6)*, an enzyme needed in the production of DA. Patients with this disease develop a characteristic combination of dystonia and parkinsonism, which are both strikingly responsive to dopaminergic medications.

A larger group of genetic defects resulting in parkinsonism is characterized by degeneration of dopaminergic neurons. The best example for this is parkinsonism owing to α-synuclein accumulation in dopaminergic cells. In fact, one of the first identified genetic defects leading to parkinsonism is the result of a mutation of the gene encoding for α-synuclein *(7)*. α-Synuclein abnormalities may also occur in "sporadic" PD. Thus, α-synuclein has been identified as one of the major components of the hallmark eosinophilic inclusion bodies that are found in the SNc of patients with the disease (Lewy bodies; *see* Subheading 2.1.).

This constellation of findings has resulted in the classification of PD as an synucleinopathy, together with less frequent diseases that also share synuclein abnormalities, including some of the multiple system atrophies, cortical Lewy body disease, olivopontocerebellar atrophy and the Hallervorden-Spatz syndrome. These clinically distinct entities differ pathologically in the location of synuclein deposits. Interestingly, some diseases, which clinically mimic PD (such as progressive supranuclear palsy) appear to be associated with aggregation of τ-protein rather than α-synuclein, and are now classified as tauopathies, a group of diseases that also include Alzheimer's disease.

The hydrophilic protein α-synuclein is a normal constituent of many neurons in the adult nervous system, including dopaminergic and other vulnerable cells *(3)*. It is preferentially found in synaptic vesicles and membranes along axons and terminals. The pathological process leading to aggregation of α-synuclein in PD appears to result from a conformational change of the α-synuclein molecule from its usual unfolded, soluble form into a β-pleated sheath, which readily aggregates with itself and with other proteins *(8)*, eventually forming large deposits that appear to be toxic to the cell.

Even under normal conditions, dopaminergic cells seem to be exposed to a high level of oxidative stress as a result of the presence of dopaminergic metabolism and other factors. This may render these neurons particularly vulnerable to nonspecific genetic or environmental insults that, by themselves, would not be sufficient to induce cell death in other cells. Interestingly, many of the factors known to be involved in neuronal damage in PD, including many of the known genetic defects, mitochondrial diseases, or toxins appear to interfere with the cell's ability to eliminate damaged or mutated proteins through the ubiquitin proteasome system *(9)*. Failure of this system may result in the accumulation of toxic proteins, such as mutated α-synuclein, in the cell, eventually leading to cell death *(9)*. Although this is still under considerable debate, the DA cell degeneration in PD is, at least in part, due to apoptosis (programmed cell death).

3. BRAIN PATHWAYS INVOLVED IN PARKINSONISM

A substantial body of research has addressed the question of how loss of dopaminergic cells in the SNc may affect the function of the basal ganglia, and related structures to eventually result in the behavioral signs of parkinsonism. The current anatomic and functional model of basal ganglia circuitry will first be introduced, followed by a discussion of the abnormalities seen in parkinsonism.

3.1. Anatomy

The neuroanatomy of the basal ganglia has been reviewed extensively in previously published comprehensive reviews *(10–12)*. In brief, the basal ganglia are a group of functionally related subcortical nuclei that include the neostriatum (comprised of the caudate nucleus and the putamen), the ventral striatum, GPe, STN, GPi, SNr, and SNc. They are anatomically connected to large portions of the cerebral cortex, thalamus, and brain stem. These nuclei appear to be organized in segregated modular re-entrant circuits, a structural setup that is thought to significantly enhance the efficiency and speed of cortical processing.

Most research focused on the dysfunction of basal ganglia circuits in parkinsonism had concentrated primarily on the "motor circuit," which will be described in some detail. In primates, this circuit is centered around the somatosensory, motor, and premotor cortices that send projections to the "motor portion" of the striatum, the postcommissural putamen, and to the STN. A second major group of inputs to striatum and STN arises from the intralaminar thalamic nuclei (i.e., the centromedian and parafascicular nucleus [CM/Pf]).

Topographically segregated cortical information is conveyed from the striatum to the output nuclei of the basal ganglia (GPi and SNr). The connections between the striatum and the basal ganglia output nuclei are thought to be organized into "direct" and "indirect" pathways *(10)*. The direct pathway arises from striatal neurons that project monosynaptically to neurons in GPi and SNr, whereas the indirect pathway arises from a different set of neurons that projects to Gpe *(11)*. Some striatofugal neurons may also collateralize more extensively, reaching GPe, Gpi, and SNr *(13)*. GPe conveys the information it receives to GPi/SNr either directly, or via the STN. The population of striatal neurons that gives rise to the direct pathway can be further characterized by the presence of the neuropeptides substance P and dynorphin, by the preferential expression of DA D_1 receptors, and by the fact that these neurons (as well as some striatal interneurons) appear to be targets of inputs from the intralaminar thalamic nuclei. The population of striatal neurons that gives rise to the indirect pathway expresses preferentially enkephalin and DA D_2 receptors *(11)*. The functionally important segregation of D_1 and D_2 receptors between the direct and indirect pathways has been most clearly demonstrated in DA-depleted animals, although several studies in normal animals have supported the existence of a degree of overlap between D_1- and D_2-positive cell populations. However, the D_1–D_2 dichotomy may still serve to explain the apparent dual actions of DA, released from the nigrostriatal pathway arising in the substantia nigra pars compacta, on striatal output. DA appears to modulate the activity of the basal ganglia output neurons in GPi and SNr by facilitation of transmission over the direct pathway and inhibition of transmission over the indirect pathway *(11)*. The net effect of striatal DA release appears to be a reduction of basal ganglia output. On the other hand, a reduction of DA release as is seen in PD will result in a net increase in basal ganglia output.

Movement-related basal ganglia output arises particularly from the caudo-ventral "motor" portion of GPi. This region of GPi projects almost exclusively to the posterior part of the ventrolateral nucleus (VLo in macaques), which in turn sends projections toward the supplementary motor area, the primary motor cortex and premotor cortical areas. Another source of movement-related output from the basal ganglia are projections from the dorsolateral sensorimotor territory of the SNr. These projections terminate in the ventral anterior (VA) nucleus and in the mediodorsal (MD) nucleus of thalamus. These nuclei, in turn, innervate premotor (and non-motor) regions of the frontal lobe. Both GPi and SNr also send projections to noncholinergic neurons in the pedunculopontine nucleus (PPN) and to the intralaminar thalamic nuclei. Additional projections from the SNr reach the superior colliculus. This connection may play a critical role in the control of saccades and orienting behaviors.

3.2. Normal Function of the Basal Ganglia

Voluntary movements appear to be initiated at the cortical level of the motor circuit. Cortical activation of those striatal neurons that give rise to the direct pathway is thought to lead to a reduction of inhibitory basal ganglia output, subsequent disinhibition of related thalamocortical neurons, and facilitation of movement. In contrast, activation of those striatal neurons that give rise to the indirect pathway will lead to increased basal ganglia output and, presumably, to suppression of movement. Because the majority of neurons in GPi increase their firing rate with movement, it has been speculated that the main role of the basal ganglia is to inhibit and to stabilize the activity of the thalamo-cortical network. The basal ganglia may also play a role in the control of specific kinematic parameters, such as amplitude, velocity, or direction of movement or may focus movements, allowing intended movements to proceed while suppressing competing motor acts *(12)*. Besides these elemental functions in motor control, the basal ganglia may also be involved in other motor functions, such as the generation self-initiated (internally generated) movements, procedural learning, and movement sequencing *(14)*.

3.3. Animal Models

The study of pathophysiological changes in the basal ganglia that result from loss of dopaminergic transmission has been greatly facilitated by a variety of animal models. Earlier models of the disease such as the reserpine-treated rodent, or treatment of animals with DA-receptor blockers are no longer in common use because of the nonspecificity and transitory nature of the symptoms they produce.

More recent models of PD utilize specific dopaminergic toxins that may induce pathological changes in the SNc that are strikingly similar to those seen in the human disorder. Thus, the 6-hydroxydopamine (6-OHDA)-treated rat has become the standard rodent model for the disease. Injections of this toxin into the SNc, or into the median forebrain bundle result in oxidative damage to dopaminergic neurons in the SNc, and large reductions of the striatal DA content. Another potentially useful rodent model can be produced by treatment of the animals with Rotenone *(15)*. In primates, by far the most faithful model of parkinsonism, both in terms of behavioral and pathological changes, is produced by treatment with 1-methyl-4-phenyl-1,2,3,6-tetrahydropyridine (MPTP) *(16)*. Like rotenone, MPTP is an inhibitor of the mitochondrial complex I.

The most recent attempts to model parkinsonism in animals have been based on overexpression of α-synuclein, either globally through the use of transgenic methods, or targeted to the SNc through the use of viral vectors *(17)*. Although these models replicate some of the neurodegenerative aspects of the disease, they do not reproduce the movement abnormalities typically observed in parkinsonism.

3.4. Pathophysiology

Current views concerning the pathophysiology of parkinsonism are in large part based on studies in the MPTP- and 6-OHDA models of the disorder. These studies focused initially on global activity changes in the basal ganglia. Thus, metabolic and microelectrode recordings of neuronal activity showed that MPTP-induced parkinsonism in primates is associated with reduced tonic neuronal discharge in GPe, and increased discharge in STN, GPi and SNr, as compared to normal controls (Fig. 1). These results, and the known anatomical connections between the different structures, have been used to develop the model shown in Fig. 2. According to this pathophysiological scheme, which remains the most widely used model for circuit dysfunction in parkinsonism, DA loss in the striatum results in a cascade of activity changes throughout the basal ganglia nuclei. On the one hand, DA loss

Normal

Parkinsonism

GPe

STN

GPi

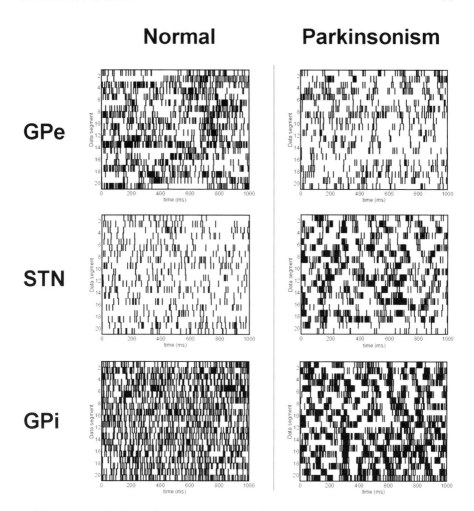

Fig. 1. Raster displays of spontaneous neuronal activity recorded in different basal ganglia structures within the basal ganglia circuitry in normal and parkinsonian primates. Shown are 10 consecutive 1000-ms segments of data from GPe, STN, and GPi. The neuronal activity is reduced in GPe, and increased in STN and GPi. In addition to the rate changes, there are also obvious changes in the firing patterns of neurons in all four structures, with a marked prominence of burstiness and oscillatory discharge patterns in the parkinsonian state.

may result in reduced activity in the direct pathway, resulting in disinhibition of the basal ganglia output nuclei. More importantly, however, it seems that DA loss in the striatum results in greater inhibition of GPe, and, consequently, in disinhibition of STN and GPi. The circuit dysfunction within the indirect pathway has been further corroborated by microdialysis studies *(18)*.

The net effect of the change, in the direct and indirect pathways is an increase in basal ganglia output to the thalamus, which may result in greater inhibition of

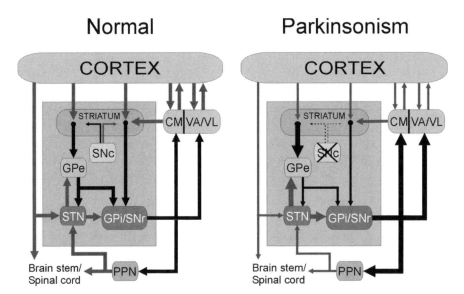

Fig. 2. Basal ganglia–thalamo-cortical circuitry. The basal ganglia circuitry (grey box) involves striatum, external and internal pallidal segment (GPe, GPi, respectively), substantia nigra pars reticulata and pars compacta (SNr, SNc, respectively), subthalamic nucleus (STN). Cortical input reaches the basal ganglia via the corticostriatal and the cortico-subthalamic connections. Basal ganglia output is directed toward the centromedian (CM) and ventral anterior/ventral lateral nucleus of thalamus (VA/VL), as well as the pedunculopontine nucleus (PPN). Excitatory connections are shown in grey, inhibitory pathways in black. In the parkinsonian state, loss of dopamine in the striatum results in activity changes throughout the basal ganglia (represented by the thickness of the connecting arrows), which lead to increased basal ganglia output to the thalamus.

thalamo-cortical neurons. Conceivably, this may reduce the responsiveness of cortical mechanisms involved in motor control. Increased tonic inhibition of thalamo-cortical neurons by increased basal ganglia output in parkinsonism may also render precentral motor areas less responsive to other inputs normally involved in initiating movements.

Brainstem areas such as the pedunculopontine (PPN) region may also be involved in the development of akinesia. It has been shown that lesions of this nucleus in normal monkeys can lead to hemiakinesia, possibly by reducing stimulation of SNc neurons by input from the PPN, or by a direct influence on descending pathways *(19)*. It remains unclear, however, whether the motor abnormalities seen after PPN inactivation are, in fact, related to parkinsonism, or represent changes in the behavioral state or other disturbances that have no direct relation to Parkinson's disease. It is noteworthy that these animals do not manifest rigidity or tremor, which appear to be critically dependent on thalamic circuitry.

Because parkinsonism is a network or circuit disease, surgical or pharmacological interventions at a variety of targets within the network could be successful. This can indeed be appreciated when considering the results of lesion studies in parkinsonian primates. One of the most important and dramatic experiments in this regard was the demonstration that lesions of the STN in MPTP-treated primates reverse all of the cardinal signs of parkinsonism, presumably by reducing GPi activity *(20)*. Similarly, GPi and SNr inactivation have been shown to be effective against at least some parkinsonian signs in MPTP-treated primates *(21,22)*.

Several important findings in animals and patients with basal ganglia lesions are not compatible with the rate-based model outlined above. For instance, lesions of the "basal ganglia-receiving" areas of the thalamus (VA/VL) do not lead to parkinsonism, as the model would suggest. Such lesions are, in fact, beneficial in the treatment of tremor and rigidity. Similarly, lesions of GPi in the setting of parkinsonism lead to improvement in all aspects of Parkinson's disease without any obvious detrimental effects. Furthermore, they are effective against both parkinsonism and drug-induced dyskinesias *(23)*. Dyskinesias are thought to arise from pathologic reduction in basal ganglia outflow, and should, thus, not respond positively to further reduction of pallidal outflow. Additionally, some of the more recent anatomical and biochemical studies have provided results, which are not in full agreement with the aforementioned model *(13)*. For instance, comparisons between MPTP-intoxicated monkeys or PD patients and their respective controls failed to reveal any significant decrease in the density of GPe output neurons expressing the messenger RNA (mRNA) coding for the γ-aminobutyric acid (GABA)-synthesizing enzyme glutamic acid decarboxylase (GAD) in the parkinsonian state. Assuming that GAD activity reflects the production and subsequent release of GABA, the lack of change in GAD activity in GPe suggests that activity changes in GPe may not be significant. Furthermore, the expression of mRNA coding for cytochrome oxidase subunit I (COI mRNA) was significantly increased in parkinsonian monkeys in neurons of STN, GPi and SNr, confirming that their activity is increased after nigrostriatal denervation, but there was no significant change in COI mRNA in GPe. Taken together, these findings suggest that the simple rate-based model of parkinsonian pathophysiology may not be sufficient to explain the circuit abnormalities in PD, and that other factors may be important as well.

Among these, alterations in discharge patterns and synchronization between neighboring neurons have been extensively documented in parkinsonian monkeys and patients. For instance, neuronal responses to passive limb manipulations in STN, GPi, and thalamus occur more often, are more pronounced and neurons have widened receptive fields after treatment with MPTP *(24)*. There is also a marked change in the degree of synchronization of discharge between neurons in the basal ganglia. Cross-correlation studies have revealed that a substantial proportion of neighboring neurons in globus pallidus and STN discharge in unison in MPTP-treated primates *(25)*, in contrast to the virtual absence of synchronized discharge of such neurons in normal monkeys. Finally, the proportion of cells in STN, GPi, and SNr with discharge in oscillatory or nonoscillatory bursts is greatly increased in the parkinsonian state *(25)*.

Although some of these abnormal discharge patterns may reflect abnormal proprioceptive input in parkinsonian individuals, it now seems that tremor and other parkinsonian abnormalities are indeed caused by synchronized oscillations in the basal ganglia. In agreement with this, lesions of the STN or GPi significantly reduce tremor in MPTP-treated monkeys and in patients with parkinsonism *(26)*. Such abnormal oscillatory activity may arise from changes in local pacemaker networks, such as a feedback circuit involving GPe and STN *(27)*, or through loss of extrastriatal DA *(28)*. Additionally, intrinsic membrane properties of basal ganglia neurons are conducive to the development of oscillatory discharge *(29)*. Increased inhibitory basal ganglia output may also contribute to the generation of oscillatory discharge in the thalamus, which may then be transmitted to cortex. It has proven to be extremely difficult to identify a single source of oscillatory discharge in the basal ganglia–thalamo-cortical circuitry. Oscillations throughout the entire basal ganglia–thalamo-cortical network may be tightly related to each other, so that no one oscillator can be identified as their sole source *(29)*.

Although tremor is perhaps the most obvious example of a parkinsonian sign that may develop as a direct consequence of abnormally patterned basal ganglia output, certain aspects of akinesia or bradykinesia may also be related to altered neuronal activity. Thus, the role of oscillatory discharge in the basal ganglia and its relationship to parkinsonian motor signs was recently re-evaluated, primarily based on results in patients in whom deep brain stimulation leads, implanted into the STN were used to record local field potentials from that nucleus *(30)*. These and other studies have lead to the concept that oscillatory interactions between basal ganglia and cortex may be a normal phenomenon, and, that high-frequency (>60 Hz) oscillations, may, in fact be prokinetic. In parkinsonism, however, low frequency oscillations (<30 Hz) dominate the cortico-basal ganglionic interaction. These oscillations are seen as antikinetic.

Nonoscillatory, phasic activity in the basal ganglia may also be deleterious to normal movement, because it may erroneously signal excessive movement or velocity to precentral motor areas, leading to a slowing or premature arrest of ongoing movements and to greater reliance on external clues during movement. Alternatively, phasic alteration of discharge in the basal ganglia may simply introduce noise into thalamic output to the cortex that is detrimental to cortical operations.

4. TREATMENT

4.1. Pharmacotherapy

4.1.1. Symptomatic Therapy

The currently available treatments for PD are in large part symptomatic, and do not alter the course of the disease. The oldest type of therapy that is still in use today, are the anticholinergic medications, such as trihexiphenidyl or benztropine. These drugs remain useful, particularly in cases of tremor-predominant PD.

However, their use is often problematic because of unpleasant side effects, such as memory disturbances, sedation, dry mouth, or urinary retention, particularly in older patients.

After its introduction in the early 1960s, DA-replacement therapy quickly became the mainstay of treatment of the disorder. The available treatments aim to replace the lost striatal DA, but may, of course, also work in other location, such as GPi, SNr, and STN, or areas outside of the basal ganglia, such as thalamus and cortex. The first agent to be introduced was the DA precursor levodopa, an amino acid, which is metabolized into DA both peripherally and centrally. It quickly became apparent that the peripheral conversion into DA results in gastrointestinal and autonomic side effects, which significantly limit the usefulness of this agent. This problem was partially remedied by combining levodopa with blockers of dopa-decarboxylase (carbidopa or benserazide). These combination treatments have had an enormous impact on the outlook of patients with PD, greatly ameliorating many of their clinical problems, and virtually normalizing their life expectancy. More recently, blockers of another enzyme, which is involved in peripheral metabolism of levodopa, catechol-*O*-methyl-transferase (COMT), was added to the therapeutic arsenal. The two available COMT inhibitors—tolcapone and entacapone—are particularly useful in patients who suffer significant fluctuations in their clinical status throughout the day. Although problems with liver toxicity forced almost complete withdrawal of tolcapone from the market, entacapone is now offered as a separate preparation, or as part of a combination drug, which also contains levodopa and carbidopa. The key to the effectiveness of both, carbidopa and entacapone, is that they do not cross the blood–brain barrier, so that their effects are strictly peripheral.

Levodopa therapy has a number of troubling side effects. The most prevalent short-term problems include autonomic disturbances, such as orthostatic hypotension and nausea. However, more troublesome are long-term complications, including drug-induced dyskinesias, hallucinations, and effect fluctuations (such as wearing-off phenomena). Although hallucinations and fluctuations are likely to be related to the acute presence of the drug, and are thus treatable by reducing the dose of levodopa, this drug appears to predispose the patient to develop involuntary movements. Additionally, it remains a possibility that levodopa may favor the production of free radicals in dopaminergic cells, and may hasten the degeneration of these neurons. Although this hypothesis is supported by some in vitro studies, it has not been convincingly demonstrated to be applicable to the human disorder. However, because of these potential problems associated with the long-term use of levodopa, many physicians recommend to delay the use of this agent as long as possible.

The most important alternatives to levodopa therapy are direct acting DA-receptor agonists, such as ropinirole, pramipexole or pergolide. Although there are significant differences in their DA-receptor subtype specificity, the clinical differences between these medications are minor. A number of studies have shown that use of these agents may help to delay the need for use of levodopa/carbidopa. This has prompted the recommendation that DA-receptor agonists should be used as first-line agents in patients with PD. It appears that these agents may also have a mild neuroprotective effect *(31)*, which has further bolstered the case for their early use, often as monotherapy. However, in all stages of the disease, the maximal benefit that can be accomplished with these agents does not reach that of levodopa, so that most patients have to use levodopa when the direct acting agonists are no longer sufficiently active. Because all of the direct acting DA agonists have a longer half-life than levodopa/carbidopa, they are also often useful as add-on agents in later stages of the disease, when the response to levodopa/carbidopa may become erratic.

The side effects of the direct-acting DA-receptor agonists are similar to those of levodopa, including nausea, cognitive side effects, and dyskinesias (although these agents do not appear to "kindle" involuntary movements). Although also described for levodopa, recent studies have shown that daytime sedation is a particularly significant side effect of these compounds that frequently limits their use. Additionally, pergolide is an ergot derivative, and, like other ergot compounds, may result in ergotism, and may also induce cardiac fibrosis. This agent should therefore only be used with caution in patients with pre-existing heart conditions. Ropinirole and pramipexole are nonergot compounds, and, therefore, do not have these side effects.

4.1.2. Neuroprotective Therapy

Based on recent insights into the pathogenesis and pathophysiology of PD, a large number of compounds have been suggested for neuroprotection in this disease. Drugs that reduce α-synuclein aggregation or inhibit apoptosis (propargylamine, caspase inhibitors), antioxidants (glutathione enhancers, tocopherol, flavonoids), anti-inflammatory drugs (nonsteroidal anti-inflammatory agents, inhibitors of cyclooxygenase-2), as well as glutamate receptor antagonists, given in an effort to reduce excitotoxicity, may all serve to provide some level of neuroprotection. Additionally, growth factors and agents to protect mitochondrial function have also been proposed as neuroprotective agents. Conceivably, cocktails of such drugs may be used to provide effects beyond those achievable with single-drug approaches.

Fortunately, some of these neuroprotective agents are already available for clinical use. One of them, the monoamine oxidase (MAO)-B inhibitor selegiline, was introduced based on the premise that PD may be caused by an (unknown) environmental toxin akin to MPTP, which requires an MAO-B dependent toxification step *(32)*. The initial studies with this medication were complicated by the fact that selegiline also has modest symptomatic effects that were not completely accounted for in these experiments. This drug remains widely used to prevent the progression of PD, and it is now thought that mechanisms independent of its MAO-B-blocking actions may contribute to its neuroprotective actions. Additionally, DA-receptor agonists such as ropinirole or pramipexole, and the glutamate receptor antagonists amantadine and riluzole, as well as Coenzyme Q-10 (CoQ_{10}), an agent that may help to protect mitochondrial function, are available to parkinsonian patients. Other agents, such as glia-derived nerve growth factor are under active investigation as new neuroprotectants.

4.2. Treatment Algorithm

It is useful to consider the use of the available pharmacotherapies in the context of an algorithm that takes into account the patient's most prominent problem (Table 2). Thus, many patients with minimal or no disabling symptoms may be best served with a recommendation to not use any medications, or to use only the neuro-protective agents, such as selegiline or CoQ_{10}. Once symptoms become more disabling, other medications can be added. In cases of tremor-predominant parkinsonism, it may be sufficient, particularly in young patients, to use one of the anticholinergic agents, otherwise, dopaminergic medications should be added in a stepwise fashion, starting with a relatively mild agent such as amantadine, then using DA-receptor agonists, and finally levodopa in combination with either carbidopa alone, or carbidopa and entacapone. Complications such as dyskinesias or cognitive impairments can often be treated with a reduction of the dose of the used medication. However, if the patient truly needs the dopaminergic medication to control otherwise disabling symptoms, it may be necessary to add other medications to treat the side effects. For instance, dyskinesias appear to respond to amantadine in many patients, likely as a result of its anti-glutamatergic effects, and drug-induced hallucinations can be treated with the newer atypical antipsychotic agents such as clozapine, quetiapine, ziprasidone, aripiprazole, or risperidone. All of these agents have a low rate of extrapyramidal side effects, and can therefore be used in parkinsonian patients. Finally, effect fluctuations (wearing-off phenomena) can be treated by shortening the interdose intervals, by using slow-release forms of levodopa/carbidopa, or by adding the COMT inhibitor entacapone or a direct agonist to the regimen.

Nonmotor signs and symptoms of PD usually require other types of treatment. Thus, depression in PD often responds readily to serotonin reuptake inhibitors such as fluoxetine and sertraline, or tricyclic antidepressants such as imipramine and amitriptyline. Symptomatic orthostasis may require the use of mineralocorticoids (fludrocortison) or the α-receptor mimetic midodrine. Finally, nonpharmacological interventions such as speech therapy or physical therapy are also often useful. Additionally, many patients and their families require extensive help through rehabilitation services or social interventions to adjust to the emerging physical or cognitive deficits.

4.3. Surgical Treatment

Many patients eventually reach a clinical state in which the commonly used antiparkinsonian pharmacotherapeutic agents are no longer effective. For these patients, functional neurosurgical approaches can be very beneficial. Neurosurgical procedures were, in fact, widely used in the 1950s and 1960s, but were essentially abandoned with the dawn of the levodopa era. After highly promising results from animal experimentation, which demonstrated reversal of parkinsonian motor signs through lesioning of the STN in MPTP-treated monkeys *(20)*, there has been renewed interest in surgical treatments of parkinsonism. This was first employed in

Table 2
Available Treatment Options for Patients With Parkinson's Disease

Clinical problem	Treatment option
No functional impairment	1. Delay symptomatic therapy 2. Start selegiline and/or Coenzyme Q-10
Mild symptoms	1. Akinesia/bradykinesia—start amantadine 2. Tremor—start anticholinergic drugs (trihexiphenidyl, benztropine) 3. Depression—start serotonin reuptake inhibitor or tricyclic antidepressant 4. Anxiety—start anxiolytic (benzodiazepine)
Disabling motor symptoms	1. Start dopaminergic therapy with dopamine receptor agonists 2. Later add levodopa/carbidopa in gradually increasing doses

Disease complications/medication side effects	1. Wearing off
	  a. Add dopamine agonist (if not taking)
	  b. Add/change levodopa/carbidopa to long-acting form
	  c. Add COMT inhibitor
	2. Dyskinesias
	  a. Reduce dopaminergic medications
	  b. Consider adding amantadine (if not taking)
	3. Hallucinations
	  a. Graded reduction of symptomatic medications (anticholinergics ? selegiline, amantadine ? COMT inhibitor ? dopamine agonists ? slow-release levodopa/carbidopa ? 'regular' levodopa/carbidopa)
	  b. Reduce psychoactive medications (sedatives, opioids, antidepressants)
	  c. Start antipsychotic agent (quetiapine, clozapine, risperidone, aripiprazole, or ziprasidone)
	4. Excessive sedation
	  a. Reduce sedatives/anxiolytics
	  b. Reduce dopaminergic medications (dopamine agonists, COMT inhibitor, levodopa/carbidopa)
	5. Autonomic failure
	  a. Add fludrocortisone
	  b. Add midodrine

Treatment-resistent motor symptoms	Functional neurosurgical treatments 1. Tremor-predominant disease—consider thalamotomy or thalamic stimulator (DBS) 2. Prominent dyskinesias or dystonia—pallidal DBS or lesions 3. Prominent akinesia/bradykinesia—STN DBS or lesions, pallidal DBS or lesions.

the form of GPi lesions (pallidotomy) *(33)* and, more recently, with STN lesions *(34)*. Additionally, high-frequency deep brain stimulation (DBS) of both the STN and GPi have been shown to reverse parkinsonian signs, probably by multiple modes of action, for instance, by inhibition of STN neurons through depolarization block, by activation of inhibitory afferents, or by true activation of STN efferents to the pallidum. Follow-up studies in patients who have been treated with these procedures have demonstrated that the disease continues to progress in patients with lesions or DBS, but that these patients get strong symptomatic benefits, which may last in excess of 5 years.

The available surgical procedures should also be tailored to the needs of the individual patient. Thus, thalamotomy or thalamic DBS implantation procedures (targeting the thalamic ventral intermediate nucleus [Vim]) are most effective against parkinsonian tremor (and, perhaps, rigidity), whereas interventions at the level of the STN appear to be effective against akinesia, bradykinesia, and tremor. GPi lesions or stimulation are particularly useful in the treatment of disabling dyskinesias and dystonia.

Through the use of modern imaging techniques and microelectrode mapping prior to lesioning or DBS lead placement, these procedures have a lesser incidence of surgical and other complications than they had in the 1950s and 1960s. Similar to other neurosurgical procedures, they may induce hemorrhages, infections, or more specific complications such as cognitive problems (likely in part due to collateral damage from probe passage through frontal areas), visual field defects owing to optic tract damage during pallidal procedures, or stroke-like symptoms as a result of vascular or mechanical damage *(35)*.

Most researchers believe that lesions and DBS procedures are either equally effective, or that DBS procedures may be (marginally) superior to pallidotomy in the treatment of PD. The advantages of lesions are that they are generally relatively straightforward and inexpensive to carry out, and that patients with lesions do not need any particular follow-up. However, these procedures are irreversible. Additionally, bilateral pallidal lesions have an increased risk of side effects, such as speech and swallowing dysfunction. DBS procedures, on the other hand, are reversible, and can be done bilaterally without significantly increased risk of side effects. However, DBS procedures carry the risk of infection and hematoma associated with any permanent introduction of a foreign body into brain matter, stimulators require battery replacements, and patients with these devices need relatively intensive follow-up because frequent adjustments of stimulation parameters are needed.

One of the persistent paradoxes in basal ganglia research remains that these invasive procedures seem to have very little effect on normal motor performance. Thus, no clear motor deficits and only subtle cognitive side effects have been demonstrated. Mood disturbances, such as depression or manic episodes have been described, but are also relatively uncommon. It appears that the brain can tolerate or compensate for a lack of basal ganglia function much more readily that for the abnormal basal ganglia output that occurs in PD.

4.4. Treatments Under Development

A variety of new treatment options are currently under development, and may become available in the near future. Among these are new dopaminergic medications such as transdermal application of short-acting dopamine agonists, or attempts to use DA-D$_1$-receptor specific agents, such as dihydrexidine and others. Nondopaminergic treatments are also under development. For instance, adenosine A2A receptors antagonists have antiparkinsonian effects in animal experimentation and humans *(36)*. There is also substantial interest in drugs that target glutamatergic system. Initial attempts have focused on antagonists that block ionotropic glutamate receptors. Preclincial and clinical studies with these medications (such as MK-801 or remacemide) have yielded mixed results, mostly because of the development of substantial side effects because such glutamate receptors are ubiquitously distributed throughout the central nervous system *(37)*. More recently, metabotropic glutamate receptors has emerged as worthwhile targets for therapeutic interventions, and several laboratories and pharmaceutical companies are actively investigating the possibility of using these drugs in parkinsonism. These compounds have the advantage of being relatively selectively distributed to certain basal ganglia loci, so that side effects may be less likely to occur than with the ionotropic glutamate receptor ligands. Although these agents are developed to provide symptomatic relief, a large number of neuroprotective treatments are under very active development, as was mentioned earlier.

Finally, other surgical procedures are also being tested. For instance, there has been a long history of using dopaminergic transplants in patients with PD. Initial transplantation studies have focused on the use of dopaminergic adrenal or fetal mesencephalic donor tissues. Owing to the mixed results of studies investigating the use of such grafts in parkinsonian patients, these procedures remain experimental. A particular problem that has become apparent is the appearance of transplantation-induced dyskinesias that may be the result of unregulated DA release from the transplanted tissue *(38)*. Because of ethical and efficacy concerns, it is likely that graft procedures will increasingly rely on stem cells or encapsulated genetically modified cells that may offer the opportunity to regulate the graft's DA production.

Another promising surgical approach is based on primate and rodent experiments that have shown that treatment of SNc cells with glia-derived nerve growth factor may protect such neurons from degeneration and may induce sprouting of dopaminergic terminals *(39)*.

GLOSSARY OF MEDICAL TERMINOLOGY

Akinesia: Inability to initiate or sustain movements.

Apraxia: Inability to perform a previously learned motor activity in the absence of motor, sensory or comprehension deficits. Apraxia is often described as an impairment of selection or sequencing of voluntary movement.

Ataxia: Uncoordinated or inaccurate movement that is not the result of paresis, alteration in tone, loss of postural sense or involuntary movements.

Basal ganglia: A group of subcortical brain structures strongly implicated in the development of movement disorders such as Parkinson's disease.

Bradykinesia: Abnormal slowness of movement, sluggishness.

Cerebellar signs: Physical signs of cerebellar disease. Ataxia is a typical cerebellar sign.

Chorea: Discrete involuntary arrhythmic movements.

Dementia: Loss of cognitive abilities; usually affects more than one area of cognition (e.g., memory and executive functions and visuospatial abilities).

Dystonia: Slow, sustained involuntary movements or postures, often associated with prominent co-contraction of antagonist muscle groups and overflow of activation to inappropriate muscle groups; severely disruptive to the execution of intended movements.

Dyskinesia: Descriptive summary term which encompasses all abnormal, nonoscillatory, nonepileptic involuntary movements (including chorea, athetosis, dystonia, ballismus, myoclonus).

Freezing: Sudden and unexpected occurrence of akinesia.

Hypophonia: Voice of low volume.

Incidence: Number of new cases of a disease diagnosed each year.

Lewy body: Pathologic abnormality found on microscopic examination of degenerating dopaminergic neurons in patients who died of Parkinson's disease.

Movement disorder: Term used either to describe a physical sign of involuntary or abnormal movement in the absence of weakness, or to describe the syndrome that causes such motor abnormalities; encompasses hypokinetic disorders (e.g., Parkinson's disease) and hyperkinetic disorders (associated with dyskinesias or nonparkinsonian tremor).

Myoclonus: Jerking, nonoscillatory movements.

Orthostasis: Precipitous fall in blood pressure on arising; a sign of autonomic failure.

Paratonia: Increased muscle tone, which has a voluntary component to it. Paratonia is a classical sign of frontal lobe dysfunction, and is seen in advanced Parkinson's disease.

Parkinson's disease: Pathological entity in which loss of dopaminergic neurons in the substantia nigra and the occurrence Lewy bodies are associated with the development of physical motor (such as akinesia, bradykinesia, rigidity and postural abnormalities) and nonmotor signs (such as orthostasis and dementia).

Parkinsonism: The behavioral syndrome associated with Parkinson's disease and other conditions.

Parkinson-plus syndrome: A condition in which patients show signs of parkinsonism in addition to physical signs that are not part of Parkinson's disease.

PET: A nuclear medical examination technique that traces the distribution of radioactive materials in the brain.

Prevalence: Total number of people in a population with a certain disease at a given time.

Rapid eye-movement sleep behavior disorder: A failure of movement suppression during rapid eye-movement (REM) sleep, associated with complex behavior although dreaming.

Retropulsion: The sensation of being pulled backward. Retropulsion is a typical form of postural instability seen in Parkinson's disease.

Rigidity: Increased muscle tone, which, on examination by passive movements of the affected limb is independent of the velocity of the imposed movement. Rigidity is a classic sign of Parkinson's disease.

Spasticity: Increased muscle tone, which, on examination by passive movements of the affected limb, is more pronounced with imposed movements of high velocity. Spasticity is seen in many diseases in which the cortical control of spinal motor neurons is disrupted.

Supranuclear gaze palsy: The inability to carry out voluntary eye movements in patients in whom the same eye movements can be elicited as a response to activation of brainstem reflexes.

Tremor: Oscillatory involuntary movement.

Micrographia: Small handwriting.

Upper motor neuron signs: Physical signs that indicate the presence of damage to the cortical or subcortical control of brain stem and spinal motor neurons. Classical upper motor neuron signs are spasticity and increased deep tendon reflexes.

Wearing-off: The premature loss of the effect of a given dose of a medication.

REFERENCES

1. Parkinson J. An Essay on the Shaking Palsy, Sherwood, Neely and Jones, 1817.
2. Hughes AJ, Daniel SE, Kilford L, Lees AJ. Accuracy of clinical diagnosis of idiopathic Parkinson's disease: a clinico-pathological study of 100 cases. J Neurol Neurosurg Psychiatry 1992;55:181–184.
3. Braak H, Del Tredici K, Rub U, de Vos RA, Jansen Steur EN Braak E. Staging of brain pathology related to sporadic Parkinson's disease. Neurobiology of Aging 2003;24:197–211.
4. Beal MF. Mitochondria, oxidative damage, and inflammation in Parkinson's disease. Ann N Y Acad Sci 2003;991:120–131.
5. Cummings JL, Masterman DL. Depression in patients with Parkinson's disease. Int J Geriatr Psychiatry 1999;14:711–718.
6. Ichinose H, Ohye T, Takayashi E, et al. Hereditary progressive dystonia with marked diurnal fluctuation caused by mutations in the GTP cyclohydrolase I gene. Nature Genetics 1994;8:236–242.
7. Polymeropoulos MH, Lavedan C, Leroy E, et al. Mutation in the alpha-synuclein gene identified in families with Parkinson's disease. Science 1997;276:2045–2047.
8. Trojanowski JQ, Lee VM. "Fatal attractions" of proteins. A comprehensive hypothetical mechanism underlying Alzheimer's disease and other neurodegenerative disorders. Ann N Y Acad Sci 2000;924:62–67.
9. McNaught KS, Olanow CW, Halliwell B, Isacson O, Jenner P. Failure of the ubiquitin-proteasome system in Parkinson's disease. Nature Reviews Neuroscience 2001;2:589–594.
10. Albin RL, Young AB, Penney JB. The functional anatomy of basal ganglia disorders. Trends Neurosci 1989;12:366–375.
11. Gerfen CR, Wilson CJ. The Basal Ganglia. In: A Björklund, T HökfeldL Swanson (Eds.), Handbook of Chemical Neuroanatomy, Integrated Systems of the CNS, Part III, Vol., Amsterdam: Elsevier, 1996:369.
12. Wichmann T, DeLong MR. Functional neuroanatomy of the basal ganglia in Parkinson's disease. Adv Neurol 2003;91:9–18.
13. Parent A, Cicchetti F. The current model of basal ganglia organization under scrutiny. Movement Disorders 1998;13:199–202.
14. Schultz W. The phasic reward signal of primate dopamine neurons. Advances in Pharmacology 1998;42:686–690.
15. Betarbet R, Sherer TB, MacKenzie G, Garcia-Osuna M, Panov AV, Greenamyre JT. Chronic systemic pesticide exposure reproduces features of Parkinson's disease. Nature Neuroscience 2000;3:1301–1306.
16. Burns RS, Chiueh CC, Markey SP, Ebert MH, Jacobowitz DM, Kopin IJ. A primate model of parkinsonism: selective destruction of dopaminergic neurons in the pars compacta of the substantia nigra by N-methyl-4-phenyl-1,2,3,6-tetrahydropyridine. Proc Natl Acad Sci USA 1983; 80:4546–4550.
17. Kirik D, Annett LE, Burger C, Muzyczka N, Mandel RJ, Bjorklund A. Nigrostriatal alpha-synucleinopathy induced by viral vector-mediated overexpression of human alpha-synuclein: a new primate model of Parkinson's disease. Proceedings of the National Academy of Sciences of the United States of America 2003;100:2884–2889.

18. Robertson RG, Graham WC, Sambrook MA, Crossman AR. Further investigations into the patho-physiology of MPTP-induced parkinsonism in the primate: an intracerebral microdialysis study of gamma-aminobutyric acid in the lateral segment of the globus pallidus. Brain Research 1991;563:278–280.

19. Kojima J, Yamaji Y, Matsumura M, et al. Excitotoxic lesions of the pedunculopontine tegmental nucleus produce contralateral hemiparkinsonism in the monkey. Neurosci Lett 1997;226: 111–114.

20. Bergman H, Wichmann T, DeLong MR. Reversal of experimental parkinsonism by lesions of the subthalamic nucleus. Science 1990;249:1436–1438.

21. Wichmann T, Kliem MA, DeLong MR. Antiparkinsonian and behavioral effects of inactivation of the substantia nigra pars reticulata in hemiparkinsonian primates. Exp Neurol 2001;167: 410–424.

22. Lieberman DM, Corthesy ME, Cummins A, Oldfield EH. Reversal of experimental parkinsonism by using selective chemical ablation of the medial globus pallidus. J Neurosurg 1999;90: 928–934.

23. Obeso JA, Rodriguez-Oroz MC, Rodriguez M, DeLong MR, Olanow CW. Pathophysiology of levodopa-induced dyskinesias in Parkinson's disease: problems with the current model. Annals of Neurology 2000;47:S22-32; discussion S32–S24.

24. Filion M, Tremblay L, Bedard PJ. Abnormal influences of passive limb movement on the activity of globus pallidus neurons in parkinsonian monkeys. Brain Res 1988;444:165–176.

25. Bergman H, Wichmann T, Karmon B, DeLong MR. The primate subthalamic nucleus. II. Neuronal activity in the MPTP model of parkinsonism. J Neurophysiol 1994;72:507–520.

26. Bergman H, Wichmann T, DeLong MR. Amelioration of Parkinsonian Symptoms by Inactivation of the Subthalamic Nucleus (STN) in MPTP Treated Green Monkeys. Movement Disorders 1990;5 (Suppl 1):79.

27. Plenz D, Kitai S. A basal ganglia pacemaker formed by the subthalamic nucleus and external globus pallidus. Nature 1999;400:677–682.

28. Bergman H, Raz A, Feingold A, et al. Physiology of MPTP tremor. Movement Disorders 1998;13, Suppl. 3:29–34.

29. Bevan MD, Magill PJ, Terman D, Bolam JP, Wilson CJ. Move to the rhythm: oscillations in the subthalamic nucleus-external globus pallidus network. Trends Neurosci 2002;25:525–531.

30. Brown P. Oscillatory nature of human basal ganglia activity: relationship to the pathophysiology of Parkinson's disease. Movement Disorders 2003;18:357–363.

31. Schapira AH. Neuroprotection and dopamine agonists. Neurology 2002;58:S9–S18.

32. Anonymous. DATATOP: a multicenter controlled clinical trial in early Parkinson's disease. Parkinson Study Group. Arch Neurol 1989;46:1052–1060.

33. Baron MS, Vitek JL, Bakay RAE, et al. Treatment of advanced Parkinson's disease by GPi pallidotomy: 1 year pilot-study results. AnnNeurol 1996;40:355–366.

34. Gill SS, Heywood P. Bilateral subthalamic nucleotomy can be accomplished safely. Movement Disorders 1998;13:201.

35. de Bie RM, de Haan RJ, Schuurman PR, Esselink RA, Bosch DA, Speelman JD. Morbidity and mortality following pallidotomy in Parkinson's disease: a systematic review. Neurology 2002; 58:1008–1012.

36. Ikeda K, Kurokawa M, Aoyama S, Kuwana Y. Neuroprotection by adenosine A2A receptor blockade in experimental models of Parkinson's disease. J Neurochem 2002;80:262–270.

37. Greenamyre JT, Eller RV, Zhang Z, Ovadia A, Kurlan R, Gash DM. Antiparkinsonian effects of remacemide hydrochloride, a glutamate antagonist, in rodent and primate models of Parkinson's disease [comment]. Annals of Neurology 1994;35:655–661.

38. Freed CR, Greene PE, Breeze RE, et al. Transplantation of embryonic dopamine neurons for severe Parkinson's disease. [comment]. N Engl J Med 2001;344:710–719.

39. Gash DM, Zhang Z, Ovadia A, et al. Functional recovery in parkinsonian monkeys treated with GDNF. Nature 1996;380:252–255.

III Psychiatric Disorders

6

Schizophrenia

Stephan Heckers and Sabina Berretta

Summary

Schizophrenia is one of the major diagnostic and treatment challenges in medicine. Although approx 1% of the population suffers from schizophrenia, available treatments remain symptomatic and rarely allow for a full functional recovery. This results in a large burden for persons afflicted with schizophrenia, their families, and the society at large.

We have made progress in reliably diagnosing schizophrenia and in exploring the neural basis of schizophrenia. Neural circuits involving dopaminergic, glutamatergic, and γ-aminobutyric acid (GABA)ergic neurons in prefrontal cortical regions, in the temporal lobe, and in the thalamus are involved in mediating the psychotic features and the cognitive deficits of schizophrenia. Studies of this emerging neural circuitry include the mapping of brain structure and function in patients, the quantification of cellular and molecular changes in postmortem specimens, and the validation of changes in animal models of schizophrenia. Recently, several risk genes for schizophrenia have been identified, providing specific targets for the development of diagnostic tests and therapeutic interventions.

In this chapter, we review basic concepts of the clinical presentation, the neural and genetic basis, and the pharmacological treatment of schizophrenia.

Key Words: Schizophrenia; psychopathology; epidemiology; genetics; neurochemistry; neuroanatomy; pathology; animal models; treatment; outcome.

1. INTRODUCTION

Schizophrenia is a severe mental illness. Although many questions remain—about the diagnostic boundaries, disease mechanisms, optimal treatment, and disease progression and outcome—there is no debate about the seriousness of schizophrenia. Schizophrenia affects about 1% of the population, typically in the second and third decade of life. A person suffering from schizophrenia often does not accept the diagnosis, which can lead to poor compliance with pharmacological and nonpharmacological treatment and unstable social relationships. The limited resources of the existing mental health care system only add to the daunting challenges a person with schizophrenia has to overcome.

From: *Current Clinical Neurology: Neurological and Psychiatric Disorders:*
From Bench to Bedside
Edited by: F. I. Tarazi and J. A. Schetz © Humana Press Inc., Totowa, NJ

In this chapter, we review the diagnostic concept of schizophrenia and its history, the signs and symptoms on which the diagnosis is based, the current status of neuroscientific and genetic investigations of schizophrenia, the currently available pharmacological and nonpharmacological treatment modalities, and the predictors of disease progression and outcome

2. DIAGNOSIS OF SCHIZOPHRENIA

The term *schizophrenia* was coined by the Swiss psychiatrist Eugen Bleuler in 1911. It was his intention to change the diagnostic term for a group of severely ill psychiatric patients, who at that time were diagnosed with *dementia praecox*, a concept introduced by the German psychiatrist Emil Kraepelin in 1886. It is important to understand the concept of *dementia praecox* first, before we can appreciate Bleuler's contribution, as well as the still ongoing debate about the boundaries of the diagnostic construct schizophrenia.

Kraepelin introduced new diagnostic entities for patients who presented with similar (but not always overlapping) signs and symptoms, and—this was the crucial criterion—showed the same course and outcome. The term *dementia praecox* captures this notion very well: it describes a group of patients who suffer a decline of function in the realms of cognition and affect regulation (i.e., dementia) at an early age (i.e., praecox). Three years after his conceptualization of *dementia praecox*, Kraepelin introduced the diagnosis *manic-depressive illness* (now referred to as bipolar disorder), to separate from *dementia praecox* a group of patients who also present with abnormalities of cognition and affect regulation, often at an early age, but who do not progress to dementia and severe impairments of social functioning.

It was exactly this dichotomy into *dementia praecox* and *manic-depressive illness* that Bleuler wanted to overcome: he felt strongly that the patients who were diagnosed with *dementia praecox* did not always progress to an end stage of dementia, but could recover some, if not all, of their skills lost during the acute episodes of their illness. Therefore, he abandoned the term *dementia praecox*, and proposed schizophrenia, which translates best into "splitting of the mind." This term is often misunderstood as a split identity (as in the concept of the multiple personalities). Instead, Bleuler felt that at the core of the illness was an inability to synchronize cognition (which leads to rational decisions) and affect (which allows for more immediate assessments and responses). This leads to abnormal associations between thoughts, to affective indifference, to an ambivalence about most life decisions, and to an uncoupling from reality to the degree that the inner life assumes pathological predominance (i.e., autism). These four cardinal symptoms—association, affectivity, ambivalence, and autism (often referred to as Bleuler's Four As)—can be accompanied by accessory symptoms, that emanate out of the cardinal symptoms. Accessory symptoms include the well-known symptoms of hallucinations and delusions, as well as other abnormalities of cognition and motor behavior.

Table 1
The DSM-IV Diagnosis of Schizophrenia

Criterion
A	>2 criteria for >1 month
	delusions
	hallucinations
	disorganized speech
	grossly disorganized/catatonic behavior
	negative symptoms
B	Social dysfunction
C	Duration: 6 months
D	Schizoaffective/mood disorder exclusion
E	Substance/general medical condition exclusion
F	Relationship to a pervasive developmental disorder

The debate about the exact definition of the diagnostic construct schizophrenia and about the boundaries between psychosis (i.e., the impairment of reality testing as seen in delusions and hallucinations) and affective illness still continues. There are some who strongly endorse the Kraepelinian dichotomy into schizophrenia and bipolar disorder, whereas others favor the unitary concept of psychosis, which encompasses all patients with schizophrenia and affective psychosis *(1)*. These debates are not just of interest for the academic psychiatrist—they impact on our ability to predict disease outcome, select the best treatment, and ultimately uncover the mechanisms and causes leading to schizophrenia.

The diagnostic system proposed in the fourth edition of the Diagnostic and Statistical Manual of Mental Disorders (DSM-IV) is currently considered to be the gold standard for the diagnosis of schizophrenia (Table 1). To be given the diagnosis schizophrenia, the person has to present with at least two of the following symptoms: delusions, hallucinations, disorganized speech, grossly disorganized behavior, and negative symptoms (such as flat affect, social withdrawal, or anhedonia) for at least 6 months, during which the symptoms have to be prominent or continuous for at least 1 month. These changes must lead to a decrease of social function (e.g., poor school or job performance, strained relationships). Once these criteria of severity and duration are met, it must be confirmed that these changes are not a result of another medical illness or the use of drugs, and that the person does not suffer from major abnormalities of affect regulation, in which case the diagnoses bipolar disorder or schizoaffective disorder (an intermediate between schizophrenia and bipolar disorder) have to be considered.

These widely used diagnostic criteria have greatly improved the reliability of the diagnosis, i.e., there is generally good agreement between clinicians in arriving at the diagnosis. However, there still remains a great deal of uncertainty, even for very experienced clinicians, when evaluating patients who straddle between nonaffective psychosis and affective psychosis. More importantly, it is not clear at all whether the reliable concept of schizophrenia guarantees a common cause and disease mechanism. For example, it is possible that distinct causes and pathologies will be uncovered for subgroups of schizophrenia patients. Evidence for such heterogeneity has been difficult to obtain, but is accumulating for dichotomous models (e.g., patients with and without prominent negative symptoms, i.e., deficit and nondeficit schizophrenia) *(2)* and for even finer parcellation into more than two subgroups.

3. THE SIGNS AND SYMPTOMS OF SCHIZOPHRENIA

The diagnosis of schizophrenia rests entirely on the observation of signs by the evaluator and the report of symptoms by the patient. There are, as of yet, no other objective markers (such as blood test, radiological exam, or physiological stress test) to assist with the diagnosis. Furthermore, the documentation of signs and symptoms is not as straightforward as in other fields of medicine, in which the physical exam and the interview often provide the data necessary to make a diagnosis.

A major challenge in the diagnostic process of schizophrenia is poor cooperation, because the person often rejects being labeled with a psychiatric illness. However, a skilled clinician is able to arrive at a tentative psychiatric diagnosis after a thorough interview of the patient. The diagnostic process can be supported by information gleaned from an inspection of available records and, most importantly, further interviews with relatives and friends. The cornerstone of the diagnosis of schizophrenia, however, is the structured patient interview, often referred to as the Mental Status Exam (MSE). The material provided by the MSE comes in three different flavors: observation of behavior (signs), report of experiences by the patient (symptoms), and inferences of abnormal mental states based on observation and report.

The initial contact can provide evidence that the person suffers from a mental illness. The attire might be inappropriate (such as three winter coats in summer time) and the grooming might be poor. Eye contact is often avoided or, at times, prohibited by wearing sunglasses. The facial expression can be flat and with little or no range throughout the interview. The attitude toward the interviewer might be guarded or suspicious and at times frankly hostile. The person's body might show very little activity and movement (so-called psychomotor retardation) and no modulation throughout the interview. This might range from a frozen facial expression, to bradykinesia or abulia, and ultimately catatonia. In contrast, some patients, especially those who feel constrained by the interview setting, might become agitated and possibly assaultive. All of these observations are not diagnostic for schizophrenia, but in aggregate with the symptoms and inferences are very helpful in making the diagnosis. They inform primarily about the item "grossly disorganized/catatonic behavior" of criterion A (see Table 1) for the diagnosis of schizophrenia.

Documenting how the person responds verbally is a crucial part of the MSE. The normal person responds logically, coherently, and with direction toward a goal. The schizophrenia patient might show a lack of coherence and no clear path when providing a narrative or when answering questions. This can vary from circumstantiality or tangentiality, over flight of ideas, to loose associations and complete derailment of the thought process. Additionally, other abnormalities such as perseveration, clang association, and thought blocking can be found. These abnormalities of thought process inform about the item "disorganized speech" of criterion A (*see* Table 1).

An important piece for making the diagnosis of schizophrenia is the patient's report of unusual sensory experiences in the form of illusions (misperceived objects) or hallucinations (a percept-like experience in the absence of an appropriate stimulus, but with the full force and impact of an actual perception, which is not under the voluntary control of the experiencer) *(3)*.

Such experiences are often in the auditory modality and typically in the form of distinct voices. If the voices provide a running commentary to the person's actions or if two voices are conversing, then this experience is considered to be of high diagnostic significance, and no additional criterion A item (*see* Table 1) is needed to make the diagnosis schizophrenia. But hallucinations are often less prominent, at times barely identifiable, and over time can become integrated into the everyday life of the patient with schizophrenia. A concerning form of auditory hallucination are command hallucinations, in which a voice orders the person to engage in a particular behavior. This can range from mundane acts, such as brushing teeth, to serious self-injury and possibly the death of others or oneself. Hallucinations occur in other sensory domains as well, especially the visual and the somatosensory realm.

The reported mood and the description of the person's life provide important information as well. Most schizophrenia patients withdraw from their friends and family members and become isolated. This almost invariably leads to a decrease of social functioning, with strains in personal relationships and poor school/work performance. Such data provide information about the item "negative symptoms" of criterion A.

The interviewer has to weigh the validity of the person's responses to questions and the free verbal production. In some cases, it is obvious that the thought content is bizarre and clearly not congruent with normal reality testing. For example, when a woman reports that she avoids her own apartment because she is convinced that her neighbors have planted metal devices into her own, her daughter's, and her dog's bowel, in order to control their movements, it is intuitively clear that this belief (and possibly her sensory experience, which would constitute a viscerosensory hallucination) is not grounded in reality. However, many other reports remain more ambiguous. What do we make of the fear that all actions are monitored by a secret agency—it is possible but is it true? How do we evaluate overvalued and rigidly held religious beliefs? To diagnose a delusion, the interviewer has to evaluate how the opinions and beliefs fit into a commonly shared sense of reality and then infer that the person is in an abnormal mental state.

The quality of delusions can vary considerably: they can be rational and highly systematized or they can be bizarre and internally inconsistent *(4)*. Delusions may lead to strong affective responses and at times violent acts or they can be well integrated into the person's life without affecting the person's feelings and decisions. Delusions may also affect the ability of the patient to accept the diagnosis of a mental illness. Such lack of insight can create a major challenge, because the patient may refuse treatment or avoid contact with treaters all together.

To summarize, the schizophrenia patient might present with a lack of function (i.e., negative symptoms such as decreased psychomotor activity, anhedonia, social withdrawal) or abnormal experiences (i.e., positive symptoms such as delusions, hallucinations, and thought disorder). Now that we have a basic understanding of the signs and symptoms of schizophrenia, how can we explain them? How does the brain give rise to positive and negative symptoms?

4. THE NEURAL BASIS OF SCHIZOPHRENIA

Kraepelin's *dementia praecox* concept was closely linked to the hypothesis that distinct brain areas and brain functions are affected, giving rise to the panoply of clinical features. At the end of his career, Kraepelin was convinced that the pathology of *dementia praecox* had been defined (i.e., specific abnormalities in the upper three layers of the cerebral cortex).

We know now that multiple, interconnected brain regions, including cortical areas such as the anterior cingulate gyrus and medial orbitofrontal cortex, and paleocortical and subcortical regions, e.g. hippocampus, thalamus, amygdala, and nucleus accumbens, are involved in the pathophysiology of schizophrenia (see Table 2). These regions are reciprocally connected with each other, with higher order association areas of the cerebral cortex such as the dorsolateral prefrontal cortex (governing cognition, judgment, and insight), and with the hypothalamus (modulating vegetative functions such heart rate, temperature control, feeding behavior, and sexual drive). This allows cortico-limbic brain circuits to play an important role in assigning emotional and motivational significance to sensory inputs. These interactions are crucial for the creation of representations and in the evaluation of the intentionality of others. Such functions are perturbed in schizophrenia. Compelling parallels can be drawn between disturbances observed following lesions of specific cortico-limbic regions (such as the amygdala or the anterior cingulate gyrus) and the clinical symptomatology of schizophrenia, particularly flat or inappropriate affect, social withdrawal and delusional thinking, loss of attentiveness, and "akinetic mutism." Furthermore, stimulation of the human amygdala evokes a variety of highly complex emotions and hallucinations and patients with temporal lobe epilepsy can develop psychotic symptoms similar to schizophrenia *(5)*. This supports the notion that pathology of limbic regions such as the amygdala and hippocampus can give rise to some of the clinical features of schizophrenia.

Support for a circuitry-based pathology of schizophrenia involving multiple, interconnected, cortico-limbic brain regions comes also from the wide array of neurotransmitters and neuromodulators, as well as synaptic proteins, that appear to be affected in this disease. The original "dopamine (DA) hypothesis" of schizophrenia originated from the observation that drugs of abuse increasing DA release (e.g., cocaine, amphetamine) can trigger psychotic symptoms and the finding that

Table 2
The Neural Basis of Schizophrenia

Brain region	Cellular pathology	Functional abnormality	Resulting deficits
Prefrontal cortex	Interneuron deficit	Abnormal activation during working memory tasks	Impaired insight, poor attention, poor working memory, delusions
Superior temporal gyrus	?	Abnormal activation during auditory hallucination	Auditory hallucinations, thought disorder
		Decreased activation during passive auditory detection (mismatch)	
Thalamus	Cell loss (?)	Impaired activation during memory tasks	Poor episodic memory
Hippocampus	Interneuron deficit	Impaired activation during memory tasks	Poor declaractive memory, delusions and hallucinations
Amygdala	?	?	Abnormal processing of emotional stimuli, negative symptoms
Cerebellum	?	Impaired activation during memory tasks	Abnormal timing
Striatum	?	Increased dopamine release	Psychomotor abnormalities

antipsychotic drugs block DA D_2-like receptors in a direct correlation with their antipsychotic efficacy. Although it has been surprisingly difficult to uncover the genetic and molecular basis for DA dysfunction in schizophrenia, there is little doubt that DA plays an important role in schizophrenia.

More recent hypotheses on DA and schizophrenia propose that altered dopaminergic transmission, and in particular the phasic increase of DA release at the time of psychosis, may result from a disruption of its regulation by other neurotransmitters, such as glutamate *(6)*. A dysfunction of glutamatergic neurotransmission, possibly with a selective decrease of *N*-methyl-D-asparate (NMDA) glutamate receptor function, is also gaining increasing support *(7)*. Glutamate is the most prevalent excitatory neurotransmitter, involved in many brain functions. A drug-induced psychosis provided some of the initial evidence for a role of glutamate in schizophrenia: the anesthetic ketamine and the illicit drug phencyclidine (also known as PCP or angel dust) block the NMDA glutamate receptor and can induce a mental state that resembles schizophrenia. As for the DA hypothesis, uncovering the exact details of glutamatergic dysfunction in schizophrenia has been challenging, although recent postmortem and genetic findings *(see* Section 6) have supported the notion that glutamatergic neurotransmission is perturbed in schizophrenia.

A role for serotonin in the pathogenesis of schizophrenia had been originally proposed on the basis of the similarity between LSD, which is psychotomimetic, and serotonin *(8)* and was lately supported by the finding that LSD activates 5-hydroxytryptamine (5-HT)$_{2A}$ receptors. Furthermore, the atypical antipsychotics clozapine, olanzapine, risperidone, and quetiapine exhibit antagonistic activities at multiple serotonin receptors and have been found to downregulate cortical 5-HT$_{2A}$ following chronic treatment in animal studies *(9)*. Although the actual occurrence of disruptions of the serotoninergic system in schizophrenia is still a matter of debate, recent findings seem to support its role in this disease *(10)*. Interestingly, a number of serotoninergic receptor families have been shown to modulate the effect of other neurotransmitters, such as glutamate, GABA, acetylcholine, and DA *(11)*.

Abnormalities of GABAergic transmission in schizophrenia appear to be among the most consistent findings in postmortem studies and strongly suggest involvement of specific interneuronal subpopulations in multiple limbic regions *(12)*. Altered numbers of GABAergic interneurons, as well as changes in the expression of several markers for GABAergic transmission, have been reported in most of the brain regions currently believed to be involved in schizophrenia. GABA is an inhibitory neurotransmitter broadly expressed throughout the central nervous system. Intrinsic GABAergic circuits in cortical and subcortical regions tightly regulate the activity of glutamatergic projection neurons. Thus, alterations of glutamatergic and GABAergic transmission are inextricably linked to each other. It has been hypothesized that the overinclusive (unable to filter out extraneous information), disorganized thought processes typical of schizophrenia may reflect, at least in part, a disruption of GABAergic transmission resulting in failure of appropriate gating mechanisms. On a highly speculative level, it is intriguing to note that specific subpopulations of interneurons have been shown to generate and support oscillatory patterns of brain activity, which play an important role in information processing and storage.

Within the context of circuit-based hypotheses of schizophrenia, it may be of interest to understand how specific anatomic models of schizophrenia could link distinct signs and symptoms to specific brain areas or neural circuits. For example, how does the brain give rise to hallucinations? It had long been proposed that the same brain areas that are engaged in normal perception also give rise to an abnormal hallucinatory experience. Recent neuroimaging studies have now convincingly shown that this is indeed the case *(13)*.

Let us review this for the auditory domain. Information arrives from the inner ear via the brainstem and the thalamus to tonotopically organized regions in the primary auditory cortex, located in a region of the superior temporal gyrus called Heschl's gyrus. The highly segregated auditory information is then processed in the surrounding auditory association cortex and integrated with all other sensory modalities (i.e., vision, somatosensory) in the large areas of the prefrontal and parietal cortices. When a person experiences auditory hallucinations in form of voices, the region of the primary auditory cortex is significantly activated, indicating that the experience of hearing the voices is similar to the perception of "real" voices at the level of the brain *(13)*. Similar findings have also been reported for the visual system and the experience of hallucinating colors and shaped objects. Many questions still remain unanswered: how is the primary auditory cortex information integrated into the larger mental representation, including the ability to remember previously stored information and the ability to identify the person behind the voice experience? How is it possible, for most schizophrenia patients, to gain insight into the nonveridical nature of the hallucinatory experience?

In summary, we are steadily gaining insight into the specific neuropathology of schizophrenia, affecting distinct cortico-limbic regions such as the anterior cingulate gyrus, the dorsolateral prefrontal cortex, the hippocampus and limbic thalamus. It is now obvious that schizophrenia is the result of a disruption of information processing within multiple, interconnected circuits linking these regions. Such disruption involves complex interactions among numerous neurotransmitters (GABA, glutamate) and neuromodulators (DA, several neuropeptides such as cholecystokinin, neuropeptide Y, neurotensin). To explore the cellular basis of schizophrenia further, animal models have proven to be a fruitful area of investigation.

5. ANIMAL MODELS

As for other diseases, modeling schizophrenia in experimental animals serves a necessary, indispensable role. The main purpose and advantage is to allow experimental testing of specific hypotheses regarding schizophrenia. However, the design of heuristic models for schizophrenia, with adequate face, construct, and predictive validity has represented an enormous challenge and has met, at least until recently, with limited success. Construct validity has been restricted by our incomplete understanding of the pathophysiological mechanisms of schizophrenia and by its heterogeneous etiology involving complex interaction among genetic, epigenetic, and environmental factors. Convincing face validity is hampered by the fact that schizophrenia is a disorder of the highest human functions (e.g., hallucinations, delusions, thought disorder, lack of speech content), so that reproducing the full clinical spectrum of this disease is not a meaningful goal. Predictive validity, particularly considered in relationship to neuroleptic treatment, has been somewhat more successful.

Despite these difficulties, increasingly sophisticated animal models of schizophrenia have contributed useful and much needed information to the understanding of this disease. These models have naturally developed in parallel with our understanding of this disease. For instance, initial hypotheses postulating excessive dopaminergic transmission in schizophrenia prompted a generation of animal models designed to mimic such condition. We know now that such models, by themselves, hold little construct validity. More recently, however, dopamine-based models have been used in combination with other experimental manipulations, such as NMDA receptor blockade, to test the role of DA in the context of more complex, circuit-based, abnormalities. In turn, postmortem findings indicating abnormalities in glutamatergic transmission in several brain regions support the basic assumption of NMDA receptor antagonist-based models but point to subtle, neurochemically and anatomically selective, changes rather than the generalized disruption induced by systemic administration of NMDA receptor antagonists.

These recent phases of the evolution of animal models of schizophrenia indicate that the emerging strategy has shifted from models designed to reproduce the disease as a whole to what has been defined as "component" or "partial" modeling (12,14). The basic idea is to focus on specific aspects of the disease with the ultimate goal of recomposing the complex, multifaceted puzzle that schizophrenia still represents. A specific example of this strategy is to consider the multiple, interconnected brain circuits involved in this disease and investigate how a distinct abnormality within a specific brain region, as detected in schizophrenia, can affect downstream target regions. Recently, this approach has been used to dissect out, from a complex network of cortico-limbic circuitry, one potential source of abnormal afferent activity to the hippocampus. In these experiments, a broad set of changes detected in the hippocampus of schizophrenic patients, involving specific subpopulations of hippocampal interneurons, was reproduced in experimental animals in which a local disruption of GABAergic transmission within the amygdala was induced pharmacologically (15).

Another interesting example of "component" modeling is the study of specific behavioral responses known to be impaired in schizophrenia that can be tested in experimental animals. These include behavioral paradigms such as prepulse inhibition of startle, auditory sensory gating, latent inhibition and social isolation (16). These behavioral paradigms are used as models for psychophysiologic constructs of schizophrenia and are particularly useful in combination with other experimental manipulations as a way to test the face validity of specific models.

Table 3
Lifetime Expectancy (Morbid Risk) Estimates of Schizophrenia

	Lifetime expectancy (%)
If no relative has schizophrenia	1
If the following relative has schizophrenia:	
One parent	10
Both parents	46
Sibling	10
Child	6
	Proband-wise concordance (%)
For twin if co-twin has schizophrenia:	
Dizygotic twin	14
Monozygotic twin	46

Finally, recent animal models have been developed to investigate the etiology of schizophrenia with respect to genetic abnormalities, prenatal and postnatal events, epigenetic factors, and disrupted neurogenesis and stress. Some of these models successfully reproduce neurochemical and behavioral changes similar to those found in schizophrenia and, in some cases, have a degree of predictive validity, i.e., changes can be reversed by neuroleptics. Other animal models, involving neonatal brain lesions, are aimed at disrupting the development of specific brain regions involved in schizophrenia in order to test their effects on cortical and subcortical regions connected to them. Interestingly, neonatal lesions of the hippocampus induce schizophrenia-related behaviors and molecular changes that emerge only after puberty, thus mimicking the typical course of this disease *(17)*.

6. CAUSES OF SCHIZOPHRENIA

Schizophrenia is caused by genetic as well as nongenetic factors. Genetic factors include mutations in the DNA, abnormalities of DNA transcription into RNA, and abnormal translation of mRNA into protein. Nongenetic factors vary from insults during early brain development (e.g., *in utero* infection/hypoxia and birth trauma), postnatal developmental phases (e.g., viral infections and malnutrition), as well as social stressors during adolescence and adulthood (e.g., leaving home, migration to another country, urban environment). How these factors work together to create devastating changes of behavior in the second or third decade of life remains a puzzle. Here, we briefly review the genetics of schizophrenia.

The search for the genetic causes of schizophrenia dates back 100 years. It became clear early on, that the risk to develop schizophrenia is increased if another family member is already affected with schizophrenia (Table 3). The highest rates are reported for monozygotic twins, who have a 50% concordance rate for the development of schizophrenia. The family studies of schizophrenia have been confirmed

Table 4
Novel Genes for Schizophrenia

Gene	Abbreviation	Locus	Protein function
Neuregulin	NRG1	8p12-p21	Modulates glial cells and glutamate NMDA receptors
Dysbindin	DTNBP1	6p22	Synaptic function (?)
G72	G72	13q34	Interacts with DAAO
D-amino acid oxidase	DAAO	12q24	Modulates D-serine
RGS4	RGS4	1q21-22	Regulates G protein signal
Catechol-O-methyl transferase	COMT	22q11	Catabolic enzyme of dopamine
Proline dehydrogenase	PRODH	22q11	Degrades proline, affects glutamate

and extended by adoption studies, which helped to decrease the confounding effect of the shared environment on the genetic factors in schizophrenia. Taken together, there is now convincing evidence that a combination of risk genes contributes to the development of schizophrenia. However, it is also obvious that schizophrenia is not completely determined by genes (as in an autosomal dominant disease with full penetrance, such as Huntington's disease).

The exact genetic mechanisms of schizophrenia have remained elusive. The introduction of molecular biology techniques and the access to large patient populations has resulted in many links between the diagnosis of schizophrenia and a polymorphism in the human genome, thereby allowing researchers to home in on specific stretches of one of the chromosomes. Unfortunately, linkage to chromosomal regions has been hard to confirm in independent replication studies.

More recently, several genes have been implicated in the disease mechanism of schizophrenia (Table 4). The identification of individual genes and their products (i.e., proteins) is a significant step forward in identifying the genetic determinants of schizophrenia *(18)*. Several genes code for proteins known to affect pathways relevant for schizophrenia. For example, the newly found protein neuregulin 1 (NRG1), a protein coded for by the gene *G72* on chromosome 13q34, and the enzyme D-amino acid oxidase (DAA) are all in the position to affect glutamatergic neurotransmission.

On the other hand, a mutation in the gene coding for catechol-*O*-methyl transferase (COMT), the catabolic enzyme of DA, is associated with impaired brain function in schizophrenia. The COMT gene contains a missense mutation, which translates into a substitution of Met for Val at codon 108y158 (Val108/158 Met). The enzyme containing Met is unstable and has only one-fourth of the activity of the enzyme containing Val. This means that the Val/Val phenotype is associated with increased DA catabolism, resulting in impaired brain function in regions that depend on proper COMT function. A recent study found that the COMT Val allele, which was more common in schizophrenic offspring, predicted a less efficient physiological response in prefrontal cortex *(19)*.

Taken together, there is now compelling evidence for specific risk genes for schizophrenia, which will lead to a better understanding of the disease mechanisms and the discovery of targets for drug development.

7. TREATMENT OF SCHIZOPHRENIA

So far, the pharmacological treatment of schizophrenia has been guided by serendipity. The first generation of antipsychotic drugs was introduced in the 1950s, after French researchers discovered their calming and sedating properties (which explains why they are also referred to as neuroleptics). Only after the clinical efficacy of these drugs was established, did it become clear that they all modulate the DA neurotransmitter system by blocking preferentially the D_2 DA-receptor subtype. Following this discovery, the search for antipsychotic drugs focused on spe-

Table 5
Antipsychotic Medication

Compound	TM	FDA approval	Manufacturer	CPZ (mg/d)	Daily dose (mg)
Clozapine	Clozaril®	1989	Novartis	50	300–900
Risperidone	Risperdal®	1994	Janssen	2	2–6
Olanzapine	Zyprexa®	1996	Lilly	5	10–20
Quetiapine	Seroquel®	1998	AstraZeneca	75	300–750
Ziprasidone	Geodon®	2000	Pfizer	60	120–160
Aripiprazole	Abilify®	2002	Otsuka/ Bristol-Myers Squibb	7.5	10–30
Chlorpromazine	Thorazine®		Generic	100	100–1000
Thioridazine	Mellaril®		Generic	100	30–800
Perphenazine	Trilafon®		Generic	10	2–60
Fluphenazine	Prolixin®		Generic	2	5–40
Haloperidol	Haldol®		Generic	2	3–50

cific neurotransmitter systems: first the dopaminergic system, then the serotonergic system, and most recently the glutamatergic system.

Two classes of antipsychotic drugs are currently available on the US market for the treatment of psychosis in general and schizophrenia specifically (Table 5). The first generation antipsychotic drugs range from low-potency drugs such as chlorpromazine to high-potency drugs such as haloperidol and fluphenazine. All mediate their antipsychotic effects primarily via blockade of DA receptors, which is directly related to their propensity to cause adverse effects in the motor system. These motor side effects are referred to as extra-pyramidal side effects (EPS), because striatal neurons rather than the motor cortex pyramidal neurons are primarily affected. EPS range from those that present within hours or days (dyskinesias and akathisia), to months (parkinsonian symptoms), and possibly years (tardive dyskinesia). One potentially lethal adverse event is the neuroleptic malignant syndrome (NMS), which includes fever, extrapyramidal symptoms (typically with muscle rigidity), and autonomic dysfunction. NMS is rare, can occur with any type of first-generation antipsychotic, and requires immediate medical attention. The patient should be taken off the antipsychotic drug that caused NMS, but can be tried on another antipsychotic drug.

Although first-generation antipsychotic drugs are effective in many patients, a substantial number of patients do not respond adequately or suffer debilitating side effects. This explains the continued search for better treatment of schizophrenia, which resulted in the introduction of the second-generation antipsychotics. The first and most significant advance in the treatment of schizophrenia was clozapine, which is superior to first-generation antipsychotics in the treatment of psychosis and causes little, if any, EPS. However, clozapine is associated with a potentially lethal adverse event, agranulocytosis, which requires regular blood testing. Furthermore, clozapine can cause NMS, excessive sedation, and a dose-dependent risk of epileptic seizures.

The introduction of clozapine was followed by *five* second-generation antipsychotics (olanzapine, risperidone, quetiapine, ziprasidone, and aripiprazole) within the last 10 years. These compounds differ in their receptor-binding profile, their half-life time, their side-effect profile, and potentially their ability to improve cognition, but all are effective in the treatment of psychosis. The receptor profile of the second-generation antipsychotics differs from the traditional compounds, by targeting receptors other than the DA D_2 receptor, including serotonin receptors (primarily the 5-HT_{2A} receptor subtype), histaminergic receptors, and muscarinic receptors. They all share with clozapine its higher affinity for 5-HT_{2A} over D_2 receptors, which may contribute to their benign extrapyramidal profile. Some of these drugs (i.e., clozapine, quetiapine, and ziprasidone) also have direct 5-HT_{1A} agonist activity, although others (i.e., olanzapine and risperidone) can interact indirectly with 5-HT_{1A} receptors to improve symptoms of schizophrenia *(9)*.

The newest addition to the armamentarium of antipsychotic drugs is aripiprazole, a partial agonist at the D_2 and 5-HT_{1A} receptors, and an antagonist at 5-HT_{2A} receptors. The mechanism of D_2 partial agonist (i.e., blockade of D_2 receptors in the setting of a hyperdopaminergic state, and stimulation of the D_2 receptor when intrasynaptic DA levels are low) tends to stabilize dopaminergic neurotransmission and holds the promise that the drug might alleviate symptoms of psychosis, improve cognitive deficits, minimize sedation, and avoid extrapyramidal side effects and the observed increase in metabolic activities and body weight. The question, which of the available antipsychotic drugs should be chosen as first-line treatment is currently a matter of intense debate *(20)*. Most experts recommend one of the newer second-generation antipsychotic drugs and reserve clozapine and a combination of second- and first-generation antipsychotic drugs for those patients who have failed adequate trials (i.e., 6 weeks) of two or three of the newer second-generation antipsychotic drugs.

In addition to the two classes of antipsychotic drugs, many patients with schizophrenia also benefit from other classes of psychotropic medication. First, several drugs have been shown to augment the efficacy of antipsychotic drugs *(21)*. These drugs include mood stabilizers such as valproic acid and lithium, tranquilizers such as benzodiazepines, and novel (still experimental) approaches, such as glycine, D-cyclo-serine and AMPAkines, which facilitate glutamatergic function. Second, patients with schizophrenia often suffer from other psychiatric conditions (such as panic attacks, obsessive-compulsive disorder, posttraumatic stress disorder, and substance abuse), which require the administration of additional psychotropic medication.

The pharmacological management of schizophrenia needs to be implemented into a comprehensive treatment plan. Poor communication between the patient and the mental health professional, the frequent occurrence of adverse effects, and the cognitive deficits lead many patients to discontinue their medication. Education about the illness and supportive programs that involve the patient's family are confirmed methods to improve the treatment of psychosis. Specific forms of psychotherapy, such as cognitive-behavioral interventions, have been shown to be effective in the treatment of positive symptoms, such as delusions and hallucinations. Finally, the reintegration of the person with schizophrenia into the society is greatly enhanced by social skills training and supportive community services, which include clubhouses, residential programs, and mobile outreach teams of mental health workers.

8. OUTCOME OF SCHIZOPHRENIA

Kraepelin was initially convinced that poor outcome is an essential part of the clinical presentation of dementia praecox/schizophrenia. At the end of his career, however, he became more cautious and questioned whether all cases always progress with severe cognitive decline. Extensive research has now shown that schizophrenia does not necessarily lead to an end stage of severe deficits. In fact, about 25% of patients will recover with little if any deficits, 25% will remain with severe deficits, and the remaining 50% cover the spectrum between these two poles. These outcome statistics remind us that we have to consider every schizophrenic patient to be eligible for recovery. However, several predictors of outcome allow us to estimate these chances. For example, female patients and those with higher levels of education and stronger cognitive skills have a better outcome. But these statistical inferences, derived from large patient samples, do not necessarily allow us to predict the course and outcome of the illness in an individual patient.

Schizophrenia is also associated with a significantly increased risk of medical morbidity. This is explained, in part, by the insufficient access to medical care, but there is compelling evidence for a link between schizophrenia and specific medical illnesses. For example, the risk for the development of cardiovascular illness is greatly increased in schizophrenia, which leads to increased morbidity and mortality. It is currently a matter of intense debate, how much this increased risk of medical morbidity in schizophrenia is caused or aggravated by the administration of antipsychotic drugs.

The worst outcome of schizophrenia is suicide. Approximately 6% of all schizophrenic patients die by their own hands, an eightfold increased risk compared to the general population *(22)*. Suicide in schizophrenia, however, can be prevented. A comprehensive treatment plan, including antipsychotic medication (especially clozapine), has proven to reduce the risk of suicide.

9. CONCLUSION

The clinical presentation of schizophrenia can be complex, but most patients are accurately diagnosed using standardized criteria. The signs and symptoms of schizophrenia often appear in the second or third decade of life and may persist for short periods (e.g., 6 months) or can result in a lifelong struggle. Although the disease mechanisms and ultimate causes of schizophrenia remain unknown, we have seen great progress in unraveling the neural and genetic basis of schizophrenia. Pharmacological and nonpharmacological treatments of schizophrenia can provide significant relief for most patients and extensive periods of remission for some. The outcome of schizophrenia varies between complete recovery of function to persistent cognitive impairments and psychiatric disability. Future research will uncover the neural basis of the clinical heterogeneity, the variable response to treatment, and the range in outcome.

GLOSSARY OF MEDICAL TERMINOLOGY

Abulia: Abnormal reduction in speech, movement, thought, and emotional reaction.

Accumbens, nucleus: Forebrain region corresponding to the ventral portion of the corpus striatum.

Akathisia: A condition of motor restlessness, an urge to move about constantly and an inability to sit still; a common extrapyramidal side effect of neuroleptic drugs.

Akinetic mutism: Subacute or chronic state of altered consciousness, in which the patient appears alert intermittently, but is not responsive, although descending motor pathways appear intact; as a result of lesions of various cerebral structures.

Amygdala: Subcortical brain region located within the temporal lobe. It is one of the components of the limbic system that is most specifically involved with emotional experience.

Anhedonia: Absence of pleasure from the performance of acts that would ordinarily be pleasurable.

Antipsychotic: A drug that is effective in the treatment of psychosis.

Autosomal gene: A gene located on any chromosome other than the sex chromosomes (X or Y).

Bradykinesia: An abnormal slowness of movement, sluggishness of physical and mental responses.

Brainstem: The lowest part of the brain, which merges with the spinal cord. It consists of the medulla oblongata, midbrain, and pons.

Clang association: Specific type of formal thought disorder, i.e., use of two words with a similar sound.

Catatonia: A syndrome of psychomotor disturbances, characterized by mutism (inability to talk), stupor (inability to move), muscular rigidity, and excitement.

Delusion: A fixed, false belief, seen most often in psychosis.

Dopamine: A catecholamine neurotransmitter.

Dopamine D_2-like receptor: One of the two families of dopamine receptors (i.e., D_1 and D_2). It includes dopamine receptors D_2, D_3, and D_4.

Dyskinesia: Impaired (fragmentary or incomplete) voluntary movement.

Hallucination: A percept like experience in the absence of an appropriate stimulus.

Hippocampus: Allocortical structure situated beneath the cortical mantle. Together with the amygdala constitutes the core of the limbic system.

Interneuron: Short axon neurons mostly forming local circuits within a specific brain region.

Limbic (system): a heterogeneous array of cortical and subcortical brain structures, including the anterior cingulate gyrus, hippocampus, amygdala, and portions of the thalamus, that are involved in the processing of emotion.

NMDA glutamate receptor: One of the four ion channel-coupled glutamate receptor subtypes, named after one of the most selective agonists N-methyl-D-aspartate. These receptors are implicated in memory and learning, neuronal cell death, ischaemia, and epilepsy.

Paleocortex: The phylogenetically oldest part of the cortical mantle of the cerebral hemisphere.

Perseveration: The constant repetition of a word or phrase.

Polymorphism (of genes): A difference in DNA sequence among individuals, groups, or populations.

Psychotomimetic: A drug or substance that produces psychological and behavioral changes resembling those of psychosis; e.g., LSD.

Psychotropic medication: A drug or substance capable of modifying mental activity.

Serotonin: A monoamine neurotransmitter, also called 5-hydroxytryptamine (5-HT).

Serotonin 5HT$_{2A}$ receptor: A subtype of the 5HT$_2$ receptor group.

Subcortical: Brain region situated beneath the cortical mantle.

Superior temporal gyrus: A longitudinal gyrus on the lateral surface of the temporal lobe between the lateral (sylvian) fissure and the superior temporal sulcus.

Synaptic proteins: Proteins in the synapse, involved in the regulation of neurotransmitter release.

Temporal lobe epilepsy: Seizures with elaborate and multiple sensory, motor, and/or psychic components. A common feature is the clouding of consciousness and amnesia for the event.

Thalamus: Large, ovoid masses, consisting chiefly of grey substance, situated one on each side of and forming part of the lateral wall of the third ventricle. It is divided into two major parts: dorsal and ventral, each of which contains many nuclei.

REFERENCES

1. Kendler KS, Karkowski LM, Walsh D. The structure of psychosis: latent class analysis of probands from the Roscommon Family Study [see comments]. Arch Gen Psychiatry 1998;55: 492–499.
2. Kirkpatrick B, Buchanan RW, Ross DE, Carpenter WI. A separate disease within the syndrome of schizophrenia. Archives of General Psychiatry 2001;58:165–171.
3. Slade PD, Bentall RP. Sensory Deception. A scientific analysis of hallucination. 1 ed. Baltimore & London: The Johns Hopkins University Press, 1988.
4. Sims A. Symptoms in the mind. An introduction to descriptive psychopathology. London: W.B. Saunders, 1999.
5. Gloor P. The temporal lobe and limbic system. New York, NY: Oxford University Press, 1997.
6. Grace AA. Phasic versus tonic dopamine release and the modulation of dopamine system responsivity: a hypothesis for the etiology of schizophrenia. Neuroscience 1991;41:1–24.
7. Konradi C, Heckers S. Molecular aspects of glutamate dysregulation: implications for schizophrenia and its treatment. Pharmacology & Therapeutics 2003;97:153–179.
8. Wooley D, Shaw E. A biochemical and pharmacological suggestion about certain mental disorders. Proc. Natl. Acad. Sci. 1954;40:228–231.
9. Tarazi FI, Zhang K, Baldessarini RJ. Long-term effects of olanzapine, risperidone, and quetiapine on serotonin 1A, 2A and 2C receptors in rat forebrain regions. Psychopharmacology 2002;161: 263–270.
10. Lopez-Figueroa AL, Norton CS, Lopez-Figueroa MO, et al. Serotonin 5-HT1A, 5-HT1B, and 5-HT2A receptor mRNA expression in subjects with major depression, bipolar disorder, and schizophrenia. Biol Psychiatry 2004;55:225–233.
11. Roth BL, Hanizavareh SM, Blum AE. Serotonin receptors represent highly favorable molecular targets for cognitive enhancement in schizophrenia and other disorders. Psychopharmacology (Berl) 2003;174:17.
12. Benes FM, Berretta S. Gabaergic interneurons: Implications for understanding schizophrenia and bipolar disorder. Neuropsychopharmacology 2001;25:1–27.

13. Weiss AP, Heckers S. Neuroimaging of hallucinations: a review of the literature. Psychiatry Research: Neuroimaging 1999;92:61–74.
14. Kilts CD. The changing roles and targets for animal models of schizophrenia. Biol Psychiatry 2001;50:845–855.
15. Berretta S, Lange N, Bhattacharyya S, Sebro R, Garces J, Benes FM. Long Term Effects of Amygdala GABA Receptor Blockade on Specific Subpopulations of Hippocampal Interneurons. Hippocampus 2004;14:876–894.
16. Swerdlow NR, Braff DL, Geyer MA. Animal models of deficient sensorimotor gating: what we know, what we think we know, and what we hope to know soon. Behav Pharmacol 2000;11: 185–204.
17. Lipska BK, Weinberger DR. To model a psychiatric disorder in animals: schizophrenia as a reality test. Neuropsychopharmacology 2000;23:223–239.
18. O'Donovan MC, Williams NM, Owen MJ. Recent advances in the genetics of schizophrenia. Human Molecular Genetics 2003;12:R125–R133.
19. Egan MF, Goldberg TE, Kolachana BS, et al. Effect of COMT Val108/158 Met genotype on frontal lobe function and risk for schizophrenia. Proceedings of the National Academy of Sciences of the United States of America. 2001;98:6917–6922.
20. Davis JM, Chen N, Glick ID. A meta-analysis of the efficacy of second-generation antipsychotics. Archives of General Psychiatry 2003;60:553–564.
21. Goff DC, Freudenreich O, Evins AE. Augmentation strategies in the treatment of schizophrenia. CNS Spectrums 2001;6:904–911.
22. Harris EC, Barraclough B. Suicide as an outcome for mental disorders: a meta-analysis. British Journal of Psychiatry 1997;170:205–228.

7

Autism Spectrum Disorders

Evdokia Anagnostou and Eric Hollander

Summary

Autism is a developmental disorder, characterized by repetitive behaviors and by deficits in social skills and communicative abilities. Autism spectrum disorders affect 60 out of 10,000 individuals, resulting in significant costs to families and society. Neuropathological and imaging studies point to abnormalities in the limbic system and the cerebellum, and accelerated brain grown in the first 2 years of life. Abnormalities in serotonin function have been identified in affected patients and their families. Genetic studies document high concordance in monozygotic twins and genome screens have identified multiple loci as possibly associated with autism, with the strongest evidence pointing to regions $2q$ and $7q$. Although there is a relative lack of well-controlled treatment studies, selective serotonin reuptake inhibitors and atypical antipsychotics are useful in the treatment of repetitive behaviors and aggression. Nonpharamacological interventions include intensive early childhood educational programs, and interventions targeted at problem behaviors and social skills improvement.

Key Words: PDD; autism; Asperger's; neurobiology; genetics; phenomenology; treatment.

1. AUTISM SPECTRUM DISORDERS

Autism is a devastating developmental disorder classified under the pervasive developmental disorders. It affects social interaction, communication, and repetitive/compulsive behaviors. Autism, Asperger's syndrome, and pervasive developmental disorder not otherwise specified (PDD-NOS), collectively known as autism spectrum disorders (ASD), cause lifelong functional impairment and severely impact both affected individuals and their families. This chapter emphasizes the neurobiology, phenotypes, and current treatments for autism.

2. BRAIN PATHWAYS

Abnormalities in almost every neural system in the brain have been causally linked to autism. Studies of the small number of autistic brains currently available

From: *Current Clinical Neurology: Neurological and Psychiatric Disorders: From Bench to Bedside*
Edited by: F. I. Tarazi and J. A. Schetz © Humana Press Inc., Totowa, NJ

have revealed abnormalities mostly in forebrain limbic structures, cerebellar circuits, and the growth patterns of the brain. New imaging techniques have started to corroborate data from pathology studies.

2.1. Limbic System

In the limbic system, the most consistent histological abnormality is the presence of small, densely packed neurons in the amygdala, hippocampus, and mammillary bodies *(1,2)*, and large neurons in the diagonal band of Broca in the septum in young children. These brain structures are part of the circuit of Papez, which is important in memory and emotions. Cortical malformations are also occasionally observed, which indicates abnormalities in neuronal migration and points to injury during fetal development.

Volumetric studies of the limbic structures have produced some conflicting data that probably reflects heterogeneity within the autistic population. In contrast, functional imaging studies are somewhat more consistent. For instance, transient frontal hypoperfusion at 2 to 4 years of age has been demonstrated by regional cerebral blood flow (rCBF) studies. Marked bitemporal hypoperfusion has been reported by two independent groups *(3,4)* using single photon emission computed tomography (SPECT) or positron emission tomography (PET). Neuronal hypofunction also has been suggested by magnetic resonance spectroscopy (MRS). Functional magnetic resonance imaging (fMRI) studies have shown decreased activation of the left amygdala during "theory of mind" tasks. Overall, functional imaging techniques offer preliminary data to support amygdala dysfunction in autism.

2.2. The Cerebellum

In the cerebellum, the most consistent abnormality is that of a decreased number of Purkinje cells in the cerebellar cortex *(1,2,5)*. This change is associated with small neurons in the inferior olive and deep cerebellar nuclei, as well as with a decreased neuronal density in deep nuclei. Given that the Purkinje and inferior olive cells develop a tight synaptic relationship by 28 weeks gestation, the above findings imply that the Purkinje cell loss takes place prenatally. Furthermore, the postnatal changes in number and size of the deep nuclei and inferior olive neurons suggest that these pathological processes continue into the postnatal period. Inconsistent findings include hypoplasia of vermal lobules VI and VII, malformations of the inferior olive, and prominent arcuate nuclei *(2,6)*.

Structural imaging studies of the cerebellum and posterior fossa have failed to reveal consistent abnormalities. Reduced brainstem, midbrain, and pons size, and cerebellar atrophy, particularly of vermal lobules VI and VII, have all been reported. Functional imaging studies have recently demonstrated increased cerebellar motor activation and decreased cerebellar attention activation in autistic patients. The correlation of clinical findings and observed cerebellar abnormalities remains problematic, because the reported anomalies are not observed across studies and may be present in other non-autistic neurological disorders.

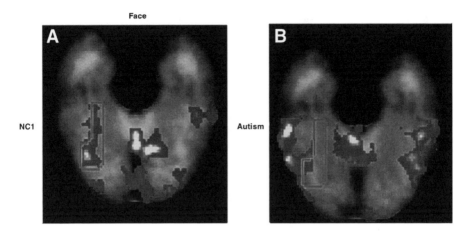

Fig. 1. Composite activation maps superimposed on averaged anatomic images. The region of interest (fusiform gyrus) is outlined in green. Note that the fusiform gyrus is activated during face discrimination in the control group (NC1) **(A)** but not in the autistic group **(B)**. *See* color insert preceding p. 51. (From ref. *8*. Copyright 2000, American Medical Association. All rights reserved.)

2.3. Brain Growth

Alterations in brain size is the most consistently replicated finding. Autistic children tend to have small heads at birth followed by an excessive increase in head size between 1 and 2 months and 6 and 24 months of age *(7)*. Megalencephaly during childhood has been suggested by MRI and pathology studies. In a recent volumetric study, the white matter was shown to be disproportionately large compared to controls. Increased brain size may be associated with altered functional connections between specialized neural systems as a result of disorganization. Further support for this hypothesis comes from analysis of the corpus callosum, the major fiber pathway interconnecting the two cerebral hemispheres, which is found to be smaller in autistic patients than in controls. Less neural integration is actually consistent with the theory of "lack of central coherence" as an explanation for autistic symptoms. Abnormalities in other cortical and subcortical areas have been reported but not replicated.

2.4. Other Clues From Functional Imaging

In terms of functional imaging, auditory stimulation studies have shown decreased perfusion of the left superior temporal gyrus indicating that autism is associated with an abnormal pattern of activation of the left temporal cortex. Given that the left temporal cortex is implicated in the organization of language, the language impairment observed in autistic patients may be linked to this abnormality. In studies in which patients were asked to perform tasks looking at faces, the face perception area in the fusiform gyrus was not activated *(8)* (Fig. 1). This is in keeping with clinical observations of autistic patients having difficulty recognizing and discriminating amongst facial expressions. Decreased activation in the dorsolateral prefrontal cortex and posterior cingulate cortex during spatial memory tasks has been observed and may explain the impairment in executive function seen in autistic patients.

In summary, neuropathological and imaging studies point to anatomic abnormalities, and dysfunction of the amygdala and limbic forebrain structures. These findings seem to be consistent with the social deficits observed in autism. Abnormalities noted in the cerebellum are still somewhat difficult to interpret clinically. Acceleration of brain growth in early childhood followed by a dramatic deceleration is the most consistent finding in this population, possibly suggesting poor cortical organization and supporting the theory of "lack of central coherence."

3. MOLECULAR TARGETS

Abnormalities in multiple systems have been postulated, including serotoninergic, noradrenergic, dopaminergic, opioid, and oxytocin/vasopressin systems. The evidence so far does not support primary involvement of the noradrenergic and opioid systems, although the evidence for the involvement of the dopaminergic system is rather conflicting. In contrast, there is significant evidence implicating serotoninergic and oxytocin/vasopressin systems in the pathophysiology of autism.

3.1. Serotonin

There are multiple studies implicating serotonin in the pathophysiology of autism, and serotonin seems to be critical in neurodevelopment. The first serotoninergic neurons in the brain are evident by 5 weeks of gestation and by 15 weeks typical serotonin bodies are seen in the cells of raphae nuclei. All serotonin receptors and transporters are present by 4 months of gestation. The fact that serotonin arrives in target regions earlier that other monoamines may mean that it regulates the terminal maturation of other monoamine systems, such as dopamine, and therefore, it may be key for further development.

Evidence for low serotonin in the synapses in the central nervous system has been reported. A PET study using a radiolabeled serotonin precursor found decreased serotonin synthesis in the cortex, thalamus, and dentate nucleus. The loss of serotonin terminals can lead to altered developmental processes in the target areas described above. Additionally, increased 5-hydroxytryptamine (5-HT)1d inhibitory autoreceptor sensitivity in adult autistic patients has been demonstrated, which is consistent with decreased 5-HT synthesis. Furthermore, the severity of these 5-HT1d abnormalities has been correlated with the severity of repetitive behaviors in autism *(9)*.

Pharmacological manipulation of serotonin systems in the autistic population has shown that acute depletion of the 5-HT precursor tryptophan can exacerbate anxiety, self-injurious behaviors, and stereotypies in autistic subjects. Decreased central serotonin responsiveness was demonstrated by a blunted prolactin response to the 5-HT releasing agent fenfluramine. Recent data suggest that serotonin reuptake inhibitors may be useful in controlling global severity and repetitive behaviors.

Platelet hyperserotonemia has been also documented in multiple studies. In some studies, there is a correlation between elevated serotonin levels in the platelets and the severity of cognitive impairment, stereotypies, and behavioral disturbances, but these findings have not always been replicated. Additionally, it seems that serotonin abnormalities in autistic patients are shared by other asymptomatic, non-autistic family members. This seems to imply that elevated blood serotonin levels may be associated with a genetic liability to certain subtypes of autism.

3.2. Oxytocin/Vasopressin System

There has been an abundance of evidence linking the vasopressin/oxytocin system to social attachment, mate preference, and repetitive movements in animal studies *(10,11)*. Children with autism seem to manifest lower plasma oxytocin levels than their normal peers, and they fail to show the expected increases in plasma oxytocin levels with age. Deficits in oxytocin-processing peptides in autism have also been reported. Finally, a significant reduction in repetitive behaviors was demonstrated after oxytocin infusion in a group of patients with autism *(12)*, which suggests a possible role for intervention with oxytocin agonists.

4. ANIMAL MODELS

Although no animal model exists that adequately explains all the features of autism, several studies have explored structural, genetic, toxic, or infectious etiologies of autism in mice, rats, and pigs (Table 1). The most promising ones involve lesions of the limbic system resulting in deficits in social interaction and repetitive behaviors in monkeys and rats. Additionally, eliminating the disheveled gene by genetic manipulation has produced a mouse with limited social interaction. This gene functions in the Wnt pathway, which is a pathway important for cell-to-cell interaction during embryogenesis. A different gene (WNT_2) in this pathway has been found to be mutated in some autistic families. In a cohort of 160 families with no autism, the mutated gene was not found. Knock-out mice for the oxytocin gene show an inability to develop social memory, and a Fragile X Mental Retardation 1 (*FMR1*) knock-out mouse demonstrates increased perseveration. Furthermore, maternal infection during pregnancy has been cited as the "principal non-genetic cause" of autism *(13)*. Neonatal or fetal inoculation with the borna or the influenza virus results in impaired play and exploratory behavior and deficits in social interaction in rat and mouse models. Several attempts at creating autism models by teratogen exposure, i.e., thalidomide or valproate, look promising but behavioral studies have not been done yet.

Table 1
Selected Autism Animal Models

Author	Species	Model	Behavioral phenotype
Bechavalier et al., 1996	Monkey	Middle temporal lobe lesions	Social deficits, stereotypies
Woltemink et al., 2001	Rat	Central and lateral amygdalae lesions	Social deficits
Bobee et al., 2000	Rat	Medial cerebellar lesions, day 10	↑ spontaneous activity, ↓ anxiety in novel situations
Lijam et al., 1997	Mouse	Dvl1 or disheveled gene knockout	Social deficit, abnormal sensorimotor gating
Ferguson et al., 2000	Mouse	Oxytocin gene knockout	No social memory
Engelmann et al., 1994	Brattleboro rat	Spontaneous mutation leading to Vasopressin knockout	Social & cognitive deficits Diabetes insipidus
Pletnikov et al., 1999 Horning et al., 1999	Lewis rat	Neonatal borna infection, leading to limbic & cerebellar malformations	Impaired play behavior & emotional reactivity
Shi et al., 2003	Mouse	Fetal influenza infection	Deficits in social interaction, decreased exploratory behavior
Comery et al., 1997	Mouse	FMR1 knockout, resulting in abnormal dendrites of layer V neurons	Increased perseveration

136

5. GENETICS

Although Kanner and Asperger felt that autism is a disorder of neuropathological origin, the psychiatric community of the 1950s questioned the heritability of the syndrome. In the late 1960s, a case series of families who had more than one autistic child was published. The incidence of autism in these families was reported to be two to three times greater than that of the general population and it was argued that this would support a genetic etiology.

5.1. Twin and Family Studies

In the late 1970s, the first twin study indicated a higher concordance for autism among monozygotic (MZ) vs dizygotic (DZ) twins. Subsequent twin studies have revealed a MZ concordance rate of 70% vs a rate of 0% in the DZ twins. When milder cognitive or social deficits were included, the MZ concordance rate was 82% vs a rate of 10% in the DZ pairs. Several studies of the non-autistic family members followed. Social reticence, pragmatic language deficits, and difficulty adjusting to changes in environment are present with increased frequency in the parents of affected children compared to controls, and are known as the broader autistic phenotype.

5.2. Genome Screens

There have been seven genome screens for autism susceptibility loci in autistic siblings. Possible loci associated with autism have been mapped to chromosomes 1, 2, 3, 5, 6, 7, 13, 15, 16, 17, 19, and X with chromosomes 2 and 7 being the most consistent.

On the long arm of chromosome 2, a region approx 35 megabases long and containing approx 100 genes shows a strong association with autism. The association becomes even stronger if phrase speech delay (PSD) is included in the phenotype *(14)*. Similarly, region *7q* shows a strong association with autism that becomes even stronger if PSD is used as an endophenotype *(15,16)*. Interestingly, chromosomal region *7q* includes the AUTS1 gene, which is responsible for severe familial expressive aphasia *(17)*. AUTS1 has been found in siblings and unrelated individuals with either autism or language disorder. In one screen, chromosomal region *6q* was also shown to strongly associate with autism. A mutation of the glutamate receptor gene in *6q21* has been identified in 8% of autistic subjects vs 4% of controls and appears to be transmitted from mothers to autistic sons.

5.3. Other Candidate Gene Regions

5.3.1. 15q11-q13

An increased frequency of cytogenetic abnormalities of the region *15q11-13* has been reported in the autistic population *(18)*. These include a variety of anomalies such as maternally derived interstitial duplications, submicroscopic deletions and a supernumerary chromosome 15. Chromosomal region *15q11-13* is of particular interest for two main reasons. First, it harbors genes for several subunits of the

GABA$_A$ receptor and some association has been found between one marker and autism. Second, abnormalities in the same region also result in Angelman syndrome, which is a childhood neurological disorder with autistic features. Angelman syndrome usually results from a lack of maternal gene expression, but also from a mutation in the *UBE3A* gene. However, mutations of the *UBE3A* gene have not been found in autistic individuals without Angelman syndrome.

5.3.2. Serotonin Transporter and Reelin

Given the considerable evidence for abnormalities in the serotonin system in autism, attempts have been made to identify an abnormality in the serotonin transporter genes. Several polymorphic variants of the *5-HTTLRP* (a polymorphism of the serotonin transporter gene) have been reported to show preferred transmission in families of autistic probands. Despite this, the evidence remains conflicting with different polymorphisms associating with autism in different studies.

Reelin is an extracellular matrix protein that is responsible for correct lamellar formation of the fetal brain. Reelin is also important for cell signaling and synaptic plasticity in the adult brain. Abnormalities of brain reelin mRNA have been reported in multiple psychiatric disorders, including autism, and consequently, reelin polymorphisms remain an area of active research.

5.4. Immunogenetics

There is some evidence for an association between autoimmunity and autism. Families of autistic children have a higher number of individuals with autoimmune diseases than families of nonaffected children. Some autistic children or their mothers have major histocompatibility complex (MHC) haplotypes that predispose to autoimmunity. In twin studies, autistic children are more likely to have auto-antibodies to myelin basic protein, neurofilament protein, and vascular endothelium than controls. The question of a functional deficit of the MHC molecules in autism has been raised as a result. However, none of the genome screens has had any signals near the MHC locus on *6p* so far. Our group has demonstrated increased antibodies to heat shock protein 90 *(19)* and increased expression of D8/17, an immune marker on B-cells *(20)*, in autistic patients.

5.5. Other Chromosomal and Genetic Disorders

Genetic conditions associated with autism include tuberous sclerosis, neurofibromatosis, Down syndrome, and Fragile X syndrome. The reported prevalence rates of autism in these disorders varies widely because of small sample sizes, but they collectively represent less than 6 to 7% of autistic individuals and this figure includes other nongenetic medical disorders, such us congenital rubella.

In summary, autism has a large genetic contribution, although this does not exclude environmental factors in the pathogenesis of the disorder. Twin, cytogenetic, and genome screens studies have been invaluable and identification of pathogenetic genes is expected in the near future. Among patients with autism, only a small percentage also has another identifiable genetic disorder.

6. EPIDEMIOLOGY

The first epidemiological studies of autism took place in England in the mid-1960s. Since then, 32 large surveys of autism have been published in English *(21)*. The studies vary significantly in sample size, approach to identifying subjects, screening methodology, and the diagnostic instruments employed. Furthermore, the diagnostic criteria have changed over time from Kanner's criteria in the 1960s to DSM-IV and ICD-10 in the 1990s. Accordingly, the prevalence estimates vary greatly. When prevalence data is limited to studies after 1987, the prevalence is estimated to be 10 of 10,000. In 12 recent studies, patients meeting criteria for PDD-NOS were also included. The estimated prevalence of PDD-NOS is 15 per 10,000. Additional efforts have been made to calculate the prevalence of Asperger's syndrome, which is estimated to be 2.5 per 10,000. However, the number of patients diagnosed as such remains small in the current studies making the prevalence rate calculation difficult. By combining the above data, the collective prevalence of ASDs is calculated to be 27.5 per 10,000. Despite this, recent epidemiological surveys have reported rates on the order of 60 per 10,000.

This apparent increase in prevalence rates has stimulated a debate over whether the incidence of autism is increasing. It is worth noting that there is very little incidence data in the literature and most approaches to answer this question have used prevalence data. Incidence refers to the number of new cases diagnosed per year, whereas prevalence refers to the number of cases both old and new at a given time. The increasing numbers of children referred to a specialist have been used as evidence of increasing incidence of PDD. However, there were no controls for confounders such as changes in diagnosis, availability of services, public awareness and decreasing age at diagnosis. Comparing cross-sectional studies is also plagued by differences in design, diagnostic criteria, and identification methods of autistic subjects. Repeat surveys over time in the same geographic region could control for some of these variables, but still improved detection over time and a dynamic population may skew the results. Successive birth cohort studies have failed to show a change in prevalence so far. Incidence studies would be more useful in assessing the perceived increased rate of autism in the general population, although controlling for changes in diagnostic criteria and case detection methods would still be necessary. Two current incidence studies currently showed an upward trend, but no attempt was made to investigate the above cofounders. Everything considered, there is currently no adequate evidence to support the hypothesis of an increase in the incidence of autism.

Regarding other epidemiological features of autism, the mean male to female sex ratio is calculated to be 4.3 to 1. There is no correlation between socioeconomic status or intellectual level and autism in the studies conducted after 1980. Rates of medical conditions associated with autism vary greatly among studies. Epilepsy, Down syndrome, Fragile X syndrome, sensory deficits, congenital rubella, and cerebral palsy have all been evaluated in this population. Only 6% of autism cases have been associated with another medical condition that is potentially linked to the etiology of autism. Of the above disorders, the most frequent is epilepsy with a co-prevalence rate of up to 42%. Approximately 30% of patients with autistic spectrum disorders have normal intelligence, 30% have mild deficits, and 40% are profoundly retarded. The rates of mental retardation are considered to be lower in Asperger's syndrome and PDD-NOS.

In conclusion, epidemiological surveys to date estimate PDD prevalence to be up to 60 per 10,000 with PDD-NOS being the most common form. It predominately affects boys, and is frequently associated with mental retardation. A small percentage of affected patients have another medical disorder whose cause may be possibly linked to autism. The available data has not yet provided firm evidence that the incidence of autism is rising.

7. PHENOMENOLOGY

The DSM-IV lists autism, Asperger syndrome, PDD-NOS, childhood disintegrative disorder (CDD), and Rett syndrome under the broader category of pervasive developmental disorders (PDD). The first three are commonly referred to as ASDs, whereas Rett syndrome and CDD should be considered distinct entities. The clinical characteristics of ASDs are social interaction and communication deficits, and repetitive stereotyped movements. By definition, onset is before 3 years of age.

7.1. Social Impairment

The most characteristic deficit in autism is the impairment in social interaction, which often presents itself as the inability to form relationships and to reciprocate. The social deficits in autism are found in basic social communicative behaviors, i.e., lack of eye contact and facial expression, in contexts in which coordination of these behaviors results in a "social-cognitive event," such as pointing, and in reciprocal relationships. Three forms of social phenotypes have been reported in the literature: aloof, passive, and active but odd. Retrospective studies and a systematic review of videotapes recorded at birthdays have shown that eye contact abnormalities, joint attention and imitative behaviors can be identified as early as 12 months of age. In a large prospective study, 83% of children with abnormalities in pointing, gaze monitoring, and pretend play that presented at 18 months had a diagnosis of autism at 3.5 years of age. However, the sensitivity of this finding drops when children with severe mental handicaps are included.

7.2. Communicative Deficits

Impairments in communication include both verbal and nonverbal language. There is an overlap between social skills and communication. Nonverbal communicative behaviors, such as facial expressions and eye contact are classified under the social domain. However, use of gestures, such as pointing, nodding, and showing are considered communicative behaviors. Deficits in nonverbal communication have been repeatedly reported in the autistic population. About half of autistic children are considered to be nonverbal, but this number seems to be decreasing with early intervention programs. For verbal autistic persons, there is a multitude of deficits reported, including deficits in pragmatics, variable expressive, and receptive difficulties, semantic impairments, and occasionally phonology abnormalities. Autistic patients may initiate conversation about preoccupations or routine details and some children are quite talkative, but their speech output is more like a monologue than directed communication. In other words, their language lacks a social quality. Additionally, echolalia, reversing pronouns, neologisms, abnormalities in the rhythm, and intonation have all been observed. In autistic patients, verbal IQ is usually lower than performance IQ. However, patients with Asperger's syndrome may have verbal IQ in the same range or higher than performance IQ. Verbal apraxia or dyspraxia is often noted and it is usually accompanied by some degree of receptive language deficit.

7.3. Repetitive Behaviors

Restrictive and/or repetitive behaviors are the third category required by DSM-IV and ICD-10 to make the diagnosis of ASD. Repetitive motor behaviors such as arm flapping, rocking, bouncing, and spinning are quite common. However, they are probably not specific to autism, as such behaviors are commonly observed in normally developing infants and young children and they are also seen in other developmental and psychiatric disorders. Importantly, the rates of these repetitive behaviors seem to correlate with mental age in non-autistic individuals, but not in autistic patients. Higher level repetitive behaviors, such as restricted interests, are more characteristic of autistic behavior. Rigid routines and rituals are seen in autism, but are also present in obsessive-compulsive disorder (OCD), Tourette's syndrome, and learning disabilities; however, they are more prevalent and elaborate in the autistic population and changes to routines cause much more distress. There are several theories explaining repetitive behaviors in autism: repetitive behaviors as a homeostatic mechanism, as an operant behavior, as a result of impaired mentalizing ability, as a consequence of weak central coherence, or as a symptom of impaired executive function. Although all of these theories have significant shortcomings, different theories may explain different types of behavior. For example, the homeostatic mechanism may explain how high levels of arousal lead to increased repetitive movements, although the central coherence hypothesis may be more useful in explaining the circumscribed content of some of these behaviors.

PDD-NOS represents a category of patients with autistic features too mild to meet the criteria for autism. According to DSM-IV and ICD-10, Asperger's is defined by significant social deficits and repetitive behaviors and interests, in the absence of language or cognitive delay. Some have postulated that Asperger's syndrome is somewhat qualitatively different from autistic disorder, although others feel that it is similar to high-functioning autism. This controversy remains an area of active research.

8. TREATMENT

Although several classes of medications have been used to target specific symptoms in autism *(22)*, there are no medications approved for the treatment of autism. With few exceptions, most drug treatment studies have been open label studies or based on clinical experience. The evidence currently points to the use of serotonin reuptake inhibitors (SRIs), atypical antipsychotics, and possibly anticonvulsants as most beneficial in this population.

8.1. SRIs

As discussed previously, there is significant evidence for the involvement of the serotonin system in the development of symptoms in autism. Hence, the use of SRIs is quite promising. One of the original SRIs to be studied in this population was clomipramine. Clomipramine has been shown to be superior to placebo in ratings of certain autistic symptoms, namely compulsive ritualistic behavior and anger *(23,24)*. However, severe side effects have been reported in some patients, such as QT prolongation, urinary retention, sedation or insomnia, and grand mal seizures. Thus, the development of selective serotonin reuptake inhibitors (SSRIs) has been of great interest given that the side-effect profile is more favorable. For example, fluoxetine and fluvoxamine have been shown to improve ritualistic behavior, social interaction, temper outbursts, OCD symptoms, and global severity in uncontrolled trials *(25,26)*. Side effects reported for both medications include hyperactivity and agitation or sedation, insomnia, elation, and nausea. Open label studies have shown sertraline to be useful in improving anxiety, aggression, self-injury, repetitive behaviors, and global severity, and to be well tolerated. Citalopram has been used successfully in OCD, anxiety disorder, and school phobia. In a retrospective review, it was associated with significant improvement in PDD, anxiety, and mood General Cognitive Index scores. Mixed serotonin and norepinephrine reuptake inhibitors, such as venlafaxine, have also been shown to improve irritability and repetitive behaviors in small studies *(27)*.

8.2. Atypical Antipsychotics

Atypical antipsychotics block both serotonin and dopamine receptors. Two double-blind placebo trials, one in children and one in adults, and multiple open-label studies have shown risperidone to improve irritability, anxiety, aggression, and self-injurious behaviors, repetitive behaviors, and global severity. Common side effects include sedation and weight gain in children. The incidence of dyskinesia and dystonia could not be assessed in theses studies given their relative short course *(28,29)*. Other atypical antipsychotics currently under investigation include olanzepine and quetiapine.

8.3. Anticonvulsants

There are several case reports of valproic acid being effective in the treatment of autistic individuals who also had a seizure disorder. A group of autistic children and adults showed improvement in repetitive behaviors, social relatedness, aggression, and affective liability in an open-label study, with 4 out of 10 responders having abnormal electroencephalograms (EEGs) *(30)*. An open-label study and a case report with patients who had comorbid symptoms of mania showed valproate to be effective and safe in this population. A double-blind, placebo-controlled trial of lamotrigine showed no effect in the PDD population.

8.4. Other Drug Treatments

Although typical antipsychotics are effective in improving stereotypies and attention, they are associated with significant side effects including dyskinesias, acute dystonic reactions, and sedation, and therefore are not considered to be first line of treatment. There is evidence that lithium may be useful as an adjunct to treat aggression, but it puts patients at risk for iatrogenic diabetes insipidus *(31)*. Psychostimulants such as methylphenidate have been shown to reduce hyperactivity and irritability, but autistic children seem to be more prone to its side effects. Clonidine, an α2-adrenergic receptor agonist, improves global severity, irritability, and stereotypies, but produces side effects like sedation and hypotension. Buspirone, an anxiolytic medication that is a partial agonist of the 5-HT1A receptor may improve anxiety, but may also worsen aggression. There is anecdotal evidence of efficacy for donepezil, a cholinesterase inhibitor, famotidine, an antihistamine, and amantadine, an antiparkinsonian agent. Controlled trials are needed to evaluate open label preliminary results.

8.5. Natural Products and Dietary Restrictions

Despite the public attention that secretin *(32)* and dimethylglycine (DMG) have received, carefully controlled studies have failed to demonstrate any benefit in this population. Controlled studies with multivitamin supplementation such as pyridoxine or pyridoxine–magnesium combination are negative or have not yet been completed. Dietary interventions have also been controversial in autism. The most commonly used one is a low casein and/or gluten diet. The rational is supposedly related to removal of proteins from the diet that may produce toxic brain metabolites. Moderate improvements have been reported, but large well-controlled trials are needed. There is also some preliminary evidence that the ketogenic diet may be used in this population as an additional or alternative treatment.

In summary, there is evidence that supports the use of SSRIs and atypical antipsychotics in autistic children for the treatment of repetitive movements and aggression. There is also preliminary data that suggests that valproic acid may be beneficial in this population. Other medications discussed need to be further investigated before general recommendations can be made. Current pharmacological treatment approaches involve either recruiting stratified populations who score high for a particular symptom to determine efficacy for that particular symptom (i.e., aggression or repetitive behaviors) or early intervention to determine the impact on the developmental of symptoms *(22)*.

8.6. Nonpharmacological Interventions

8.6.1. Comprehensive Early Intervention Programs

A striking feature of autism is variability in the final outcome. Some young children with autism make impressive gains, speak almost normally, and function in normal classrooms although others remain aloof, never speak, or never integrate in peer groups. Autism researchers have felt that there is a window of opportunity to intervene in early childhood, in order to possibly modify the ultimate outcome. Encouraging data first arose in the 1980s, when it was reported that about half the patients enrolled in an intensive early intervention program were in regular classrooms in elementary school and maintained this effect through adolescence. However, most researchers cannot agree on what type of intervention is the most appropriate and what are the underlying mechanisms that are responsible for success. Currently, there are several early intervention programs used. Behavioral programs, i.e., Applied Behavioral Analysis (ABA), the Walden program, and Life skills and Education for students with Autism and other Pervasive developmental disorders (LEAP) all focus on the acquisition of discrete skills. Newer behavioral methods are better at using more naturalistic interventions as the children improve. Developmental programs such as Greenspan and Wieder's Developmental intervention and the Denver model recognize the interplay among cognitive, communicative, social, and emotional development. These interventions are child-centered. Treatment and Education for Autistic and related Communication handicapped Children (TEACCH) is a program that combines behavioral and developmental approaches and emphasizes individual functioning in a group setting. All programs report back with encouraging results. However, none of these studies have compared programs against each other, the sample sizes are small, most did not randomize their subjects and most used different assessment methods pre- and post-intervention making interpretation of the results difficult *(33)*. Large multicenter studies are needed to address which interventions are effective in which patients, and what are the critical ingredients of a program that make it a successful intervention.

8.6.2. Problem Behavior Interventions

The most commonly identified problem behaviors in the research literature are aggression, tantrums, self-injury, and stereotypy *(34)*. Stimulus or instruction-based interventions (teaching alternative prosocial skills), as well as systems change (ecological interventions, e.g., staff ratios) and extinction (reducing maladaptive behaviors by removing rewarding stimuli) are used more often in recent studies, although punishment and reinforcement are more commonly found in the older studies. Although there is a significant decrease in the problem behaviors reported in almost all studies (at least 80% reduction of target behavior in 50% of subjects), interventions developed using functional assessment information seem to be the most effective. While the above data is encouraging, gaps remain and more studies are needed to address how to prevent problem behaviors, whether the acquired skills can be generalized to other settings, and whether the typical intervention agents (teachers, parents) can implement the intervention with similar efficacy.

8.6.3. Sensory and Motor Interventions

The rationale for sensorimotor interventions in the autistic population is based on the fact that these children are known to have sensory and motor deficits. A comprehensive review of the literature has been published by Baranek *(35)*. The available studies are plagued with problems, such as methodological issues, failing to establish a link between the assumed mechanism and the functional outcome, and interventions that are based on older neurological theories that have been disproved (e.g., sensorimotor handling). Most categories of intervention have shown mixed results in poorly controlled trials, including sensory integration and stimulation approaches, auditory integration training, and prism lenses. Because there is no evidence that these programs can substitute for the available educational interventions, they should be used only as supplementary interventions.

8.6.4. Interventions Facilitating Social Interaction

Difficulties in social interactions and relationships are one of the core features of autism. Several interventions target specifically social skills, especially in light of limited success in this domain with pharmacological intervention *(36)*. There are several types of social interventions. Ecological interventions, which are manipulations of the physical and social environment, produce weak to moderate improvements in young adults, and variable results in children. They are mostly viewed as necessary, but not sufficient, for producing significant changes in social development. Collateral skill interventions are those in which autistic children improve socially as a result of training in another seemingly unrelated skill. This probably works by bringing autistic children in contact with typically developing peers, thus activating natural processes of social development. These interventions seem to be effective when incorporated in more comprehensive programs. Non-autistic peer-mediated intervention procedures offer social skills training to other non-autistic children that are designed to change social interaction for children with autism. A number of studies have demonstrated a robust treatment effect, but these studies are limited by the fact that the results need to be extended to "untrained" peers.

In summary, there is evidence to suggest that early nonpharmacological intervention is effective in the autistic population. However, well-controlled studies with adequate sample sizes are needed, as well as studies that compare the individual methods. Behavioral interventions are successful for problem behaviors, and also seem to improve social skills. The evidence for the effectiveness of sensorimotor interventions is weak and such interventions should be used only as a supplementary tool.

9. FUTURE DIRECTIONS

At this time, our understanding of the neurobiology of autism remains limited. Substantial progress has been made in our ability to accurately diagnose ASD. However, work remains to be done in further delineating the boundaries among autistic disorder, PDD-NOS, and Asperger's syndrome. Better methods for quantifying aspects of ASD will be necessary for advancing neurobiological and genetics studies. The explosion of knowledge in genetics has brought much enthusiasm to the field. A further delineation of candidate chromosomal regions and the identification of genes responsible for the symptoms of autism is imminent. The recent availability of postmortem tissue from autistic patients has enabled neurochemical and cytological investigations. The analysis of presynaptic and postsynaptic serotonergic measures across cortical and subcortical regions will be of great value. Imaging modalities promise to better elucidate the neural basis of autism. For example, fMRI will be helpful in identifying the dynamic processes involved in the generation of symptom domains in autism. The use of large and homogenous samples is necessary in future functional imaging studies. A challenge will be to adapt in vivo neuroimaging techniques to infants and toddlers, because the disorder evolves to its full form in the first few years of life. Significant progress has also been made in the psychopharmacology of autism, and preliminary studies have demonstrated the efficacy of SSRIs and atypical antipsychotics for controlling some symptoms. It is unlikely that one drug will significantly impact all signs of autism, and large placebo-controlled trials in populations stratified for severity in a specific target domain are underway. Therapeutic agents affecting other systems, such as glutamatergic, oxytocin, or immune systems, may offer other avenues for treatment. Finally, a careful study of behavioral and educational techniques will allow available treatments to be compared, and will enable the development of specific treatments for individual patients.

GLOSSARY OF MEDICAL TERMINOLOGY

Childhood disintegrative disorder (CDD): Pervasive developmental disorder in which apparently normal development in the first 2 years is followed by developmental regression and behavioral change, often accompanied by loss of coordination and loss of bowel and bladder control.

Congenital Rubella: Syndrome caused by maternal rubella infection during pregnancy. It is associated with multisystem abnormalities and autism.

Down syndrome: The most common cause of mental retardation, it is caused by duplication of chromosome 22. It gives rise to characteristic dysmorphology, as well as, multisystem abnormalities.

Echolalia: A disorder of speech in which the subject repeats the words or phrases of others; usually present in patients with PDD and organic mental disorders

Endophenotype: A subgroup of subjects from the population being studied that share a unique characteristic in addition to the phenotype being studied.

Fragile X: Aa syndrome caused by mutations of the FMR1 gene, leading to an unstable CCG repeat and an unstable X chromosome. It is the second most common cause of mental retardation affecting boys more that girls. It is associated with characteristic dysmorphic features.

Homeostatic mechanism as related to repetitive behaviors: Theory based on the hypothesis that the reticular activating system in autistic patients is overactive and that repetitive behaviors serve as displacement activities to block further sensory input relating to the arousing situation.

Hypoplasia: Decreased growth

Incidence: Tthe number of new cases of a disease occurring in a defined period over the number of people at risk.

Magnetic resonance spectroscopy (MRS): Functional brain-imaging technique that can provide information on concentrations of endogenous substances that contain naturally occurring paramagnetic nuclei.

Megalencephaly: Large brain size

Neologism: New word invented by the subject or word to which new idiosyncratic meaning has been given, or distorted word

Prevalence: Frequency of cases both old and new in the population at a given time.

Rett Syndrome: Neurodevelopmental disorder, caused by mutations of the MECP2 gene on X-chromosome. It is classified under the pervasive developmental disorders. It is characterized by progressively decreasing brain and body organ growth, autistic features, seizures, dementia, and early death.

Perseveration: Continuation of a response after it is no longer appropriate; often associated with frontal lobe dysfunction.

Polymorphism: Occurrence of two or more gene structures in the same population

Pragmatics: The effective use of language appropriate to a given context

Semantics: The meaning of words

Speech apraxia: The inability to produce speech in the absence of any primary motor or sensory deficits

Theory of central coherence: The ability to interpret stimuli in a global way dependent on the context

Theory of mind: The ability to recognize that others have minds apart from their own mind, and understand the mental state of others

REFERENCES

1. Kemper TL, Bauman ML. Neuropathology of infantile autism. J Neuropathol Exp Neurol 1998;57:645–652.
2. Bailey A, Luthert P, Dean A, et al. A clinicopathological study of autism. Brain 1998;121:889–905.
3. Zilbovicius M, Boddaert N, Belin P et al. Temporal lobe dysfunction in childhood autism: a PET study. Am J Psychiatry 2000;157:1988–93.
4. Ohnishi T, Matsuda H, Hashimoto T et al. Abnormal regional blood flow in childhood autism. Brain 123:1838–1844.
5. Ritvo ER, Freeman BJ, Scheibel AB et al. Lower Purkinje cell counts in the cerebella of four autistic subjects: initial findings of the UCLA-NSAC autopsy research report. Am J Psychiatry 1984;143(7):862–866.
6. Courchesne E, Yeung-Courchesne R, Press G et al. Hypoplasia of cerebellar vermal lobules VI and VII in autism. N Engl J Med 1998;318:1349–1354.
7. Courchesne E, Carper R, Akshoomoff N. Evidence of brain overgrowth in the first year of life in autism. JAMA 2003;290(3):393,394.
8. Schultz RT, Gauthier I, Klin A et al. Abnormal ventral temporal cortical activity during face discrimination among individuals with autism and Asperger syndrome. Arch Gen Psych 2000;57:331–340.
9. Hollander E, Novotny S, Allen A, Aranowitz B, Cartwrite C, DeCaria C. The relationship between repetitive behaviors and growth hormone response to sumatriptan challenge in adult autistic disorder. Neuropsychopharmacology 2000;22:163–167.
10. Popik P, Vetulani S, Van Ree JM. Low dose of oxytocin facilitates social recognition in rats. Psychopharm 1992;106(1):71–74.
11. Popik P, Van Ree JM. Long term facilitation of social recognition in rats by vasopressin related peptide: a structure-activity study. Life Sci 1992;50(8):567–72.
12. Hollander E, Novortny S, Hanratty M et al. Oxytocin infusion reduces repetitive behaviors in adults with autistic and Asperger's disorders. Neuropsychopharmacology 2003;28:193–98.

13. Ciaranello AL, Ciaranello RD. The neurobiology of infantile autism. Annu Rev Neurosci 1995;18:101–128.
14. Buxbaum JD, Silverman JM, Smith CJ et al. Evidence for susceptibility gene for autism on chromosome 2 and for genetic heterogeneity. Am J Hum Genetics 2001;68:1514–1520.
15. International Molecular Genetics Study of Autism Consortium. A full genome screen for autism with evidence for linkage to a region on chromosome 7q. Human Mol Genetics 1998;7:571–578.
16. Barrett S, Beck JC, Bernier R et al. An autosomal genomic screen for autism. Collaborative Linkage study of Autism. Am J Med Genet 1999;88:609–615.
17. Koch A, Wolpert CM, Menold MM et al. Genetic studies of autistic disorder and chromosome 7. Genomics 1999;61:227–236.
18. Lamb JA, Moore J, Bailey A, Monaco AP. Autism: recent molecular genetic advances. Hum Mol Genet 200;9:861–868.
19. Evers M, Cunningham-Rundles C, Hollander E. Heat shock protein 90 antibodies in autism. Mol Psych 2002;7(Suppl2):S26–S28.
20. Hollander E, DelGiudice-Asch G, Simon L et al. B lymphocyte antigen D8/17 and repetitive behaviors in autism. J Am Psych 1999;156:317–20.
21. Fombonne E. Epidemiology of the pervasive developmental disorders. TEN 2003;5(1):29–36.
22. Hollander E, Phillips AT, Yeh CC. Targeted treatments for symptom domains in child and adolescent autism. Lancet 2003;362:732–734.
23. Gordon CT, State RC, Nelson JE et al. A double blind comparison of clomipramine, desipramine and placebo in the treatment of autistic disorder. Arch Gen Psychiatry 1993;50:441–447.
24. Brasic JR, Barnett JY, Kaplan D et al. Clomipramine ameliorates adventitious movements and compulsions in pre-pubertal boys with autistic disorder and mental retardation. Neurology 1994;44:1309–1312.
25. DeLong GR, Teague LA, McSwain KM. Effects of Fluoxetine treatment in young children with idiopathic autism. Dev Med Child Neurol 1998;40:551–562.
26. McDougle CJ, Naylor ST, Cohen DJ, et al. A double-blind, placebo controlled study of fluvoxamine in adults with autistic disorder. Arch Gen Psychiatry 1996;53:1001–1008.
27. Hollander E, Kaplan A, Catwrite C, Reichman D. Venlafaxine in children, adolescents and young adults with autism spectrum disorders: an open retrospective clinical report. J Child Neurology 2001;14:132–135.
28. McDougle CJ, Holmes JP, Carlson DC et al. A double blind placebo controlled study of risperidone in adults with autistic disorder and other pervasive developmental disorders. Arch Gen Psych 1998;55:663–641.
29. Research Units on Pediatric psychopharmacology autism network. Risperidone in children with autism and serious behavioral problems. N Engl J Med 2002;347(5):314–321.
30. Hollander E, Dolgoff-Kaspar R, Cartwrite C et al. An open trial of divalproex sodium in autism spectrum disorders. J Clin Psychiatry 2001;62:530–534.
31. Malone RP, Delaney MA, Luebbert JF, Cater J, Cambell M. A double-blind placebo-controlled study of lithium in hospitalized aggressive children and adolescents with conduct disorders. Arch Gen Psychiatry 2000;57:649–54.
32. Corbett B, Khan K, Czapansky-Beilman D et al. a double blind placebo controlled crossover study investigating the effect of porcine secretin in children with autism. Clin Pediatr 2001;40:327–331.
33. Kasari C. Assessing Change in early intervention programs for children with autism. J autism Dev Dis 2002;32:447–461
34. Horner RH, Carr EG, Strain PS, Todd AW, Reed HK. Problem behavior interventions for young children with Autism: A research synthesis. J autism Dev Dis 2002;32:423–446.
35. Baranek G. Efficacy of sensory and motor interventions for children with autism. J Autism Dev Dis 2002;32:397–422.
36. McConnell S. Interventions to facilitate Social Interaction for young children with autism: Review of available research and recommendations for educational intervention and future research. J Autism Dev Dis 2002;32:351–372.

FURTHER READING

Andres C. Molecular Genetics and animal models in autistic disorder. Brain Res Bull 2002;57:109–119.

Deuel RK. Autism: A cognitive Developmental Riddle. Pediatr Neurol 2002;26:349–357.

Cody H, Pelphrey K, Piven J. Structural and functional magnetic resonance imaging of autism. Int J Devl Neuroscience 2002;20:421–438.

Schultz R, Klin A. Genetics of childhood disorders: XLIII. Autism, Part 2: Neural foundations. J Am Acad Child Adolesc Psychiatry 2002;41:1259–1262.

Klin A, Jones W, Schultz R, Volkmar F, Cohen D. Defining and quantifying the social phenotype in autism. Am J Psych 2002;159:895–908.

8

Tourette's Syndrome and Tic Disorders

From Molecules and Cells to Symptoms and Management

James E. Swain, Robert A. King, and James F. Leckman

Summary

Tourette's syndrome (TS) is a neuropsychiatric disorder characterized by motor and phonic tics such as eye-blinks and grunts, respectively. It usually manifests in the first decade of life, and may be a considerable source of morbidity as it waxes and wanes. Advances in neuroscience, psychopharmacology, and psychotherapy are improving our understanding and the treatment of TS. Multimodal interventions that include focused treatment of comorbid conditions as well as educational and long term supportive relationships are usually the best approach.

Key Words: Tourette; tics; dopamine; basal ganglia; motor control; habits.

1. BRAIN PATHWAYS

Despite the lack of evidence for a discrete explanatory pathogenetic pathway or lesion for Tourette's syndrome (TS), clinical and research data point to neurochemical and functional abnormalities in the neural substrates of habit formation *(1)*, especially motor control loops involving the basal ganglia circuits, motor cortex, limbic nuclei, and their interconnecting pathways. Habits may be defined as assembled routines that link sensory cues with motor action. The ability to learn and subsequently perform complex behaviors through coordination of such routines underlies the phenomenon of improvement with practice. Thus, habits are an enormously adaptive part of a common evolutionary heritage that we share with other vertebrates as we engage in goal-directed behavior. The mechanisms of habit acquisition, regulation, and coordination—whether part of an adaptive response or an inappropriate movement such as a tic—are poorly understood, but likely involve the basal ganglia and functionally related areas of the cortex and thalamus *(2,3)*.

The basal ganglia comprise several richly interconnected subcortical nuclei: the striatum (caudate and putamen), globus pallidus, subthalamic nucleus (STN), and substantia nigra (SN). The striatum serves as the primary input structure, while the pars interna of the globus pallidus and the pars reticulata of the SN serve as the

From: *Current Clinical Neurology: Neurological and Psychiatric Disorders:*
From Bench to Bedside
Edited by: F. I. Tarazi and J. A. Schetz © Humana Press Inc., Totowa, NJ

151

primary output structures of the basal ganglia. Intermediate structures within the basal ganglia include the STN, pars externa of the globus pallidus, and the pars compacta of the SN. Motor, sensorimotor, association, and limbic neural circuits course through the basal ganglia forming multiple, partially overlapping, but largely "parallel" circuits that direct information from the cerebral cortex to the subcortex and then back again to specific regions of the cortex for further processing. Although various anatomically and functionally related cortical regions provide input into a particular circuit, each circuit in turn refines and refocuses its projections, sculpting the information and feeding back into discrete subsets of the cortical regions that initially contributed to that circuit's input. Within the basal ganglia and thalamus, these subcircuits appear to be anatomically segregated from others that pass through the same macroscopic structure, hence the conceptualization of these overlapping pathways as being "parallel." Despite controversy, the current consensus holds that cortical-basal ganglia circuitry has at least three reciprocal loops: those originating from, and projecting back to sensorimotor, association, and limbic cortices.

Cortical neurons projecting to the striatum outnumber striatal neurons by roughly a factor of ten. These cortical projection neurons to the striatum segregate into two structurally similar, but neurochemically distinct, compartments: striosomal and matrisomal. Each of these compartments contains large numbers of medium spiny γ-aminobutyric acid (GABA)ergic neurons that project to the basal ganglia output system (pars interna of the globus pallidus and the pars reticulata of the SN) either directly (the so-called "direct" pathway) or indirectly via the globus pallidus, pars externa (the so-called "indirect" pathway).

One model for the neural origins of tics is that proposed by Mink *(3)*, which invokes the intricate internal organization of basal ganglia circuitry, but postulates that the organizing principle for involuntary motor behavior corresponds most closely to dysregulated firing of so-called medium spiny projection (MSP) neurons of the striatum. These matrisomes receive motor and somatosensory cortical inputs and project to basal ganglia output nuclei. According to Mink, a mechanism invoking repeated inappropriate activation of discrete matrisomes is the most parsimonious explanation for the pattern of stereotyped motor output seen with tics *(3)*. Experimental evidence in support of this comes from Alexander and DeLong *(4)*, who showed that microstimulation of discrete striatal foci in conscious monkeys evoked tic-like stereotyped movements of individual body parts. These foci were presumed to be striatal output neurons, because the effect of microstimulation was abolished following microinjection of ibotenic acid into striatum, which produces fiber-sparing lesions.

Another model of tics (stereotypies) proposed by Graybiel and colleagues, postulates that they are the consequence of an imbalance of striosomal vs matrisomal activity. This model is supported by evidence that the major cortical inputs to the striosomes arise from stress-sensitive limbic regions, which could account for the increase in tics seen during periods of emotional stress or excitement, and the report that gene expression imbalances between the two compartments is related to tic severity *(2)*. However, recent data raise questions about aspects of this hypothesis. In particular, data from Graybiel's group have shown that the selective destruction of certain intercompartmental cells along with a marked shift in the striosome-matrix balance does little to alter the number of stereotypies seen in response to psychostimulants and dopamine (DA) agonists in rats *(5)*.

Because lesions to the STN, globus pallidus, SN, and prefrontal cortex can produce unwanted motor output, they must also be candidates for TS pathobiology. For example, lesions of the STN produce involuntary movements of contralateral limbs (hemiballism and hemichorea). However, the movement patterns thus produced typically do not have the same stereotyped character as seen in TS and this may favor a mechanism that leads to the discrete over activity of a specific set of striatal matrisomes.

Magnetic resonance (MR) imaging volumetric studies of basal ganglia do show alterations in caudate, putamen, and globus pallidus volume in subjects with TS. In the largest and most recent MR study of basal ganglia structure involving 154 subjects with TS and 130 healthy controls *(6)*, regional asymmetries across groups did not differ; but there were significant decreases in caudate volumes in patients with TS compared with control subjects in both children and adults. Lenticular nucleus volumes were also smaller in adults and children with TS who were diagnosed as having comorbid obsessive-compulsive disorder (OCD). However, there was no correlation between symptom severity and volume, suggesting that other brain regions are more critical for the modulation of disease severity, or that they act as target structures for therapy.

Thus far, there has only been one high-resolution study using functional MR imaging of blood oxygenation of brain tissue in a relatively small group of adults with TS *(7)*. In this study, subjects were asked to alternately suppress their tics, or release them voluntarily over 40-second blocks. Tic suppression was associated with activation of regions of prefrontal cortex and caudate nucleus, which were correlated with deactivation of the putamen and the globus pallidus. Furthermore, it was found that these state-related brain activation changes were highly inter-correlated with one another as well as being correlated with tic symptom severity during the week prior to the scan as rated by an expert clinician. These findings suggest that prefrontal cortex linked to portions of the caudate are crucially involved in tic suppression.

Metabolism and blood-flow studies have also generally implicated disturbances in cortico-striato-thalamo-cortical circuits in the pathophysiology of TS. The most consistent findings in these positron emission tomography (PET) and single photon emission computed tomography (SPECT) studies have involved decreases in basal ganglia activity. Similarly, most blood-flow studies have reported reduced perfusion either of the globus pallidus and putamen, or of the basal ganglia as a whole suggesting that metabolism and blood flow in the basal ganglia are probably reduced in adults with TS relative to healthy control subjects. However, it is also possible that this finding may be as a result of the efforts of the patients to suppress their tics in the scanner *(9)*. A number of these reports also describe regions of cortical activation or deactivation, but there has been little consistency across studies. Investigators have also examined the functional coupling of various brain regions and found that changes in the coupling of the putamen and ventral striatum with a number of other brain regions differentiated TS patients from controls. For example, the motor and lateral orbitofrontal circuits in both patients with TS and controls appear to be functionally connected *(9)*, however, the nature of the connections differed between the two groups. In controls, activity in these circuits was negatively correlated (i.e., increased activity in one is associated with relative inactivity the other), although among patients with TS activity in the motor and lateral orbitofrontal circuits was positively coupled. These results lend further credence to the hypothesis that altered limbic-motor interactions are a hallmark of this disease.

Other investigators have sought to correlate state-dependent regional activations with tic occurrence. Increased activity as measured by PET has been highly correlated with tic behavior in a set of neocortical, paralimbic, and subcortical regions, including supplementary motor, premotor, anterior cingulate, dorsolateral-rostral prefrontal, and primary motor cortices, Broca's area, insula, claustrum, putamen, and caudate *(9)*. Not surprisingly, in the one patient with prominent coprolalia, the vocal tics were associated with increased activity in prerolandic and postrolandic language regions, insula, caudate, thalamus, and cerebellum.

In vivo neurophysiological research in TS has led to two potentially important studies of individuals with TS. The first concerns the use of a startle paradigm to measure inhibitory deficits by monitoring the reduction in startle reflex magnitude when the startling stimulus is preceded 30 to 500 milliseconds by a weak stimulus, or prepulse. This prepulse inhibition (PPI) of the startle response is an operational measure of sensorimotor gating, which refers to the brain's ability to "protect" incoming information for a very brief time period. TS patients have well-established deficits in the gating or inhibiting of intrusive sensory, motor, and cognitive information, such as electrical and mechanical stimuli *(10)*. Because PPI abnormalities have been observed across a variety of neuropsychiatric populations including schizophrenia, OCD, Huntington's disease, nocturnal enuresis, attention deficit disorder, Asperger's syndrome, and TS, some final common pathways might mediate abnormal movements associated with all of these diseases. Hypotheses to account for abnormal PPI include hypofunctioning GABAergic output of the pallidum and excess dopaminergic input from limbic cortex. These deficits in inhibitory gating are consistent with the idea that TS involves some diminished ability to appropriately inhibit or gate intrusive emotional, cognitive, and sensory drives that are needed to execute motor programs and that are released as tics in TS. Second, motor system excitability has been investigated in vivo by means of single and paired pulse transcranial magnetic stimulation (TMS). Following a single TMS pulse to the motor cortex and the corresponding muscle contraction, the electromyography is silent for a very brief period of time reflecting the general degree of inhibitory control within the sensorimotor loop. However, a paired pulse TMS measures intracortical excitability and reflects the degree of inhibitory and facilitatory control within the motor cortex following a subthreshold prepulse. Studies to date in groups of patients with TS have indicated that the cortical silent period is shortened in TS and that intracortical excitability is frequently seen in children with attention deficit hyperactivity disorder (ADHD) comorbid with a tic disorder *(11)*.

Although the cortico-striato-thalami-cortical circuits have been consistently implicated in TS, the precise mechanisms in TS remain elusive. Why do tics appear when they do? Why do they wax and wane? Why do they reach a worst-ever point in early adolescence, for a majority, and become even more severe in adulthood for an unlucky few? These developmental issues are likely crucial for a full understanding of this disorder (or set of disorders). Prospective longitudinal studies are needed to explore the developmental and compensatory processes at work, and the possible effects of treatments. It will also be important to determine if any of the volumetric findings are predictive of later clinical outcomes. Ideally, future studies will combine imaging techniques with real-time neurophysiological techniques.

2. MOLECULAR TARGETS/NEUROCHEMICAL PATHWAYS

Superimposed on the brain pathways involved in TS, is a complex neurochemical organization such that neurotransmitter-specific compartments exist allowing for multiple integrative and regulatory controls of cerebral cortical input. The various neurotransmitters and neuromodulators in the basal ganglia, particularly in the striatum, appear to facilitate learning and habit formation on the basis of sensorimotor, memory-related, conditional, or reward-based cues. Understanding the neurochemistry of these integrated influences on habit formation will likely provide more elegant and effective treatments for TS.

As with habits and stereotypies, ascending dopaminergic pathways likely play a key role in the consolidation and performance of tics. Evidence for abnormal DA neurotransmission comes from the seminal clinical observations that although blockade of DA receptors using neuroleptic drugs suppresses tics in a majority of patients, the use of DA-releasing drugs may precipitate or exacerbate tics *(12)*. Indeed, it appears that some adult patients with TS release more DA intrasynaptically in response to amphetamine compared to normal controls *(13)*. However, simple theories involving the absolute amount of DA, which do not address intercompartmental balance, are unlikely to provide a complete explanation for all cases of TS, as dramatically evidenced by the co-occurrence of Parkinson's disease and TS. Studies of monozygotic twins indicate that developmental shifts in the balance of tonic-phasic dopaminergic tone occur as a result of epigenetic differences and the density of DA D_2 receptors may influence or be influenced by the severity of TS *(14)*. Dopaminergic tone could potentially be altered by wide spread activation of dopaminergic projections from the SN following limbic activation through inhibition of GABAergic interneurons (or pars reticulata cells) that terminate on dopaminergic cells *(15)*. Dopaminergic inputs on cholinergic striatal interneurons also play a key role in the crafting of habits. All these factors suggest that ascending dopaminergic pathways may be important neural circuits in tics, habits, and stereotypies.

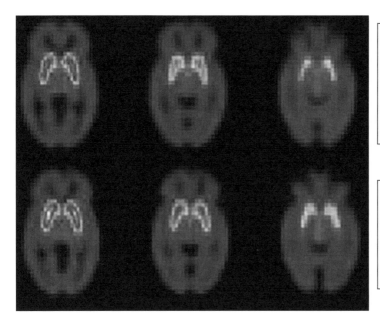

Fig. 1. This figure depicts a false-color signal proportional to dopaminergic terminal innervation in axial views through the striatum using positron emission tomography. *See* color insert preceding p. 51. (Reprinted with permission from ref. *17.*)

Radioligand binding studies of TS have primarily focused on characterizing the dopaminergic system in TS adults. This focus is based on the established efficacy of DA antagonists in the treatment of TS, the ability of DA agonists to provoke tic symptoms in some TS patients, and the unequivocally important role DA plays in modulating cortico-striato-thalamo-cortical circuits. With the exception of studies showing exaggerated synaptic DA release in response to amphetamine *(13)* and an increased number of transporter sites *(16)*, most results from studies of the dopaminergic system have been variable and inconsistent. The differences in DA levels between control and TS groups may represent medication-induced regulation of terminal marker expression, or may result from intrinsic differences in striatal dopaminergic synaptic function as suggested by the work of Albin and colleagues *(17)* shown in Fig. 1. This figure shows greater dopaminergic terminal innervation in the ventral striatum of TS patients in the lower three images compared to the upper three images of control subjects.

The literature on TS postmortem molecular neuropathology is limited to no more than seven presumed TS cases, and it is limited by a lack of specific indicators of the neurotransmitter systems involved. Although these studies generally implicate cortico-striato-thalamo-cortical circuits and the data are far from definitive, two findings deserve comment. First, four cases were reported using markers for DA transport to suggest an increased dopaminergic innervation of the striatum *(18).*

This finding has been replicated in vivo in two small series of patients using SPECT *(16)*. If there is indeed a dopaminergic hyperinnervation of the striatum, this could potentially contribute to a general increased vulnerability for subsets of matrisomes to become selectively activated in response to specific stimuli. However, dopaminergic hyperinnervation of the striatum may not be a universal finding in TS as one subsequent report could not replicate this finding despite using the same SPECT ligand and similar procedures *(19)*. Second, a series of additional neurochemical findings in the same four cases *(18)* were reported *(20)*. The most striking finding was a dramatic reduction in the levels of glutamate in the globus pallidus and the SN pars reticulata that was interpreted as reflecting a loss of input from the STN. Because the STN input to these basal ganglia output structures is excitatory and because increased activity in the GABAergic output neurons leads to inhibition of the thalamocortical projections, a loss of glutamatergic input from the STN would lead to a general tendency for the thalamocortical projections to become disinhibited and thus facilitate tic-like behaviors.

3. ANIMAL MODELS OF TS

True animal models that represent the multiplicity of TS etiologies and symptoms have been elusive. However, one possible source of animal models is the hypothesis that postinfectious autoimmune mechanisms contribute to the pathogenesis of some cases of TS as well as OCD. The reemergence of this line of reasoning is remarkable because speculation concerning a postinfectious etiology for tic disorder symptoms dates from the late 1800s. It is well established that group A β hemolytic streptococci (GABHS) can trigger immune-mediated disease in genetically predisposed individuals. Rheumatic fever (RF) is a delayed sequela of GABHS, occurring about 3 weeks following an inadequately treated upper respiratory tract infection. Inflammatory lesions involving the joints, heart, and/or central nervous system (CNS) characterize RF. The CNS manifestations are referred to as Sydenham's chorea (SC). In addition to chorea, some patients with SC display motor and phonic tics as well as OCD and ADHD symptoms, suggesting the possibility that at least in some instances these disorders may share a common etiology. Pediatric autoimmune neuropsychiatric disorder associated with streptococcal (PANDAS) infection has been proposed to represent a distinct clinical entity and includes cases of TS and OCD *(21)*. In PANDAS it is postulated that although GABHS is the initial autoimmunity-inciting event, viruses, other bacteria, or non-infectious immunological responses are capable of triggering subsequent symptom exacerbations. Recently, it has been demonstrated that antibodies produced by a 14-year-old female with RF specifically recognized mammalian neuron markers including lysoganglioside and *N*-acetyl-β-D-glucosamine (a carbohydrate epitope of GABHS) *(22)*. More importantly, these antibodies also targeted the surface of human neuronal cells and triggered the calcium/calmodulin-dependent protein kinase II cascade. Convalescent sera and sera from individuals with other GABHS disorders in the absence of chorea did not activate this kinase. If confirmed, this could provide evidence of how specific matrisomal MSP neurons might be activated in SC and may lead to a better understanding of other, possibly antibody-mediated neuropsychiatric disorders, such as TS. The recent report, that human sera from patients with high levels of auto-antibodies significantly increased oral stereotypies in rats *(23)*, has raised hopes that an autoimmune animal model of tic may be developed. A number of prospective longitudinal studies are underway to examine the relationships between newly acquired GABHS infections and other immune activators. If confirmed, the link between common childhood infections and certain neuropsychiatric disorders is tantalizing and may lead to the development of novel treatments based on intercellular immune signaling, or intracellular second messenger cascade modulation.

Another approach to modeling TS has been to generate transgenic mice, which express proteins (e.g., a cholera toxin subunit) that alter dopaminergic and glutamatergic orbitofrontal, sensorimotor, limbic, and efferent striatal circuits *(24)*. In such transgenic mice, frequent bursting, complex twitches are observed, which are reminiscent of tics in humans. Features of these behaviors, which lend credence to this animal model of TS include juvenile onset, ability to temporarily suppress, preponderance in males, and responsiveness to the human anti-tic medication clonidine. Thus far, the model suggests that excess glutamate from cortical-limbic output neurons may trigger tics.

It is likely that the next 10 years will see the refinement and integration of these kinds of animal models with human studies to account of the neural substrate of tics in all their varieties. Until the mechanisms of abnormal movements are better understood, mathematical modeling of stereotypical movements will allow meaningful extrapolation of animal model findings to human tic disorders. Thus far, animal models and research suggest that, although activation of specific, anatomically distinct subcircuits in the direct pathway that involve matrisomal MSP neurons may be key to the expression of simple tics, the execution of complex movements and vocalizations in humans may well require the coordinated participation of different striatal compartments.

4. ETIOLOGY/PHYSIOLOGY

Etiological theories for TS have ranged from "hereditary degeneration" to "irritation of the motor neural systems by toxic substances" to "a constitutional inferiority of the subcortical structures …[that] renders the individual defenseless against overwhelming emotional and dynamic forces." Predictably, each of these etiological explanations prompted new treatments and new ways of relating to families. Current theories focus on the interaction of genetic vulnerabilities with early developmental insults and hormonal exposures, psychosocial stress and the possible involvement of postinfectious autoimmune processes *(1)*.

4.1. Psychology

Neuropsychological studies of TS have focused on a broad array of functions. Although motor and phonic tics constitute the core diagnostic criteria for TS, perceptual, cognitive, and motor regulation difficulties are also common. These psychological symptoms are potentially informative about the pathobiology of the disorder. Moreover, these associated difficulties can be much more problematic for school and social adjustment than the primary motor symptoms.

Review of the literature suggests that the most consistently observed deficits in TS occur with tasks requiring the accurate copying of geometric designs, i.e., "visual-motor integration" or "visual-graphic" ability *(25)*. Even after statistically controlling for visual-perceptual skill, intelligence, and fine motor control, children with TS continued to perform worse than controls on the visual-motor tasks, suggesting that the integration of visual inputs and organized motor output is a specific area of weakness in individuals with TS. More recent reports have made a case for deficits in executive functions predominantly in the areas of response inhibition and action monitoring suggesting impairment of the frontal-striatal-thalamic-frontal circuits *(26)*.

4.2. Environmental Factors

In addition to psychosocial stress, many other stressors have been implicated in the pathogenesis of TS, including gestational and perinatal insults, sex hormones, and postinfectious autoimmune mechanisms *(1)*. For example, perinatal hypoxic/ischemic events appear to increase the risk of developing TS *(27)* by altering DA signaling. Male sex is also a risk factor and transmission within families is frequently male-to-male. The increased prevalence of TS in males has led to the hypothesis that the presence of androgenic steroids during critical periods in fetal development may play a role in the later development of the illness.

A stress-related model of pathogenesis is frequently invoked to help explain the emergence or variable expression of tic disorders, as a result of the strong clinical association between TS symptom severity and stressful life events. Such problems may find a common final pathway in the hypothalamic–pituitary–adrenal-gonadal axis, and their associated stress-related neurotransmitters and hormones, and their targets. In support of this, data suggest that TS patients may have a heightened stress reactivity of the hypothalamic–pituitary–adrenal and noradrenergic sympathetic systems as compared to healthy control subjects *(28)*.

5. GENETICS

Genetic vulnerability factors have been convincingly implicated in the transmission of TS and related disorders. The pattern of hereditary transmission in affected family members suggests major gene effects, and the results of segregation analyses are in accord with models of autosomal transmission set against a polygenic background *(1)*. Historically, efforts to identify susceptibility genes within highly affected families with traditional linkage strategies have met with limited success. However, investigators studying a large French-Canadian family have reported evidence for linkage at 11q23c. Nonparametric approaches with families in which two or more siblings are affected with TS have also been undertaken. This sib-pair approach is suitable for diseases with an unclear mode of inheritance, and has been used successfully in studies of other complex disorders, such as type 1 diabetes mellitus and essential hypertension. In one sib-pair study of TS, two areas were suggestive of linkage, one on chromosome 4q, and another on chromosome 8p.

Identity-by-descent approaches have been applied to South African and Costa Rican populations. These techniques assume that a few founder individuals contributed the vulnerability genes that are now distributed within a much larger population. The South African study implicated regions near the centromere of chromosome 2, and on 6p, 8q, 11q, 14q, 20q, and 21q. The marker in a French-Canadian family, that was associated with the highest logarithmic odds score, was the same marker (11q23c) for which significant linkage disequilibrium with TS was detected in the South African population.

Several candidate genes have been assessed in people with TS, including various DA receptors (*DRD1*, *DRD2*, *DRD4*, and *DRD5*), the DA transporter, various noradrenergic genes (*ADRA2A*, *ADRA2C*, and *DBH*), a few serotonergic genes (*5-HTT*), and a monoaminoxidase (MAO-A) gene. Genetic variation at any one of these loci is unlikely to be a major source of vulnerability to the disorder, but in concert, these alleles could have an important cumulative effect, and contribute to the phenotypic variability.

Additionally, a number of cytogenetic abnormalities have been reported in TS families at chromosomal locations 3p21.3, 7q35-36, 8q21.4, 9pter, and 18q22.3. Among the more recent findings is the report of the disruption of the contactin-associated protein 2 gene on chromosome 7. This gene encodes for a membrane protein located specifically at the nodes of Ranvier of axons. The authors hypothesized that disruption or decreased expression of this gene leads to an altered distribution of potassium channels, thereby influencing conduction of action potentials along myelinated neurons. More research is needed to confirm this finding.

Many vulnerability genes probably have a role in TS. Clarity about the nature and normal expression of even a few of the susceptibility genes in TS is likely to provide major insight concerning the pathogenesis of this disorder. Future progress could also depend on the identification of characteristic, biologically established, endophenotypes that are closely associated with specific vulnerability genes. Endophenotypes are measurable aspects of human psychiatric disorders or animal models that can be used as quantitative traits in linkage analyses. Promising endophenotypes include neurocognitive, neurophysiological, and neuroanatomical measures and patterns of treatment response.

6. PREVALENCE

Prevalence rates of TS vary according to a wide range of measures including age, sex, ethnicity, and method of assessment. Controversy between psychiatrists has raged over symptoms and their timing. Although it was thought to be a very rare disorder, current best estimates of the prevalence of TS hover around 1% of children between the ages of 6 and 17 years old *(29)*. A considerably higher percentage of children are thought to experience less severe variants of TS. Studies indicate point prevalences of tics for school-age children of 3 to 18% for boys and 0 to 11% for girls *(30)*. A recent longitudinal study of symptom exacerbation in children with TS suggests a high degree of intrasubject variability *(31)*.

TS is associated with a variety of symptoms and comorbidities *(32)*. It is generally agreed that about 50% of patients with TS also have substantial OCD symptoms, which likely involve the downstream effects of some common inherited influences. ADHD also occurs frequently among children with TS, with prevalences as high as 60 to 70%. Recent work on TS comorbidity with ADHD suggests that this dual diagnosis is associated with aggressive, delinquent, and disruptive behavior, which impacts on social, adaptive, and family functioning *(32)*. Comorbid depression, anxiety, and adjustment problems are just beginning to be systematically studied with respect to tic severity and duration, and may reflect the cumulative psychosocial burden of having tics, or else some shared biological predisposition such as abnormal cortical excitability *(11)*. Autism is another comorbidity associated with unexpectedly high rates of TS *(33)*, suggesting shared mechanisms between these disorders.

7. BEHAVIORAL PHENOTYPES IN HUMANS (SIGNS AND SYMPTOMS)

TS is a developmental neuropsychiatric disorder of childhood onset and considered a subclass of tic disorders in general. According to the Diagnostic and Statistical Manual, Fourth Edition (DSM-IV), it is characterized by brief, stereotypical but nonrhythmic "jerky" movements and vocalizations called tics. Tics, including eye-blinking, grimacing, jaw, neck, shoulder or limb movements, sniffing grunting, chirping, throat–clearing, etc., may occur over a period of months to years, or have a chronic course extending over the entire life span. Tics are infamous for following a waxing and waning pattern of severity *(1)*, making decisions regarding treatment, and the assessment of treatment interventions at times very difficult to evaluate outside of randomized, controlled clinical trials. Tics can additionally be confused with normal coordinated movements or vocalizations, or mistaken for akathisia, tardive dyskinesia, or other hyperkinetic movement disorders. Once established, however, any given tic tends to persist for a time. Tics are often exacerbated by stress and fatigue. In contrast to other movement disorders, like chorea and dystonia, tics can occur during sleep but are usually much attenuated. Some severely affected patients have atypical, soft signs on a neurological examination. These may suggest disturbances in sensory-motor integration, but their relevance is not really clear.

Motor tics often occur years before vocal tics may be noticed, and usually begin between the ages of 3 and 8. They are usually accentuated by repetitive bouts of higher frequency and intensity. In uncomplicated cases, motor and phonic tic severity peaks early in the second decade of life with many patients showing a marked reduction in tic severity by the age of 19 or 20 *(1)*, although recent data suggest that, despite their being attenuated, tics persist in most adults. The most severe cases of TS persist into adulthood. These severe cases are associated with significant interference in social and academic development and with comorbidities, such as ADHD and OCD. It remains unclear how TS and comorbid conditions may be related, but it is possible that they share common risk factors or neural substrates. These coexisting conditions can seriously detract from overall quality of life *(32)*, often causing more distress and functional impairment than the tics *per se*. Extreme forms of TS may even involve violent episodes of self-injurious motor tics involving hitting or biting, and socially stigmatizing coprolalic utterances and gestures.

Patterns of bouts of tics occurring over time scales of days to years have been described *(1)*, but have yet to be modeled in an attempt to predict likely outcome or treatment response. The bouts are characterized by brief periods of stable inter-tic intervals of short duration, typically 0.5 to 1.0 seconds and interbout intervals may last from minutes to hours over the course of a day. The frequency distribution of inter-tic interval appears to obey an inverse power law of temporal scaling, and suggest the presence of self-similar, fractal, or mathematically chaotic processes that may yield to future modeling and clinically valuable tools. Understanding the upstream processes that govern the timing of tic expression may ultimately clarify both neural events occurring in millisecond time scales as well as the natural history of tic disorders that occurs over the first two decades of life.

The simple description of tics as intermittent trains of involuntary motor discharge is quite incomplete. Indeed, tics are under partial voluntary control, as evidenced by patients' partial capacity to suppress them for brief periods of time, which is subject to many factors including stress, anxiety, and emotion. As such, tics may be thought of as part of a spectrum of partially voluntary behaviors including hair pulling, nail-biting, and other compulsions, substance abuse, pathological gambling, and our daily personal and interpersonal habits. Interestingly, activities that require focused attention and fine motor control, such as reading aloud, playing a musical instrument, engaging in certain sports, and (in one well-documented case) performing surgery are associated with transient improvements in tics.

Another feature of tics, especially evident in adolescents and adults, is that they are often associated with antecedent sensory phenomena described as faint premonitory urges, like the urge to scratch an itchy patch of skin, that are experienced as nearly irresistible and in rare cases painful. In some individuals with TS these urges are a major source of mental distress. There may also be sensory cues that prompt tics such as a cough or a particular word, suggesting the gating of motor programs by association with sensory pathways. A momentary sense of physical relief or a generalized abatement of inner tension often follows performance of a tic suggesting the addiction-like involvement of reward neurocircuitry.

8. TREATMENTS

Appropriate management of tic disorders must begin with assessment, which should involve the complete child, in the context of a rich personal and social life, and not just as someone with an abnormal motor system *(1)*. In the process of a comprehensive evaluation, the full range of difficulties and competencies should be charted. During the process of evaluation, the clinician, family, and child collaborate in the reconstruction of the child's history, tic symptomatology (onset, progression, waxing and waning, and factors that have worsened or ameliorated tic status), presence of comorbid conditions, treatment history, and current functioning. A critical question is the degree to which tics are interfering with the child's emotional, social, familial, and school functioning. To determine this, it is useful to monitor symptoms over a few months in order to assess their severity and fluctuation, impact on the family, as well as the adaptive capacity. This monitoring can often be accomplished with the family keeping records or using standard forms.

A neurological examination of a child with TS can also be of considerable value, to rule out movement disorders, although electroencephalography and structural magnetic resonance imaging are generally normal and are not yet of proven clinical use (except where there are other neurological suspicions). Similarly, laboratory studies may establish a child's general health profile and assist in differential diagnosis of other movement disorders, but there are no laboratory tests for the positive diagnosis of TS or other tic disorders.

Diagnostic criteria currently in use include the International Classification of Disease and Related Health Problems, 10th Revision (ICD-10) and DSM-IV Text Revision. Although clear differences exist comparing these classification schemes, they are broadly congruent with each other. However, although the criterion of functional impairment is consistent, it is not a useful criterion from the point of view of genetic or epidemiological studies. In order to minimize error in case ascertainment and to produce an instrument measuring the likelihood of having TS, an international team of experts has recently published a TS Diagnostic Confidence Index *(34)*. This supports the psychometric soundness of the Yale Global Tic Severity Scale *(1)* for clinicians.

Additionally, a thorough perinatal, personal, and family history along with screening for possible comorbidities including ADHD, OCD, and learning difficulties is essential. A complete review of stressors is also in order as stress is a key determinant of natural history *(28)*. Equally important is reviewing the strengths and abilities, along with an exploration of how these may be fully engaged. Psychological testing is also useful to assess and manage learning difficulties.

The decision to begin treatment is based on symptom severity and clinical presentation of each case. Many cases of TS, which are more troubling to family than the affected individual, may be managed successfully without resorting to medications. In patients presenting with comorbid ADHD, OCD, depression, or bipolar disorder, it is sometimes better to treat the comorbid condition first as treatment of such disorders will likely diminish tic severity. Similarly, it is important to address significant family, school, or social stressors as these may also exacerbate tics. Medications must be used with care as the natural, idiosyncratic, and sometimes dramatic fluctuations in tic severity in TS may be mistakenly interpreted as medication efficacy, which is purely coincidental. Likewise, fluctuations may temporarily mask a potentially useful treatment. For example, if medication is introduced during tic exacerbation, the subsequent natural coincidental improvement the tic may convince clinician and family that a medication was effective. Later, natural worsening of the symptoms may lead to reactive and sometimes dangerous increases in medication far beyond any effective anti-tic doses, with associated disabling sedation, side effects, and frustration. Often the most difficult, but wise course of treatment consists of education, reassurance, and periods of supportive, active watchful waiting, during which stressors may be addressed.

8.1. Pharmacological Treatment of Tics

No ideal anti-tic medications are currently available. Medications that have been shown to be effective in at least one positive double-blind, controlled clinical trial include α-adrenergic agonists, and atypical and typical neuroleptics. An exhaustive drug-by-drug summary of proven effects, side effects, dosing, effect size, cost, and full references may be found elsewhere *(12)*. The choice of treatment should include consideration of the side-effect profile and financial cost, and involve a full discussion involving the family.

Pharmacological treatment is usually started with low doses of α-adrenergic drugs such as clonidine *(12)*, which primarily activate presynaptic autoreceptors in the locus ceruleus to reduce norepinephrine release and turnover. This may also be responsible for sedation and reduced motor activity. It is recommended that low divided doses starting at 0.05 mg per day be given and then gradually increased to target doses of 0.2 to 0.3 mg per day. Primary side- effect considerations for adrenergic medications are mild initial sedation, blood pressure decrease, constipation, and waking during sound sleep. Transdermal patches for continuous controlled release of clonidine are now available. Another available α-2-agonist is guanfacine. It activates postsynaptic prefrontal α-adrenergic cortical receptors, which is thought to improve impulsivity, attention, and working memory. The target dose for the longer-acting guanfacine is 1.5 to 3 mg per day. Guanfacine and clonidine have also been shown to be effective in treating comorbid ADHD symptoms, although guanfacine appears to be the superior agent.

Neuroleptics have a long history of efficacy against tics. They are thought to act primarily by decreasing dopaminergic input from SN and ventral tegmentum to the basal ganglia. Of the typical neuroleptics, haloperidol, pimozide, and fluphenazine are among the most widely used and best-studied treatments of tics. Pimozide and fluphenazine appear to be less sedating than haloperidol. All of the neuroleptics carry a risk of significant potential side effects for acute dystonic reactions, tardive dyskinesia, oculogyric crises, torticollis, drug-induced Parkinsonism, akathisia, social phobia, weight gain, sedation, dry mouth, blurred vision, galactorrhea, gynecomastia, constipation, urinary retention, echocardiogram (EKG) changes including tachycardia, and loss of drive, energy, and personality. Using low doses and changing the dose gradually minimizes side effects. Medication dose reduction or discontinuation must be done very gradually, as abrupt decrements can produce withdrawal or rebound tic exacerbations.

Because of parents' and clinicians' concerns about the remote possibility of tardive dyskinesia, atypical neuroleptics are often considered before typicals. These newer, combination antidopaminergic and antiserotonergic medications carry a lower risk of tardive dyskinesia than the older typical neuroleptics, but their use in children and efficacy against tics is not as well established as for the typical neuroleptics. Double-blind, controlled trials for risperidone, olanzipine, and ziprasidone all indicate effectiveness against tics. However, like the typical antipsychotic pimozide, the atypical antipsychotics risperidone and olanzipine carry risks of dramatic weight gain, sedation, and sleep disturbance. Ziprasidone treatment requires cardiac monitoring with EKG for possible QTc interval changes. There can also be significant drug–drug interactions, especially macrolide antibiotics, which can alter the metabolism of these neuroleptics leading to serious or even fatal results. Other dopaminergic agents including tiapride and sulpiride are widely used in Europe, but are not currently available in the United States

Benzodiazepines such as clonazepam are sedative, anxiolytic drugs that act on GABA receptors to decrease excitability of nervous tissue, and they may have some antidopaminergic properties. Clonazepam is widely used for tics even though its efficacy is supported by only a few reports. Its side effects include sedation, depression, disinhibited behavior, and addiction. Tetrabenazine is a DA-depleting drug that is only approved for investigational use in the United States. Selective serotonin reuptake inhibitors (SSRIs) are not indicated for the treatment of comorbid depression, as they may either initiate or worsen tics in some individuals.

8.2. Diet and Lifestyle

Acute and chronic stress can exacerbate tics, so efforts to reduce the stress in the lives of patients with TS constitute a reasonable treatment approach. A long-term relationship with the same clinical team, who can help the patient and family deal with the changing manifestations of the disorder throughout the years, is highly recommended. Regular contact via telephone or e-mail may also be helpful. Participation in regular school and extracurricular activities is encouraged. No specific diet is known to be of particular benefit, although a balanced, healthy diet might contribute to overall well-being and stress reduction. Caffeine (e.g., cola drinks) should be minimized as it may exacerbate tics in some children. The impact of physical exercise on tic symptoms has not been systematically studied, although a regular program of exercise can be beneficial by reducing stress, increasing the child's sense of mastery, and well-being.

8.3. Educational Interventions

With the support of advocacy groups such as the Tourette Syndrome Association, TS awareness for families, educators, and peers can promote school and peer understanding, tolerance, and support, which can have a positive influence on the overall course of the illness. Active collaboration with the school by the clinician is essential, to ensure appropriate classroom management, curricular planning, strength building, and matter-of-fact teacher and community education about TS.

8.4. Psychotherapy

Although not yet well-established, a number of promising reports support the behavioral therapy of habit reversal training for isolated, troublesome tics, and to a lesser extent awareness training, especially for TS adults. A recent report *(35)* suggests that habit reversal psychotherapy in adults with TS, which consists of awareness training, relaxation training, competing response training, and contingency management, is associated with significant improvement in tic severity that persists to a 10-month follow-up.

Cognitive-behavioral treatment continues to be a mainstay of comorbid OCD, especially when there is significant anxiety or phobic avoidance. Although not rigorously supported, other formal dynamic interpersonal or supportive psychotherapeutic interventions may facilitate normal developmental tasks of friendship development, school mastery, coherent personality formation and day-to-day self-esteem and family functioning.

8.5. Other Emerging/Experimental Therapies

Plasmaphoresis and intravenous immunoglobulin administration are experimental treatments under study that have proven useful in a controlled study of children with TS and/or OCD who met rigorous criteria for the A β hemolytic streptococcus infection-associated subtype, but not in children whose TS or OCD were unrelated to streptococcus infection. Because these are often arduous procedures, the indication for their use is unclear. They should only be undertaken with experts in the context of a formal research study, because the standard treatments discussed in previous sections have proven to be effective. With certain unambiguous and sudden tic onset associated with streptococcal infection, antibiotic treatment has been occasionally remarkably effective, but antibiotic treatment is only warranted when there is clear evidence of streptococcal infection.

TMS is a new, experimental technology in which a brief, powerful magnetic field generated by a small coil positioned over the skull, induces an electrical current in the brain *(36)*. Such noninvasive brain stimulation may effect long-term changes in cortical excitability, which may be abnormal in TS *(11)*. This experimental therapy, whose stimulation parameters are still under study, will require a great deal of basic work before it may become a tic treatment.

Invasive procedures worthy of consideration for severe tics involving discrete muscle groups include botulinum toxin injections *(37)*. Botulinum toxin blocks acetylcholine release at the neuromuscular junction, and produces a reversible and temporary reduction in muscle activity, which may last weeks to months for dystonic tics. Main side effects include soreness, transient weakness, ptosis if injected for eye-blinking, and mild transient dysphagia or dysphoria if injected into the larynx.

The results of neurosurgical procedures reinforce the functional importance of thalamic regions that are part of cortical–subcortical loops *(38)*. A single case study found that high-frequency stimulation of the median and rostral intralaminar thalamic nuclei produced an important reduction of tics. This effect could either be as a result of the influence of these midline thalamic nuclei on the striatum, or on broadly distributed cortical systems and their cortico-striatal projections or both. As in other movement disorders, a deeper understanding of the circuitry involved in TS may lead to specific circuit-based therapies using deep brain stimulation to treat refractory cases. However, because TS often spontaneously resolves by adolescence, it should only be considered in the most severe and treatment refractory cases which persist into adulthood.

9. CONCLUSION

Our evolving understanding of tic disorders such as TS has been shaped by an emerging awareness of the role of basal ganglia in habit formation. Continuing neuroscience advances promise to further elucidate the functioning of these structures and the relevant neural circuits down to a molecular level, and point to the better management of TS and associated comorbidities. Research frameworks for the study of tics include neurophysiological, pharmacological, autoimmune, and genetic vulnerability in humans as well as in animal models. Work in these paradigms will also undoubtedly be relevant to other neuropsychiatric disorders of childhood onset and add to our knowledge of normal development and movement.

GLOSSARY OF MEDICAL TERMINOLOGY

Akathisia: A feeling of inner restlessness, and urge to move.
Coprolalia: Rude or obscene vocalizations.
Galactorrhea: The expression of milk from the breast.
Gynecomastia: The development of breast tissue.
Matrisomes and striosomes: Physiologically distinct grouping of cells in the striatum.
Oculogyric crisis: An acute rolling back of the eyes and loss of balance.
Plasmaphoresis: Removal of antibodies from the blood.
Ptosis: Drooping of an eyelid.
Rheumatic fever: A systemic streptococcal infection resulting in long-term autoimmune activity.
Sydenham's chorea: Movement disorder from autoimmune brain changes after rheumatic fever.
Torticollis: A twisting of the neck because of muscle contraction.

ACKNOWLEDGMENTS

This work was supported in part by NIH grants MH493515, MH61940, and RR00125 and the encouragement of the Tourette Syndrome Association.

REFERENCES

1. Leckman JF. Tourette's syndrome. Lancet 2002;360:1577–1586.
2. Graybiel AM, Canales JJ. The neurobiology of repetitive behaviors: Clues to the neurobiology of Tourette syndrome. Adv Neurol 2001;85:123–131.
3. Mink JW. Basal ganglia dysfunction in Tourette's syndrome: A new hypothesis. Pediatr Neurol 2001;25:190–198.

4. Alexander GE, DeLong MR. Microstimulation of the primate neostriatum. I. Physiological properties of striatal microexcitable zones. J Neurophysiol 1998;53:1401–1416.
5. Saka E, Iadarola M, Fitzgerald DJ, Graybiel AM. Local circuit neurons in the striatum regulate neural and behavioral responses to dopaminergic stimulation. Proc Natl Acad Sci USA 2002;99:9004–9009.
6. Peterson BS, Thomas P, Kane MJ, et al. Basal ganglia volumes in patients with Gilles de la Tourette syndrome. Arch Gen Psychiatry 2003;60:415–424.
7. Peterson BS, Skudlarski P, Anderson AW, et al. A functional magnetic resonance imaging study of tic suppression in Tourette syndrome. Arch Gen Psychiatry 1998;55:326–333.
8. Jeffries KJ, Schooler C, Schoenbach C, Herscovitch P, Chase TN, Braun AR. The functional neuroanatomy of Tourette's syndrome: An FDG pet study III: Functional coupling of regional cerebral metabolic rates. Neuropsychopharmacology 2002;27:92–104.
9. Stern E, Silbersweig DA, Chee KY, et al. A functional neuroanatomy of tics in Tourette syndrome. Arch Gen Psychiatry 2000;57:741–748.
10. Swerdlow NR, Karban B, Ploum Y, Sharp R, Geyer MA, Eastvold A. Tactile prepuff inhibition of startle in children with Tourette's syndrome: In search of an "fMRI-friendly" startle paradigm. Biol Psychiatry 2001;50:578–585.
11. Moll GH, Wischer S, Heinrich H, Tergau F, Paulus, Rothenberger A. Deficient motor control in children with tic disorder: Evidence from transcranial magnetic stimulation. Neurosci Lett 1999;272:37–40.
12. Swain JE, Leckman JF. Tourette's Syndrome in Children. Current Treatment Options in Neurology 2003;5:299–308.
13. Singer HS, Szymanski S, Giuliano J, et al. Elevated intrasynaptic dopamine release in Tourette's syndrome measured by pet. Am J Psychiatry 2002;159:1329–1336.
14. Wolf SS, Jones DW, Knable MB, et al. Tourette syndrome: Prediction of phenotypic variation in monozygotic twins by caudate nucleus D2 receptor binding. Science 1996;273:1225–1227.
15. Haber SN, Fudge JL, McFarland NR. Striatonigrostriatal pathways in primates form an ascending spiral from the shell to the dorsolateral striatum. J Neurosci 2000;20:2369–2382.
16. Muller-Vahl KR, Berding G, Brucke T, et al. Dopamine transporter binding in Gilles de la Tourette syndrome. J Neurol 2000;247:514–520.
17. Albin RL, Koeppe RA, Bohnen NI, et al. Increased ventral striatal monoaminergic innervation in Tourette syndrome. Neurol 2003;61:310–315.
18. Singer HS. Neurochemical analysis of postmortem cortical and striatal brain tissue in patients with Tourette syndrome. Adv Neurol 1992;58:135–144.
19. Stamenkovic M, Schindler SD, Asenbaum S, et al. No change in striatal dopamine re-uptake site density in psychotropic drug naive and in currently treated Tourette's disorder patients: A [(123)I]-beta-CIT SPECT-study. Eur Neuropsychopharmacol 2001;11:69–74.
20. Anderson GM, Pollak ES, Chatterjee D, Leckman JF, Riddle MA, Cohen DJ. Postmortem analysis of subcortical monoamines and amino acids in Tourette syndrome. Adv Neurol 1992;58:123–133.
21. Swedo SE, Leonard HL, Garvey M, et al. Pediatric autoimmune neuropsychiatric disorders associated with streptococcal infections: Clinical description of the first 50 cases. Am J Psychiatry 1998;155:264–271.
22. Kirvan CA, Swedo SE, Heuser JS, Cunningham MW. Mimicry and autoantibody-mediated neuronal cell signaling in Sydenham chorea. Nat Med 2003;9:914–920.
23. Taylor JR, Morshed SA, Parveen S, et al. An animal model of Tourette's syndrome. Am J Psychiatry 2002;159:657–660.
24. Nordstrom EJ, Burton FH. A transgenic model of comorbid Tourette's syndrome and obsessive-compulsive disorder circuitry. Mol Psychiatry 2002;7:617–625.
25. Schultz RT, Carter A, Gladstone M, et al. Visual-motor integration functioning in children with Tourette syndrome. Neuropsychology 1998;12:134–145.
26. Muller SV, Johannes S, Wieringa B, et al. Disturbed monitoring and response inhibition in patients with Gilles de la Tourette syndrome and co-morbid obsessive compulsive disorder. Behav Neurol 2003;14:29–37.

27. Burd L, Severud R, Klug MG, Kerbeshian J. Prenatal and perinatal risk factors for Tourette disorder. J Perinat Med 1999;27:295–302.

28. Findley DB, Leckman JF, Katsovich L, et al. Development of the Yale children's global stress index (YCGSI) and its application in children and adolescents with Tourette's syndrome and obsessive-compulsive disorder. J Am Acad Child Adolesc Psychiatry 2003;42:450–457.

29. Robertson MM. Diagnosing Tourette syndrome. Is it a common disorder? J Psychosom Res 2003;55:3–6.

30. Snider LA, Seligman LD, Ketchen BR, Levitt SJ, Bates LR, Garvey MA, Swedo SE: Tics and problem behaviors in schoolchildren: prevalence, characterization, and associations. Pediatrics 2002;110:331–336.

31. Lin HY, Yeh CB, Peterson BS, et al. Assessment of symptom exacerbations in a longitudinal study of children with Tourette's syndrome or obsessive-compulsive disorder. J Am Acad Child Adol Psychiatry 2002;41:1070–1077.

32. Sukhodolsky DG, Scahill L, Zhang H, et al. Disruptive behaviors in children with Tourette's syndrome: association with ADHD comorbidity, tic severity, and functional impairment. J Am Acad Child Adol Psychiatry 2003;42:98–105.

33. Rapin I. Autism spectrum disorders: relevance to Tourette syndrome. Adv Neurol 2001;85: 89–101.

34. Robertson MM, Banerjee S, Kurlan R, et al. The Tourette syndrome diagnostic confidence index: Development and clinical associations. Neurol 1999;53:2108–2112.

35. Wilhelm S, Deckersbach T, Coffey BJ, Bohne A, Peterson AL, Baer L. Habit reversal versus supportive psychotherapy for Tourette's disorder: a randomized controlled trial. Am J Psychiatry 2003;160:1175–1177.

36. George MS, Sallee FR, Nahas Z, Oliver NC, Wasserman EM. Transcranial magnetic stimulation (TMS) as a research tool in Tourette syndrome and related disorders. Adv Neurol 2001;85: 225–235.

37. Marras C, Andrews D, Sime E, Lang AE. Botulinum toxin for simple motor tics: a randomized, double blind, controlled clinical trial. Neurol 2001;56:605–610.

38. Vandewalle V, van der Linden C, Groenewegen HJ, Caemaert J. Stereotactic treatment of Gilles de la Tourette syndrome by high frequency stimulation of thalamus. Lancet 1999;353:724.

9

Obsessive-Compulsive Disorder

David S. Husted, Nathan A. Shapira, and Wayne K. Goodman

Summary

Obsessive-compulsive disorder (OCD) is a psychiatric illness that can be quite debilitating and historically has proven difficult to treat. Research conducted over the past decade has provided much insight into the underlying neuropathology, allowing significant advances in the treatment of these patients. Whereas psychotherapy was previously the only mode of treatment for OCD, pharmacological agents and psychosurgical procedures are proving to be effective in treating this disorder. The use of noninvasive or minimally invasive procedures to treat OCD also are currently being investigated. This chapter reviews the animal models and clinical features of OCD, as well as the neurochemicals and brain regions involved in this disorder, and the role of autoimmunity and familial inheritance. Treatment options including psychotherapy, medications, and invasive and noninvasive procedures are also discussed in detail.

Key Words: Obsessive-compulsive disorder; resistant obsessive-compulsive disorder; refractory obsessive-compulsive disorder; etiology of obsessive-compulsive disorder; treatment of obsessive-compulsive disorder; deep brain stimulation; transcranial magnetic stimulation; psychosurgery; psychotherapy; PANDAS.

1. BEHAVIORAL PHENOTYPES, PREVALENCE, AND ETHNIC AND SEX DIFFERENCES

Obsessive-compulsive disorder (OCD) is a disorder characterized by recurrent intrusive thoughts, images, or impulses (obsessions) that are typically ego-dystonic and anxiety producing. The obsessions commonly provoke the individual to engage in ritualistic behavior (compulsions) in an attempt to relieve the consequent anxiety. Compulsions that are commonly noted in OCD include repetitive handwashing (in response to contamination concerns), arranging items in a particular order (in response to concern about symmetry), hoarding (in response to concerns about saving objects), or checking/praying/asking for reassurance (in response to concern over harm, sexual behavior, or religious conflict). Compulsions are often governed by internal rules that the affected individual feels must be applied rigidly, and are not connected in a realistic way with the obsession they are designed to neutralize.

From: *Current Clinical Neurology: Neurological and Psychiatric Disorders: From Bench to Bedside*
Edited by: F. I. Tarazi and J. A. Schetz © Humana Press Inc., Totowa, NJ

They often are excessive and unreasonable, leading to marked impairment of the individual's social or occupational routine as a result of the time required to complete the compulsions.

The symptoms of OCD are similar across the spectrum of cultures and ethnicities, and have varied little in its description in the literature over the past century *(1)*. OCD is the fourth most prevalent psychiatric disorder in the United States, with a lifetime prevalence of 2.5% *(2)*. OCD has been estimated to affect almost 3% of the world's population *(2)*. Prevalence does not appear to differ across different ethnic backgrounds and populations. The male to female ratio of OCD is approximately equal, which is in contrast to other anxiety disorders that are more common in females. OCD demonstrates a bimodal age of onset, with peaks prior to puberty and in the fourth decade of life *(2)*. A statistically significant association with pregnancy, miscarriage, or parturition, as well as with streptococcal infections, has been reported *(3,4)*. OCD-like symptoms can present in acute episodes (e.g., sequelae of acute streptococcal infections in children [pediatric autoimmune neuropsychiatric disorders associated with streptococcus; PANDAS]), but it is more commonly thought of as a chronic illness. Epidemiological studies clearly demonstrate OCD has a high comorbidity with other anxiety and mood disorders, and it is associated with increased impulsivity and suicide attempts *(2)*. OCD-like symptoms are also noted to be inherent to other psychiatric disorders, including Tourette's syndrome, autism, body dysmorphic disorder, and hypochondriasis *(5)*. OCD is associated with extraordinary direct and indirect costs. This is the result of the chronic nature of the illness and the delay in diagnosis and treatment, owing to the strong desire by many patients to hide their pathology out of embarrassment. Other contributing factors are ignorance by the clinician with resultant under-diagnosis and inappropriate treatment, and the tendency of about one-third of the patients to be resistant or refractory to treatment *(2)*.

Hoarding is a subtype of OCD that is difficult to treat. Hoarding is defined as the inability to discard worthless or worn-out things, or "the acquisition of and failure to discard possessions which appear to be useless or of limited value" *(6)*. The most commonly accepted criteria for hoarding behavior to be considered pathological is the cluttering of living spaces to the extent that they are no longer usable, and a significant impairment in function because of hoarding. Prevalence appears to range from one-quarter to one-third of patients with OCD *(6)*. These patients are notoriously refractory to treatment and characteristically carry a poor prognosis.

It is not uncommon to witness patients in dermatology clinics with markedly chapped skin from excessive washing rituals, children in pediatric clinics with a recent onset of excessive checking and recurrent ear infections resulting from a group A streptococcal infection, or pregnant or postpartum females in obstetric clinics with a sudden concern about symmetry *(2–4)*. Therefore, it is important for the clinician to evaluate for OCD in settings other than just the psychiatric clinic. In evaluating patients with OCD, it is also important to assess for prevalent comorbid tics, mood disorders, anxiety disorders, and suicidal behavior *(5)*. The severity of symptoms is best measured by using the Yale–Brown Obsessive-

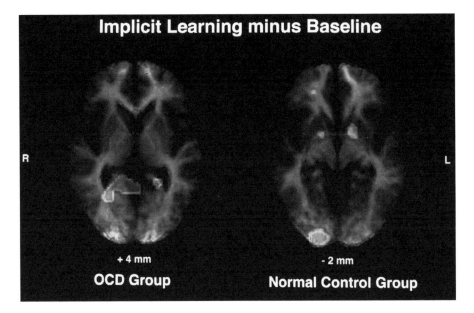

Fig. 1. Positron emission tomography demonstrates bilateral activation of the hippocampal/parahippocampal region of the brain in patients with obsessive-compulsive disorder (OCD) performing implicit learning tasks (left panel), vs bilateral activation of the inferior striatum seen in normal control patients while performing the same tasks (right panel). These findings indicate cortico-striatal dysfunction in OCD patients. *See* color insert preceding p. 51. (Reprinted from ref. *11* with permission.)

Compulsive Scale (Y-BOCS), given the reliability and validity of this scale in a number of randomized controlled trials of OCD *(7)*. The scale is relatively easy to administer, and has been adapted for use in children and adolescents *(8)*.

2. BRAIN PATHWAYS

Symptomatology of OCD is evident in a variety of disorders of the striatum, including Tourette's syndrome, Sydenham's chorea, Huntington's disease, and Parkinson's disease *(5)*. Therefore, it has been hypothesized that OCD involves pathology of the striatum and, indeed, recent brain imaging provides persuasive data to support this hypothesis. Imaging studies have demonstrated significantly decreased volume and increased grey matter density of the cortico-striatal-thalamic-cortical circuits, and increased baseline activity in the orbitofrontal cortex, cingulate gyrus, and striatum in patients with OCD *(9,10)*. These regions also are markedly more active when patient's obsessions are exacerbated. Cortico-striatal systems are known to be involved in implicit learning, which may explain the performance deficits in implicit learning tasks appreciated in neurological patients with striatal pathology (e.g., Huntington's disease) *(11)*. Imaging studies using positron emission tomography (PET) have demonstrated that patients with OCD are unable to access the cortico-striatal system when confronted with implicit learning tasks (Fig. 1), indicating cortico-striatal dysfunction *(11)*. PET studies in patients with OCD symptoms also have consistently shown increased [^{18}F]2-fluoro-2-deoxy-D-glucose uptake in the prefrontal cortex, leading to the hypothesis that this region, among others, is hyperactive in OCD *(10)*. Further studies have also indicated a role for the temporal cortex and the amygdala *(12)*. Functional imaging studies performed in patients following pharmacotherapy and behavioral therapy have demonstrated normalization of brain activity in the cortico-striatal-thalamic-cortical circuitry *(10)*.

3. NEUROCHEMISTRY AND RECEPTOR SUBTYPES

Serotonin (5-hydroxytryptophan [5-HT]) appears to be an important factor in the pathogenesis of OCD. It is postulated that OCD patients have, among other abnormalities, excessive baseline activity of the excitatory glutamatergic neurons of the orbitofrontal cortex. Serotonin is a known inhibitor of these neurons, which would lead one to postulate that increased release of 5-HT by the serotonergic neurons of the orbitofrontal cortex would lead to a diminution of symptoms clinically. Administration of meta-chlorophenylpiperazine (mCPP), a nonselective ligand that acts as an agonist of postsynaptic 5-HT$_{2C}$ receptors, has been noted to exacerbate the symptoms of OCD presumably through feedback inhibition of serotonin release. However, administration of mCPP to patients with OCD after treatment with a serotonin reuptake inhibitor (SRI) does not produce a worsening of baseline symptoms *(13)*. Studies indicate that the important 5-HT receptor subtypes in OCD appear to be the 5-HT$_{2C}$ and 5-HT$_{1D}$ receptors *(13,14)*. Studies demonstrate that desensitization of the 5-HT$_{1D}$ receptor requires a high dose and long duration of administration of SRIs, which correlates with what is clinically observed to diminish the symptoms of OCD *(14)*.

Dopamine is another neurotransmitter of the cortico-striatal-thalamic-cortical system that appears to be important in the pathology of OCD. Administration of dopamine (DA) agonists in preclinical studies has been noted to exacerbate OCD symptoms and tics when they are present *(15)*. This is consistent with the use of antipsychotics, which are DA-receptor blockers, for treating the tics associated with Tourette's syndrome.

4. GENETICS OF OCD

There is substantial evidence for a significant genetic component to OCD. Studies have shown a 70 to 80% concordance rate amongst monozygotic twins compared with 22 to 47% concordance in dizygotic twins *(16)*. Additionally, recent familial studies demonstrate a significant increase in the relative risk of developing OCD in relatives of affected probands vs relatives of controls *(16)*. Complex segregation analyses have led some investigators to propose that a major gene underlies OCD, and that a Mendelian-dominant model with significant sex effects and residual familial effects best explains the inheritance of OCD *(16)*. Further studies have demonstrated that genetic polymorphisms have a role in the pathogenesis of

OCD, with data supportive of 5-HT$_{1D}$ and 5-HT$_{2A}$ polymorphisms being a factor in mediating OCD *(17–20)*. Some data also suggest a sexually dimorphic association with low activity in catechol-*O*-methyltransferase (COMT) alleles and monoamine oxidase-A (MAO-A) alleles, but subsequent reports have been inconsistent *(20)*. Dopaminergic polymorphisms also appear to be a factor in the expression of OCD symptomatology, as dopaminergic alleles have been demonstrated to be distributed differently in patients with OCD with and without tics *(17,20)*. Other studies have demonstrated a genetic relation between OCD and Tourette's *(17,20)*. Despite significant advancements, genetic research concerning OCD is still in the early stages, as many of the initial findings have been difficult to replicate.

5. AUTOIMMUNE BASIS OF AN OCD SUBTYPE

The investigation of a potential autoimmune basis of an OCD subtype has been the focus of much recent research. More than a decade ago, an association between OCD and Sydenham's chorea was confirmed, leading many to hypothesize the presence of an autoimmune disruption of cortico-striatal-thalamic-cortical circuits in at least a subpopulation of patients with OCD *(21)*. In the past decade, a body of literature has been published describing the potential existence of a subtype of OCD that has been labeled PANDAS. PANDAS appears to be a syndrome in which children develop acute OCD-like symptoms following a clinical or subclinical streptococcal infection *(4,21)*. Systematic studies have demonstrated the onset and subsequent exacerbations of OCD and tics in this subset of children to be caused by group A β-hemolytic streptococcal (GABHS) infections *(21)*. Five clinical characteristics seem to define this OCD subgroup: the presence of OCD-like symptoms and/or a tic disorder, prepubertal symptom onset, sudden onset or abrupt exacerbations, neurologic abnormalities most prominent during exacerbations (choreiform movements, motoric hyperactivity), and streptococcal-triggered exacerbations. It has been estimated that up to 30% of OCD patients could be considered part of the PANDAS subtype based on a retrospective analysis of age of onset and clinical characteristics *(22)*. Investigators have demonstrated a significant improvement in OCD symptoms following antibiotic treatment of acute exacerbations in patients with PANDAS *(21)*. Long-term follow-up further demonstrated continued improvement in symptoms, with antibiotic prophylaxis preventing recurrent streptococcal infections. Further research is needed, however, before prophylactic antibiotic treatment in patients with PANDAS can be considered the standard of care.

It appears the autoimmune reaction in this OCD subtype is mediated by autoantibody production, as studies demonstrate increased expression of D8/17, a B-lymphocyte alloantigen, and the presence of autoantibodies in affected patients. These antistreptococcal–antineuronal antibodies appear to target the basal ganglia and other central nervous system (CNS) regions, leading to OCD symptomatology, dystonia, chorea, choreoathetosis, and encephalopathy *(21)*. Given the pathophysiology proposed for PANDAS, immunomodulatory therapies that serve to interrupt the action of auto-antibodies on the CNS would seem to be a reasonable course of treatment. Indeed, administration of intravenous immunoglobulin (IVIG) or plasmapharesis was demonstrated in a clinical trial to lead to long-term (>1 year) resolution of symptoms, with plasma exchange being better tolerated and providing greater relief in symptoms *(23)*. The use of plasma exchange or IVIG acutely for an exacerbation of neuropsychiatric symptoms in PANDAS patients requires further research, however, before being considered the standard of care.

6. ANIMAL MODELS OF OCD

The use of animal models can be a very effective tool for understanding the etiology of diseases afflicting humans and for developing new pharmacotherapeutic treatments. Investigators have suggested that symptoms of OCD are expressed in nature via animal stereotypies, which are motor behaviors in animals that are repetitive and nonfunctional in purpose. One intriguing animal stereotypy noted in nature is that of the acral lick dermatitis (ALD) observed in canines *(17,24)*. This veterinary condition is characterized by repetitive licking of the paws, which leads to dermatitis, hair loss, and discomfort. This behavior is reminiscent of the chapped skin noted in the OCD patient with germ phobia and repeated handwashing. Furthermore, the morbidity that results from the repetitive licking does not lead to any lessening of the behavior, which is similar to OCD patients who are bothered by their compulsions, yet unable to stop them. Other OCD-like behaviors that have been reported in canines are circling, tail-chasing, fly-biting, pacing, hair-biting, and spinning *(24)*. These behaviors are more commonly noted in certain canine families (e.g., Great Danes, German pointers, German shepherds, Dalmatians), with an increased prevalence amongst first-degree relatives, which lends support to the theory of it having a genetic basis *(24)*. Additionally, the pharmacotherapeutic response profile in canines is similar to that of humans, as fluoxetine (a selective serotonin reuptake inhibitor [SSRI]) and clomipramine (a tricyclic antidepressant) have been found to be beneficial in lessening these OCD-like behaviors *(17,24)*. Similarly, fluoxetine has been demonstrated to be superior to placebo in reducing stereotypical behavior in primates *(17)*.

Transgenic mice also serve as a good animal model of OCD. Researchers have engineered transgenic mice that express cholera toxin intracellularly within a cortical-limbic subset of DA D_1-receptor expressing neurons *(25)*. This neuropotentiating protein triggers glutamatergic excitation of orbitofrontal, sensorimotor, limbic, and efferent striatal circuits, leading to marked OCD-like behaviors in this mice strain. These mice are observed to engage perseveringly in all normal mouse behaviors, and to compulsively leap and groom. Furthermore, this transgenic strain exhibits a significant increase in comorbid motor tics, mimicking the association between Tourette's syndrome and OCD in humans *(26)*. Compulsive behavior also has been noted in 5-HT$_{2C}$ knockout mice, and rats treated chronically with the DA agonist quinpirole *(27,28)*.

7. TREATMENT-RESISTANT
AND TREATMENT-REFRACTORY OCD

Few patients with OCD ever experience complete resolution of symptoms. In fact, effectiveness of treatment is often gauged by the clinician as a decrease in symptoms to a level that the patient finds tolerable and at which the patient is able to function. In clinical trials, a 25 to 35% reduction of mean Y-BOCS scores is considered an adequate response to a given treatment *(29)*. Even this modest reduction in Y-BOCS scores is not achieved in 40 to 60% of patients treated with monotherapy, however *(29)*. The terms "treatment-resistant" and "treatment-refractory" (also known as "intractable") are often used interchangeably by the clinician. The synonymous use of these terms is likely a relic of the past, in which the medication options for treating OCD were limited, and resistance to first and second-line treatment exhausted the available options. With the availability of modern treatment options, it is generally accepted that the failure of at least two adequate therapeutic trials of SRIs constitutes treatment-resistant OCD *(29)*. The term treatment-refractory denotes a greater degree of resistance, but it is still debatable at which point in treatment this term becomes applicable. Based on a review of the literature and our own clinical experience, it seems reasonable to consider patients who fail a number of therapeutic trials of SRIs, standard augmentation strategies, and behavioral therapy to be treatment-refractory. Furthermore, patients who demonstrate some response to treatment yet still experience significant impairment from their residual OCD symptoms should also be considered to be treatment-refractory. This is the definition of treatment-refractory that is generally used for the selection of patients for novel treatments, such as psychosurgery. For the purpose of this chapter, therefore, treatment-refractory generally applies to patients who have failed to respond to at least three therapeutic trials of SRIs (with clomipramine being one of the SRI trials), the use of at least two atypical antipsychotics as augmenting agents, and treatment with behavioral therapy while on a therapeutic dose of an SRI. These patients have "failed" treatment by demonstrating less than a 25% reduction of Y-BOCS scores or by still experiencing significant impairment from their illness. Treatment-resistance is noted in 20 to 40% of OCD patients, although 10% of patients are noted to be refractory *(29)*.

8. TREATMENTS

8.1. Pharmacotherapies

Treatment for OCD typically requires a lifetime of medication, as OCD symptoms rarely abate over time if left untreated. Furthermore, reinstatement of a medication following a relapse can be associated with a poorer response than was seen with initial use *(29)*. Consequently, although the clinician may taper a patient's dose in order to maximize benefit while minimizing side effects, rarely will medication be entirely discontinued.

8.1.1. Serotonin Reuptake Inhibitors as a First-Line Treatment

SRIs, including clomipramine and several SSRIs (sertraline, fluoxetine, paroxetine, citalopram, and fluvoxamine), have been demonstrated in a number of rigorous randomized, double-blind placebo-controlled studies to be effective in treating OCD in both adults and children *(29–31)*. SRIs have, therefore, become the first-line agents in the pharmacological treatment of OCD. The best results often require application of SRIs for a long duration (10–12 weeks) and at a high dose (often the maximum recommended dose) *(29,30)*. Although these extreme dosing regimes only alleviate symptoms, rather than producing a complete remission, a partial diminution of symptoms can be associated with a significant improvement in quality of life and overall function *(29,30)*. In general, if the patient fails to demonstrate a significant response (at least 25% reduction Y-BOCS) to an adequate trial of a particular SRI, the clinician should switch treatment to a different SRI *(29)*. With a partial response, the clinician is best served to leave the initial maximally titrated agent in place and to add an additional agent, such as an atypical antipsychotic, to augment the effect *(29)*. Although clomipramine may be moderately more efficacious than the other SRIs, no SSRI has been clearly shown to be more efficacious than another *(31)*. However, all of the SSRIs demonstrate better safety and tolerability profiles than clomipramine, leading clinicians to more frequently utilize SSRIs rather than clomipramine.

8.1.2. Experimental Pharmacological Agents

Agents such as monoamine oxidase inhibitors, lithium, buspirone, trazodone, triiodothyronine, pindolol, anticonvulsants, and benzodiazepines have been found to be ineffective in the treatment of OCD either as monotherapies or as adjuvants *(29,30)*. Both fenfluramine and tryptophan have been found to be effective as augmenting agents in open-label studies *(29,30)*, but serious questions concerning their safety have made both medications unavailable in the United States. The role of antidepressants like venlafaxine and mirtazapine in treating OCD is not yet clear *(32–35)*. Inositol, a component of the second messenger signaling molecule inositol 1,4,5-trisphosphate, has potential as a monotherapy *(36)*, but it has been demonstrated to be ineffective when used as an augmenting agent *(37)*.

Clomipramine is metabolized in the liver to the less potent derivative desmethylclomipramine. Bypassing this first pass hepatic metabolism by administering clomipramine intravenously, therefore, floods the CNS with higher pulse concentrations of the more potent parent compound. Indeed, treatment with intravenous clomipramine has been demonstrated to be rapidly effective in a certain subset of OCD patients who are treatment-resistant to SRIs *(38,39)*. Intravenous clomipramine has been demonstrated to be effective in adults with OCD resistant to or intolerant of oral clomipramine and SSRIs in a double-blind, placebo-controlled trial *(38)*. In a double-blind, pulse-loaded study involving intravenous clomipramine, the investigators noted that subjects administered intravenous clomipramine demonstrated a more rapid response than those given oral clomipramine *(39)*. However, there was no significant difference in improvement of Y-BOCS score between the two study groups at the endpoint of the study (8 weeks). Further double-blind trials evaluating the efficacy of intravenous clomipramine are currently underway.

The role of the endogenous opioid system in the pathophysiology of OCD has been postulated by a number of researchers, given some evidence in the literature that opioid antagonists exacerbate OCD symptoms *(40)*. It was demonstrated in an open-label study that the opioid agonist tramadol (mean dose 254 mg) significantly improved symptoms when administered for a 6-week period as monotherapy in treatment-resistant OCD patients *(40)*. Additionally, researchers have performed a double-blind, placebo-controlled trial that demonstrated the benefit of oral morphine (15–45 mg/day) in treatment-resistant OCD *(41)*. It has been postulated that opiates decrease OCD symptoms via inhibition of glutamate release in the cerebral cortex, disinhibition of serotonergic neurons in the dorsal raphe, and increased DA transmission in the striatum *(41)*.

8.1.3. Atypical Antipsychotics as Augmenting Agents

Atypical antipsychotics are indicated in the treatment of OCD and comorbid tic disorders. Numerous studies document the strong relationship between tic disorders and OCD, with evidence of a greater than 35% prevalence of tic disorders in OCD patients *(15,17,29,42)*. Given that antipsychotics are a standard treatment for the tics associated with Tourette's syndrome, investigators postulated that the concurrent use of neuroleptics and SRIs in the treatment of OCD patients with tics would be an effective regimen *(42)*. Indeed, this group demonstrated in a double-blind, placebo-controlled trial that haloperidol and fluvoxamine, when used in combination, led to significant improvement in Y-BOCS scores vs the use of fluvoxamine alone in these patients *(42)*. Whereas the initial belief was that neuroleptic augmentation preferentially benefited OCD patients with comorbid tics, further research has demonstrated that OCD patients without evidence of tics also manifested significant improvement with haloperidol augmentation *(17,29,30)*. This finding has led to a large body of research concerning the use of antipsychotics in treating OCD.

The literature to date demonstrates dopamine antagonists to be the most effective agent for augmentation, with the atypical antipsychotic agents being better tolerated than the traditional neuroleptics as a result of fewer side effects *(29,30)*. It is theorized that in addition to DA blockade, the synergistic action of blockade of 5-HT_{2A} receptors by atypical antipsychotics with the simultaneous inhibition of 5-HT uptake by SRIs leads to overall greater therapeutic efficacy *(43)*. Risperidone augmentation at an average dose of 2.2 mg per day has been demonstrated in a double-blind, placebo-controlled trial to lead to a significant improvement in Y-BOCS scores vs placebo augmentation *(44)*. Similar findings have been reported subsequently in further double-blind placebo-controlled trials using risperidone augmentation *(45,46)*. Olanzapine augmentation (5–20 mg/day, mean 11.2 mg/day) of SRI treatment of refractory OCD has been demonstrated to lead to significant clinical improvement in a double-blind, placebo-controlled study *(47)*. In another double-blind, placebo-controlled trial, however, no significant difference in improvement in Y-BOCS scores was appreciated using olanzapine (mean dose 6 mg/day) as an augmenting agent *(48)*. Results from a single-blind, placebo-controlled trial have demonstrated that quetiapine augmentation of SRI therapy leads to a significant improvement in the Y-BOCS score in OCD patients *(49)*. Double-blind studies involving quetiapine as an augmenting agent are underway, as are studies involving the use of other atypical antipsychotics, such as ziprasidone and aripiprazole.

8.2. Nonpharmacological Treatments

8.2.1. Psychotherapy for Treatment of OCD

In his writings, Sigmund Freud devoted a fair amount of attention to OCD, postulating that OCD existed on a spectrum ranging from obsessive-compulsive personality disorder to psychosis. Psychoanalytic treatment was suggested by Freud, and was the accepted treatment for OCD for half a century *(1)*. At present, it appears there is little data to support such an approach. Behavioral therapy is the current focus of psychotherapy in the treatment of OCD. Behavioral therapy for treating OCD consists largely of repeated exposure to feared stimuli in order to desensitize patients and, thereby, prevent a subsequent response. A number of controlled studies demonstrate significant improvement in OCD with concurrent behavioral therapy and SSRI treatment, and meta-analyses indicate no differences between the two approaches when they are used separately *(50,51)*. OCD patients treated with behavioral therapy maintain an improved condition following discontinuation of treatment, although up to 80% of patients treated pharmacologically relapse on treatment discontinuation *(50)*. However, only one well-designed study to date has demonstrated an improvement in Y-BOCS scores using behavioral therapy in patients who are partially responsive to SRI monotherapy *(52)*. Despite the dearth of evidence in the literature, it is generally agreed that behavioral therapy should be incorporated into the treatment plan, if it is available and can be tolerated and afforded by the patient, when SRI monotherapy is inadequate *(17,50,51)*.

8.2.2. Neurosurgery for Treatment-Refractory OCD

Ablative neurosurgery (psychosurgery) has been practiced for decades for a variety of debilitating psychiatric conditions, including schizophrenia, bipolar disorder, and OCD. As the pharmacological treatment of these conditions has improved with respect to their efficacy and side-effect profiles, the role of psychosurgery has diminished. However, in the case of OCD, a condition that can be markedly impairing and commonly unresponsive to a variety of treatment regimens, psychosurgery has remained a viable option. Patients with refractory OCD typically have insight into their condition and are desperate for relief from their symptoms, which makes the risks of surgery acceptable. A variety of stereotactic neurosurgical procedures have been described in the literature for the treatment of severe, treatment-refractory OCD. In general, these procedures involve radiofrequency ablation of a portion of the cortico-striatal circuit, which consists of the orbitofrontal cortex, the caudate nucleus, the pallidum, the thalamus, and the anterior cingulate cortex *(53)*. The main regions of pathogenesis of OCD are believed to be the orbitofrontal cortex, cingulated gyrus, basal forebrain, and the caudate nucleus *(9,10,12,17)*. Differences between the various procedures mainly involve the location of the lesion and the postoperative side-effect profile. Anterior cingulotomy specifically targets the anterior cingulate cortex and the fibers of the cingulum, although anterior capsulotomy and subcaudate tractotomy interrupts the frontothalamic fibers (basal forebrain) *(53)*. Limbic leukotomy combines anterior cingulotomy and lesioning of the frontothalamic projections and is often performed in a staged manner. To date, no trial has been performed to compare the efficacy of limbic leukotomy to that of anterior cingulotomy alone.

The mechanisms by which psychosurgery improves OCD symptomatology remain poorly understood. The literature suggests persistent anatomic and metabolic changes of the anterior and posterior cingulate gyrus after lesioning the anterior cingulate, which may be the mechanism by which OCD symptoms improve following surgery *(54,55)*. There appears to be a delay in the onset of symptom improvement, suggesting the benefit of surgery is related not only to interruption of neural pathways, but also the reorganization of neural pathways following surgery *(53)*. This correlates well with the clinical finding of continuous improvement in OCD symptoms for more than 1-year postoperatively *(53,56–58)*. The different psychosurgical procedures for OCD are roughly comparable in efficacy, and appear to be relatively safe with low risk for long-term adverse effects. Given that the anterior cingulated cortex is in close proximity to the fronto-striato-pallido-thalamo-frontal circuit, there is the potential for postoperative frontal lobe abnormality and executive dysfunction. The risk of incontinence postoperatively is not surprising as the anterior cingulated gyrus is also involved in visceromotor control mechanisms. Reports of transient memory deficits and cognitive function impairments have been noted in the literature, although the incidence is rare and the changes noted are quite subtle *(53)*.

8.2.2.1. ANTERIOR CINGULOTOMY

The efficacy of stereotactic bilateral anterior cingulotomy has been demonstrated in a prospective investigation in fourteen patients with severe, treatment-refractory OCD *(56)*. Significant improvement in OCD symptoms following anterior cingulotomy was appreciated in the study, with a mean decrease in Y-BOCS scores of 12.6 at 12 months follow-up. No significant surgery-related impairments lasting over 3 months were observed. Similar efficacy with anterior cingulotomy has been demonstrated using magnetic resonance imaging (MRI) validation of lesion locations and modern diagnostic criteria for OCD *(57)*.

8.2.2.2. LIMBIC LEUKOTOMY

A retrospective chart review of 21 patients with either major depressive disorder (MDD) or OCD who underwent limbic leukotomy using MRI-guided stereotaxis has been encouraging *(58)*. Twelve of the patients had previously undergone bilateral anterior cingulotomy and, therefore, required only lesioning of the frontothalamic fibers (in essence, a "staged" limbic leukotomy), whereas the remaining six patients underwent concurrent anterior cingulotomy and lesioning of the frontothalamic fibers. Postoperative Y-BOCS values demonstrated a 36% "response" rate when compared to preoperative Y-BOCS scores. *Post hoc* analysis demonstrated a significant benefit to those who underwent a staged vs single procedure limbic leucotomy. Persistent complex partial seizures, short-term memory problems, and incontinence were reported in less than 5% of the patients. Some authors have reported even greater efficacy, with 62% of study subjects with severe OCD rated as responders following limbic leucotomy although, arguably, the investigators used liberal criteria for improvement *(59)*. Another retrospective review of the outcome of limbic leukotomy in 12 patients with severe OCD (mean Y-BOCS score 34) demonstrated similar findings *(60)*. Postoperatively, the mean Y-BOCS score was noted to be 3, and these results were appreciated to persist for the mean 45 months of postoperative follow-up. Except for one case of mild transient urinary incontinence, no significant morbidity was observed.

8.2.2.3. VAGUS NERVE STIMULATION

Vagus nerve stimulation (VNS) is predicated on the belief that the tenth cranial nerve has reciprocal influences on the limbic system and higher cortical activity as a result of it being predominantly an afferent nerve, its extensive arborization within the brain, and its widespread distribution in the body. The vagus cell bodies convey information centrally to the nucleus tractus solitarius which then projects to the remainder of the brain via three pathways: an autonomic feedback loop, direct projections to the medullary reticular formation, and ascending projections to the forebrain. The ascending projections have connections to the locus coeruleus, parabrachial nucleus, thalamus, hypothalamus, amygdala, and stria terminalis, which are all regions thought to be involved in the modulation of mood and anxiety disorders *(61)*.

VNS involves stimulation of the left vagus nerve in the cervical region using a bipolar pulse generator. This generator is implanted in the left chest wall and delivers electrical signals to the electrode that is wrapped around the vagus nerve in the neck. Surgical adverse effects include pain, coughing, left vocal cord paralysis, hoarseness, nausea, and rare infection. Of note, no alteration of normal pulmonary or cardiac function has been reported postoperatively *(62)*.

Initial reports of mood changes in patients receiving VNS for the treatment of treatment-resistant epilepsy prompted speculation that VNS would have psychiatric uses *(62)*. Later research demonstrated central increases in noradrenergic and serotonergic neurotransmission following VNS *(62)*. An open-label pilot study involving seven adults with treatment-refractory OCD was performed to explore the efficacy of VNS *(63)*. These patients were treated with 10 weeks of VNS with concurrent psychotropic medication. Overall, a 17% mean reduction from baseline in the Y-BOCS score was noted at 6 months, although one patient withdrew from the study at 3 months as a result of lack of response. Further investigation of VNS as a treatment of OCD appears warranted, especially given its minimally invasive nature and low side-effect profile.

8.2.2.4. DEEP BRAIN STIMULATION

Deep brain stimulation (DBS), which is currently an accepted treatment for movement disorders such as Parkinson's disease, is a potentially promising alternative to traditional psychosurgery for the treatment of severe, treatment-refractory OCD. Unlike traditional surgical approaches for OCD that involve irreversible lesioning of the involved circuitry, DBS offers the benefit of a potentially reversible procedure that can be utilized in a graded fashion by adjusting stimulus intensity. Consequently, treatment can be modified to fit the individual patient's needs and side-effect profile. DBS involves delivering a current via an implanted quadripolar electrode that is connected to a battery-powered impulse generator that is implanted beneath the skin in the subclavicular region. Abnormalities of neuronal activity can be suppressed by either lesioning or chronic electrical stimulation. Although the mechanism of action of DBS is not fully clarified, it is hypothesized that neuronal inactivation occurs secondary to direct disruption of neuronal firing or increased γ-aminobutyric acid (GABA) production *(62)*. The electrical current may inhibit cells and stimulate fibers depending on the stimulation parameters chosen. This therapy electrophysiologically alters abnormal patterns of neuronal firing in diseases such as Parkinson's disease and it is likely that it has a similar effect on behavioral disorders such as OCD. Using positron computed tomographic studies in patients following treatment with DBS for 3 months, a significant reduction in frontal metabolism is observed *(64)*. The DBS device may induce an "informational lesion" and disrupt one of the many nonmotor circuits of basal ganglia. These induced changes in the nonmotor circuits may be the mechanism by which frontal lobe metabolism is affected. Much research is needed to clarify the mechanisms by which DBS is effective in treating OCD, and to further elucidate the optimal target location in the CNS.

Researchers have reported marked improvement in function and symptoms in patients with severe, debilitating OCD treated with long-term electrical anterior capsular stimulation *(64)*. In a follow-up of four of the six patients originally treated with DBS, three demonstrated a significant postoperative decrease in Y-BOCS scores (>35% decrease) during stimulator-on conditions. This improvement was sustained for greater than the 21-month postoperative follow-up period. The fourth patient, who was noted to be nonresponsive was discovered to have an implant with malfunctioning batteries.

DBS is attractive from a research perspective as it allows for randomized, blinded research as a result of the reversible nature of the electrical stimulation. Intracerebral hemorrhage is the most serious adverse outcome from surgery *(61,63)*. Confusion, speech disturbance, parasthesia, oculomotor abnormalities, and muscle contractions are the most common complications of stimulation, although they are often transient and not generally disturbing to the patient *(64)*.

8.2.3. Transcranial Magnetic Stimulation

Transcranial magnetic stimulation (TMS) is the least invasive form of physical treatment of OCD. This procedure involves the induction of a magnetic field over the scalp by passing an electric current through a coil. The resultant electrical field causes depolarization of the surface cortex, which leads to either net stimulation or disruption of the neurons in the brain region targeted by the stimulator. Repeated application of TMS to a given region is termed repetitive TMS (rTMS), and the repetitive use of frequencies greater than one Hertz is termed fast-frequency rTMS (FF-rTMS). Most studies of TMS in the treatment of OCD use FF-rTMS. Although no significant effect on obsessions was noted following a single session of right prefrontal rTMS on 12 patients with OCD, a significant and sustained (>8 hours) decrease in compulsive behavior was noted *(65)*. Later studies demonstrated no difference in outcome between real and sham rTMS, although the researchers used a technique that differs from that which is used in most other rTMS studies *(66,67)*. Adverse effects, such as a severe headache or a temporary shift in auditory threshold, are mainly related to the intensity and frequency of stimuli applied, and seizures are rare *(65–67)*. The recently reported ineffectiveness of rTMS in treating OCD may be related to the magnet field strength being inadequate to reach the deeper brain regions implicated in OCD. Given the encouraging results thus far with the use of TMS in treating depression and the relative safety of this procedure, further evaluation of the efficacy of TMS in treating OCD appears warranted.

9. CONCLUSION

OCD is a disorder characterized by recurrent intrusive ego-dystonic thoughts, images, or impulses (obsessions) that tend to provoke compulsive behavior in an attempt to relieve the anxiety. OCD affects approx 3% of the population of the United States, and has a similar prevalence worldwide. The male to female ratio of OCD is approximately equal, and onset of this disease is bimodal, with peaks prior to puberty and in the fourth decade of life. The association of other disorders of the striatum with OCD, as well as the results of recent brain imaging studies, suggest that OCD is related to striatal pathology. Abnormalities of the orbitofrontal cortex and cingulate gyrus are also thought to be involved in OCD. The results of recent research strongly suggest a familial component to OCD. Genetic polymorphisms of certain serotonin receptor subtypes may play a role in the pathogenesis of OCD. Animal models and clinical research also suggest a role for serotonergic, glutamatergic, and possibly dopaminergic systems in OCD. As a result, serotonin reuptake inhibitors and antipsychotics have become the mainstay of pharmacologic treatment. Behavioral psychotherapy also has been shown to be effective in treating OCD. A variety of stereotactic neurosurgical procedures have been described in the literature for the treatment of severe, treatment-refractory OCD. The different psychosurgical procedures for OCD are roughly comparable in efficacy, and appear to be relatively safe with low risk for long-term adverse effects. DBS, which is currently an accepted treatment for movement disorders such as Parkinson's disease, is a potentially promising alternative to traditional psychosurgery for the treatment of severe, treatment-refractory OCD. VNS and TMS, likewise, are less invasive procedures that may also have a role in the treatment of OCD.

GLOSSARY OF MEDICAL TERMINOLOGY

Ego-dystonic: Aspects of a person, such as behavior or thoughts that are viewed by the self as repugnant, incompatible, or unacceptable with one's personality.

Obsessive-compulsive disorder (OCD): An anxiety disorder characterized by intrusive, recurrent thoughts (obsessions) that patients find senseless and often disturbing plus ritualistic behaviors (compulsions), usually in response to the obsessive thoughts, that interfere with psychosocial function and well-being; most patients experience both symptoms.

Parturition: The act or process of giving birth.

Plasmapharesis: The separation of the cellular components of whole blood from plasma in order to remove toxins from the blood. The plasma, which contains the undesired toxins, is disposed of while the cellular components are re-infused into the patient combined with normal saline or a plasma substitute.

Syndenham's chorea: A nonprogressive neurological movement disorder characterized by spontaneous movements, lack of coordination of voluntary movements, and muscular weakness. This disorder may occur following a streptococcal infection such as rheumatic fever, meningitis, or scarlet fever.

REFERENCES

1. Stein DJ, Stone MH. Essential papers on obsessive-compulsive disorders. New York, New York: New York University Press, 1997.
2. Bebbington PE. Epidemiology of obsessive-compulsive disorder. Br J Psychiatry 1998;35 (Suppl):2–6.
3. Williams KE, Koran LM. Obsessive-compulsive disorder in pregnancy, the puerperium, and the premenstruum. J Clin Psychiatry 1997;58:330–334.
4. Swedo SE, Leonard HL, Garvey M, et al. Pediatric autoimmune neuropsychiatric disorders associated with streptococcal infections: clinical description of the first 50 cases. Am J Psychiatry 1998;155:264–271.
5. Hollander E. Obsessive-compulsive related disorders. Washington, D.C.: American Psychiatric Press; 1993.
6. Frost RO, Steketee GS. Hoarding: clinical aspects and treatment strategies. In: Jenicke MA, Baer L, Minichiello WE, eds. Obsessive-compulsive disorders: practical management, 3rd Ed. St Louis, Missouri: Mosby, 1998, Chapter 23.
7. Goodman WK, Price LH, Rasmussen SA, et al. The Yale-Brown obsessive compulsive scale. I: development, use, and reliability. Arch Gen Psychiatry 1989;46:1006–1011.
8. Scahill L, Riddle MA, McSwiggin-Hardin M, et al. Children's Yale-Brown obsessive compulsive scale: reliability and validity. J Am Acad Child Adolesc Psychiatry 1997;36:844–852.
9. Rauch SL, Baxter LR Jr. Neuroimaging in obsessive-compulsive disorder and related disorders. In: Jenicke MA, Baer L, Minichiello WE, eds. Obsessive-compulsive disorders: practical management, 3rd Ed. St Louis, Missouri: Mosby;1998:289–317.
10. Hugo F, van Heerden BB, Zungu-Dirwayi N, Stein DJ. Functional brain imaging in obsessive-compulsive disorder secondary to neurological lesions. Depress Anxiety 1999;10:129–136.
11. Rauch SL, Savage CR, Alpert NM, et al. Probing striatal function in obsessive-compulsive disorder: a PET study of implicit sequence learning. J Neuropsych Clin Neurosci 1997;9:568–573.
12. Szeszko PR, Robinson D, Alvir JMJ, et al. Orbital frontal and amygdala volume reductions in obsessive-compulsive disorder. Arch Gen Psychiatry 1999;56:913–919.
13. Baumgarten HG, Grozdanovic Z. Role of serotonin in obsessive-compulsive disorder. Br J Psychiatry 1998;35 (Suppl):13–20.
14. Mundo E, Richter MA, Sam F, Macciardi F, Kennedy JL. Is the 5-HT(1Dbeta) receptor gene implicated in the pathogenesis of obsessive-compulsive disorder? Am J Psychiatry 2000;157: 1160–61.

15. Goodman WK, McDougle CJ, Lawrence LP. Beyond the serotonin hypothesis: a role for dopamine in some forms of obsessive-compulsive disorder. J Clin Psychiatry 1990;51 (suppl):36–43.

16. Nestadt G, Lan T, Samuels J, et al. Complex segregation analysis provides compelling evidence for a major gene underlying obsessive-compulsive disorder and for heterogeneity by sex. Am J Hum Genet 2000;67:1611–1616.

17. Stein DJ. Obsessive-compulsive disorder (seminar). Lancet 2002;360:397–405.

18. Enoch MA, Kaye WH, Rotondo A, Greenberg BD, Murphy DL, Goldman D. 5-HT2A promoter polymorphism −1438G/A, anorexia nervosa, and obsessive-compulsive disorder. Lancet 1998;351:1785–1786.

19. Enoch MA, Greenberg BD, Murphy DL, Goldman D. Sexually dimorphic relationship of a 5-HT2A promoter polymorphism with obsessive-compulsive disorder. Biol Psychiatry 2001; 49:385–388.

20. Hemmings SMJ, Kinnear CJ, Niehaus DJH, et al. Investigating the role of dopamine and serotonergic candidate genes in obsessive-compulsive disorder. Eur Neuropyschopharmacol 2003;13:93–98.

21. Leonard HL, Swedo SE: Pediatric autoimmune neuropsychiatric disorders associated with streptococcal infection (PANDAS). Int J Neuropsychopharmacol 2001;4:191–198.

22. Singer HS, Loiselle C. PANDAS: a commentary. J Psychosom Res 2003;55:31–39.

23. Perlmutter SJ, Leitman SF, Garvey MA, et al. Therapeutic plasma exchange and intravenous immunoglobulin for obsessive-compulsive disorder and tic disorder in childhood. Lancet 1999;354:1153–1158.

24. Overall KL. Natural animal models of human psychiatric conditions: assessment of mechanism and validity. Prog Neuropsychopharmacol Biol Psychiatry 2000;24:727–776.

25. Campbell KM, de Lecea L, Severynse DM, et al. OCD-like behaviors caused by a neuro-potentiating transgene targeted to cortical and limbic D1+ neurons. J Neuroscience 1999;19:5044–5053.

26. Nordstrom EJ, Burton FH. A transgenic model of comorbid tourette's syndrome and obsessive-compulsive disorder circuitry. Mol Psychiatry 2002;7:617–625.

27. Chou-Green JM, Holscher TD, Dallman MF, Akana SF. Compulsive behavior in the 5-HT2C receptor knockout mouse. Physiol Behav 2003;78:641–649.

28. Szechtman H, Sulis W, Eilam D. Quinpirole induces compulsive checking behavior in rats: a potential animal model of obsessive-compulsive disorder (OCD). Behav Neurosci 1998;112: 1475–1485.

29. Goodman WK, Ward HE, Kablinger AS, Murphy TK. Biological approaches to treatment-resistant obsessive-compulsive disorder. In: Goodman WK, Rudorfer MV, and Maser JD (eds). Obsessive-compulsive disorder: contemporary issues in management. London, UK: Lawrence Erlbaum Associates; 2000:333–369.

30. Dougherty DD, Rauch SL, Jenike MA. Pharmacological treatments for obsessive compulsive disorder. In: Nathan PE and Gorman JM (eds). A guide to treatments that work, 2nd Ed. London, UK: Oxford University Press; 2002:387–410.

31. Geller DA, Biederman J, Stewart SE, et al. Which SSRI? A meta-analysis of pharmacotherapy in pediatric obsessive-compulsive disorder. Am J Psychiatry 2003;160:1919–1928.

32. Albert U, Aguglia E, Maina G, Bogetto F. Venlafaxine versus clomipramine in the treatment of obsessive-compulsive disorder: a preliminary single-blind, 12-week, controlled study. J Clin Psychiatry 2002;63:1004–1009.

33. Denys D, Van Der Wee N, Van Megen HJ, Westenberg HG. A double-blind comparison of venlafaxine and paroxetine in obsessive-compulsive disorder. J Clin Psychopharmacol 2003; 23:568–575.

34. Koran LM, Quirk T, Lorberbaum JP, Elliott M. Mirtazapine treatment of obsessive-compulsive disorder (letter). J Clin Psychopharmacol 2001;21:537–539.

35. Koran LM, Chuong HW. Mirtazapine treatment for adult OCD (poster). Presented at the 156th Annual Meeting of the American Psychiatric Association, May 17-22, 2003, San Francisco, CA.

36. Fux M, Levine J, Aviv A, Belmaker RH. Inositol treatment of obsessive-compulsive disorder. Am J Psychiatry 1996;153:1219–1221.

37. Fux M, Benjamin J, Belmaker RH. Inositol versus placebo augmentation of serotonin reuptake inhibitors in the treatment of obsessive-compulsive disorder: a double-blind cross-over study. Int J Neuropsychopharmacol 1999;2:193–195.

38. Fallon BA, Liebowitz MR, Campeas R, et al. Intravenous clomipramine for obsessive-compulsive disorder refractory to oral clomipramine: a placebo-controlled study. Arch Gen Psychiatry 1998;55:918–924.

39. Koran LM, Sallee FR, Pallanti S. Rapid benefit of intravenous pulse loading of clomipramine in obsessive-compulsive disorder. Am J Psychiatry 1997;154:396–401.

40. Shapira NA, Keck PE, Goldsmith TD, McConville BJ, Eis M, McElroy SL. Open-label pilot study of tramadol hydrochloride in treatment-refractory obsessive-compulsive disorder. Depression and Anxiety 1997;6:170–173.

41. Koran LM, Bullock KD, Franz BE, Elliot MA. Double-blind oral morphine in treatment-resistant OCD. Presented at the 156th Annual Meeting of the American Psychiatric Association, May 17-22, 2003, San Francisco, CA.

42. McDougle CJ, Goodman WK, Leckman JF, Lee NC, Heninger GR, Price LH. Haloperidol addition in fluvoxamine-refractory obsessive-compulsive disorder: a double-blind, placebo-controlled study in patients with and without tics. Arch Gen Psychiatry 1994;51:302–308.

43. Marek GJ, Carpenter LL, McDougle CJ, Price LH. Synergistic action of 5-HT2A antagonists and selective serotonin reuptake inhibitors in neuropsychiatric disorders. Neuropsychopharmacology 2003;28:402–412

44. McDougle CJ, Epperson CN, Pelton GH, Wasylink S, Price LH. A double-blind, placebo-controlled study of risperidone addition in serotonin reuptake inhibitor-refractory obsessive-compulsive disorder. Arch Gen Psychiatry 2000;57:794–802.

45. Hollander E, Ross NB, Sood E, Pallanti S. Risperidone augmentation in treatment-resistant obsessive-compulsive disorder: a double-blind, placebo controlled study. Int J Neuropsychopharmacol 2003;6:397–401.

46. Arias F, Soto JA, Garcia MJ, Rodriguez-Calvin JL, Morales J, Salgado M. Efficacy and tolerance of risperidone addition in serotonin reuptake inhibitors (SRI) treatment for refractory obsessive-compulsive disorder. Eur Neuropsychopharmacol 2002;12:S341.

47. Bystritsky A, Ackerman DL, Rosen RM, et al. Augmentation of SSRI response in refractory OCD using adjunct olanzapine: a placebo-controlled trial. APA Annual Meeting, New Research Abstracts; 2001; New Orleans, LA:171,172.

48. Shapira NA, Ward HE, Mandoki M, et al. Placebo-controlled trial of fluoxetine versus fluoxetine plus olanzapine in obsessive-compulsive disorder. Paper presented at: New Clinical Drug Evaluation Unit (NCDEU) Annual Meeting; May 29, 2003; Boca Raton, Florida.

49. Atmaca M, Kuloglu M, Tezcan E, Gecici O. Quetiapine augmentation in patients with treatment resistant obsessive-compulsive disorder: a single-blind, placebo-controlled study. Int Clin Psychopharmacol 2002;17:115–119.

50. Foa EB, Kozak MJ. Psychological treatment for obsessive-compulsive disorder. In: Mavissakalian MR, Prien RF (eds). Long-term treatments of Anxiety Disorders. Washington, DC: American Psychiatric Press;1996:285–309.

51. Cox BJ, Swinson RP, Morrison B, Lee PS. Clomipramine, fluoxetine, and behavior therapy in the treatment of obsessive-compulsive disorder: a meta-analysis. J Behav Ther Exp Psychiatry 1993;24:149–153.

52. Albert U, Maina G, Forner F, Bogetto F. Cognitive-behavioral therapy in obsessive-compulsive disorder patients partially unresponsive to SRIs (abstract). J Eur Neuropsychopharm 2003;13: S357–S358.

53. Cosgrove GR, Rauch SL. Psychosurgery. Neurosurg Clin N Am 1995;6:167–176.

54. Rauch SL, Markris N, Cosgrove GR, et al. A magnetic resonance imaging study of regional cortical volumes following stereotactic anterior cingulotomy. CNS Spectrums 2001;6:214–216,221,222.

55. Sachdev P, Trollor J, Walker A, et al. Bilateral orbitomedial leuocotomy for obsessive-compulsive: a single-case study using positron emission tomography. Aust N Z J Psychiatry 2001;35: 684–690.
56. Kim CH, Chang JW, Koo MS, et al. Anterior cingulotomy for refractory obsessive-compulsive disorder. Acta Psychiatr Scand 2003;107:283–290.
57. Dougherty DD, Baer L, Cosgrove GR, et al. Update on cingulotomy for intractable obsessive-compulsive disorder: prospective long-term follow-up of 44 patients. Am J Psychiatry 2002; 159:269–275.
58. Montoya A, Weiss AP, Price BH, et al. Magnetic resonance imaging-guided stereotactic limbic leucotomy for treatment of intractable psychiatric disease. Neurosurgery 2002;50:1043–1052.
59. Hay P, Sachdev P, Cumming S, Smith JS, Lee T, Kitchener P, Matheson J. Treatment of obsessive-compulsive disorder by psychosurgery. Acta Psychiatr Scand 1993;87:197–207.
60. Kim MC, Lee TK, Choi CR. Review of long-term results of stereotactic psychosurgery. Neurol Med Chir (Tokyo) 2002;42:365–371.
61. Van Bockstaele EJ, Peoples J, Valentino RJ. Anatomic basis for differential regulation of the rostrolateral peri-locus coeruleus region by limbic afferents. Biol Psychiatry 1999;46:1352–1363.
62. Malhi GS, Sachdev P. Novel physical treatments for the management of neuropsychiatric disorders. J Psychosom Res 2002;53:709–719.
63. Ward H, Ninan PT, Pollack M, et al. Treatment-refractory obsessive-compulsive disorder: potential benefit of VNS therapy. Poster presented at 23rd Annual Conference of the Anxiety Disorders Association of America, Toronto, Canada; March 27–30, 2003.
64. Nuttin BJ, Gabriels LA, Cosyns PR, et al. Long-term electrical capsular stimulation in patients with obsessive-compulsive disorder. Neurosurgery 2003;52:1263–1274.
65. Greenberg BD, George MS, Martin JD, et al. Effect of prefrontal repetitive transcranial magnetic stimulation (rTMS) in obsessive-compulsive disorder: a preliminary study. Am J Psychiatry 1997;154:867–869.
66. Alonso P, Pujol J, Cardoner N, et al. Right prefrontal repetitive transcranial magnetic stimulation in obsessive-compulsive disorder: A double-blind, placebo-controlled study. Am J Psychiatry 2001;158:1143–1145.
67. Martin JLR, Barbanoj MJ, Clos S. Transcranial magnetic stimulation (TMS) for the treatment of obsessive-compulsive disorder (OCD). Cochrane Database Syst Rev 2003;3:CD003387.

10

Unipolar Depression

Julie A. Blendy and Irwin Lucki

Summary

Unipolar depression is characterized by mood dysregulation that is manifested in recurrent affective episodes over the lifetime of an individual. This chapter covers the epidemiology, pathology, genetics, and brain circuitry associated with unipolar depression. In addition, animal models of depression that have been useful in characterizing neurobiological causes for depression and development of new treatments are reviewed. Effective treatments exist for antidepressant treatment. The efficacy, side effects, toxicity, and mechanisms of action of various classes of these drugs are discussed. Finally, it has been shown that long-term use of antidepressants is effective in preventing recurring episodes of depression; cellular and molecular mediators that may underlie this effect are covered.

Key Words: Unipolar depression; noradrenaline; serotonin; antidepressant; animal models.

1. EPIDEMIOLOGY OF MAJOR DEPRESSION

Unipolar depression, also known as major depression, is the leading cause of disability in the world when measured by the number of years lived with a disabling condition. It is second only to heart disease in disease burden, which is calculated by healthy life-years lost to disability, including premature death *(1)*. Major depression has an overall life prevalence rate of 21% in women and 13% in men in the United States according to recent epidemiological studies *(2)*. The prevalence of depression has reportedly increased 6% over the past 15 years, and it currently affects nearly 20 million American adults. Additionally, the average age of onset for depression has sharply decreased from 40–50 years to 25–35 years of age and it affects individuals from all socioeconomic and ethnic backgrounds. This apparent increase in prevalence and decrease in the age of onset is probably a result of improved recognition and diagnosis of depression and an increase in individuals seeking treatment. However, these statistics likely underestimate the incidence of depression as the disease often presents with other comorbid psychiatric disorders such as panic disorder, obsessive-compulsive disorder (OCD) and posttraumatic stress disorder (PTSD).

From: *Current Clinical Neurology: Neurological and Psychiatric Disorders:*
From Bench to Bedside
Edited by: F. I. Tarazi and J. A. Schetz © Humana Press Inc., Totowa, NJ

Table 1
DSM-IV Criteria for Diagnosis of Major Depression

1. Depressed mood
2. Loss of interest or pleasure in almost all activities
3. Significant weight loss or gain or an increase or decrease in appetite nearly every day
4. Insomnia or hypersomnia
5. Objective psychomotor agitation or retardation
6. Fatigue or loss of energy
7. Feelings of worthlessness or excessive or inappropriate guilt
8. Diminished ability to think or concentrate, or indecisiveness (either by subjective account or observation of others)
9. Recurrent thoughts of death (not just fear of dying), or suicidal ideation, or a suicide attempt, or a specific plan for committing suicide.

At least 2 weeks of five or more of the above features, which are present most of the day, or nearly every day and must include depressed mood or loss of interest or pleasure in almost all activities.

2. DEPRESSION AND BEHAVIOR

In his book, the *Noonday Demon,* Andrew Solomon writes of his struggles with depression in a way that clearly characterizes the symptoms of this disease: " . . . the slippage was steady. I worked less and less well. I had begun to feel that no one could love me and that I would never be in a relationship again. I had no sexual feeling at all. I began eating irregularly because I seldom felt hungry."

As evident from this description, signs of depression include depressed mood, diminished interest or pleasure in activities, feelings of worthlessness, and a loss of energy and ability to concentrate. Additionally, patterns of sleep, appetite, and activity can be affected in depression, often in opposite directions. For example, the individual can exhibit insomnia or hypersomnia, hypophagia or hyperphagia, psychomotor agitation, or reduction *(3)*. In addition to feelings of worthlessness, or inappropriate guilt, recurrent thoughts of death or suicide are common depressive symptoms. A diagnosis of unipolar depression is made if an individual has five or more of these symptoms occurring in a 2-week period. Typically, these symptoms occur throughout a depressed person's lifetime in discrete recurring episodes (Table 1).

Milder forms of depression that do not meet the full criteria for major depression are often associated with significant anxiety symptoms, such as exaggerated worry and tension. Dysthymia produces symptoms that are less intense than in major depression and can last for years, but the low mood and associated symptoms must be present on most days for at least 2 years to qualify for this diagnosis. This dysthymic form of depression is present in about 6% of the general population *(3)*.

High rates of depression in certain neurological diseases such as Parkinson's and Huntington's diseases provide some evidence linking the dysfunction of motor and mood behaviors. Additionally, depression can occur as a biological reaction to certain physical illnesses (e.g., cardiovascular disease, diabetes, strokes affecting the left frontal cerebrum, hypothyroidism, pancreatic cancer) or to chemical substances (e.g., alcohol, methamphetamine, β-blocking antihypertensive medications). The relationship between these comorbid factors and depression is unknown, but it could result from the pathology of the primary disease, or from a response to the specific psychological stress associated with the disease.

3. DEPRESSION AND STRESS

Psychiatric morbidity that is associated with depression can often be accompanied or even precipitated by stress. There is a close clinical and biochemical resemblance between depressive symptoms and the response to stressful experiences, which suggests that depression involves activation of the primary mediators of the stress response. In fact, stressors, such as those associated with a serious loss, difficult relationship, financial problem, or change in life patterns, are associated with greater initial severity of depressive symptoms both in adults and adolescents *(4)*. Recent studies have generated substantial evidence that alterations of the stress hormone system also plays a major, causal role in the development of depression *(5)*.

The body's complex hormonal response to stress is regulated by the hypothalamic–pituitary–adrenalcortical (HPA) axis. Corticotropin-releasing factor (CRF) and arginine vasopressin (AVP) are synthesized and released from the paraventricular nucleus of the hypothalamus. This results in expression and release of adrenocorticotropic hormone (ACTH) from the anterior pituitary, which then stimulates glucocorticoid secretion from the cortex of the adrenal gland. Glucocorticoids exert a negative feedback on the synthesis and release of ACTH and CRF. Clinical data indicate that a subset of patients with depression secrete excessive glucocorticoids from the adrenal gland or exhibit hyperactivity of the HPA axis *(6)*. Furthermore, HPA axis disturbance is normalized following successful antidepressant therapy in clinically depressed patients *(7)*.

4. PATHOLOGY

In addition to hormonal alterations, clinically depressed patients exhibit distinct histopathological changes in selective brain regions, including such limbic structures as the hippocampus and the prefrontal cortex (PFC) *(8)*. Specifically, imaging studies indicate that PFC, ventral striatal, and hippocampal volumes are decreased in patients with depression *(9)*. Similarly, distinct reductions in hippocampal volume are observed in patients with HPA hyperactivity *(6)*. Preclinical studies have focused on examining stress-induced changes in the hippocampus, as this region is particularly susceptible *(6)*. In animal models, these stress-induced structural impairments can be reversed by chronic antidepressant treatment *(10)*. Furthermore, recent studies suggest that reduced hippocampal volume in depressed patients may be related to the duration of untreated episodes, in that treated patients shown significantly less damage than untreated controls *(9,11)*. Although the precise pathobiology of stress and depression remain unclear, the role of antidepressants in mediating cellular and structural repair may be an important aspect of antidepressant efficacy.

Table 2
**Therapeutic Targets and Generic and Trade Names
of Some Commonly Prescribed Antidepressants**

Generic	Category	Trade
Buproprion	NRI/DRI	Wellbutrin
Citalopram	SSRI	Celexa
Fluoxetine	SSRI	Prozac
Fluvoxamine	SSRI	Luvox
Sertraline	SSRI	Zoloft
Paroxetine	SSRI	Paxil
Venlafaxine	SSRI/NRI	Effexor
Tranylcypromine	MAOI	Parnate
Phenelzine	MAOI	Nardil

NRI, norepinephrine reuptake inhibitor; DRI, dopamine reuptake inhibitor; SSRI, selective serotonin reuptake inhibitor; MAOI, monoamine oxidase inhibitor.

5. BRAIN PATHWAYS

All antidepressant drugs currently approved for the treatment of unipolar depression affect two neurotransmitter systems: the noradrenergic and the serotinergic systems. The majority of noradrenergic cell bodies in the brain are found in the locus ceruleus, which is located on the floor of the fourth ventricle in the rostral pons. The neurons emanating from the locus ceruleus project to virtually every area of the brain and spinal cord. Alterations in neuronal firing in the locus ceruleus can alter norepinephrine release to postsynaptic sites throughout the brain. The other noradrenergic neurons in the brain are scattered through out the brainstem in loose collections of cells referred to as the lateral tegmental regions. These cells also project to the spinal cord and brain but are not as widely distributed as locus ceruleus neuronal projections.

In contrast to the relatively small numbers of noradrenergic neurons in the brain, the number of serotonergic neurons is far greater. These neurons are located in several discrete nuclei along the midline of the brain stem, which are collectively referred to as the raphe nuclei. The dorsal raphe is located in the midbrain and is part of the ventral periaqueductal gray matter, and projections from this nucleus innervate the cerebral cortex, thalamus, striatum, the substantia nigra, and the ventral tegmental area. The median raphe is located ventral to the dorsal raphe along the midbrain and innervates the hippocampus, septum, and other limbic structures. The diffuse and overlapping projections of serotinergic neurons has led to the belief that they modulate virtually all neurons in the brain.

Neuroimaging studies reveal abnormal regional cerebral blood flow (CBF) and glucose metabolism in limbic and PFC structures in mood disorders, although some disagreement exists regarding the specific locations and the direction of these changes *(12)*. The most consistent findings are that CBF and metabolism are increased in the amygdala, orbital cortex, and medial thalamus, and decreased in the PFC and the anterior cingulate cortex of depressed patients relative to healthy control subjects. The overall pattern of these metabolic changes suggests that the structures mediating emotional and stress responses are pathologically activated in depression. During antidepressant drug treatment, some of these neurophysiological abnormalities are reversed in those patients that respond well to treatment.

6. NEUROTRANSMITTER SYSTEMS

The monoamine hypothesis of depression postulated that a functional deficiency of serotonin (5-HT) or norpeinephrine (NE) in the brain is key to the pathology and or behavioral manifestations associated with depression. Reduced levels of the 5-HT metabolite 5-hydroxyindole acetic acid (5-HIAA) in cerebrospinal fluid have been reported in patients with mood disorders and suicidal behavior *(13)*. In contrast, no consistent relationship between levels of the dopamine metabolite homovanillic acid (HVA) or the NE metabolite 3-methoxy-4-hydroxy-phenylglycol (MHPG) and affective disorders has been reported over studies. However, other studies reveal a complex pathology of the noradrenergic system in major depression, especially in the NE-containing cells of the locus ceruleus, and there is some evidence for dysfunctional dopaminergic and glutamatergic systems as well. Although the ultimate neurochemical mechanism underlying the therapeutic efficacy of antidepressant drugs is still under investigation and is likely to involve multiple brain regions and neurotransmitter systems, antidepressant drugs are known to produce acute increases in 5-HT and NE levels or signaling through a variety of mechanisms. This widespread release of NE and 5-HT allows for the activation of disparate biological systems regulating stress pathology, which are likely to account for the range of behavioral symptoms observed in depression, such as changes in affect, cognition, anxiety, food intake, sleep, and norendocrine secretion.

7. GENETICS OF DEPRESSION

As a result of the high degree of symptom variation and treatment response among patients with depression, it is likely that depression results from a variety of complex and interacting causes. As in the case of many psychiatric diseases, genetic factors may play a role in the vulnerability to depression. Unipolar depression carries a familial risk, as relatives of individuals diagnosed with depression have a significantly greater chance of developing depression (11–18%) than relatives of nondepressed controls (0.7–7%) *(14–16)*. Several twin studies have established high concordance rates for unipolar depression. These studies indicate that if one monozygotic twin is affected, the other has a 60 to 80% lifetime chance of developing the disorder. In contrast, if one dizygotic twin has major depression, the other has only an 8% chance of being affected *(17–19)*. Despite evidence for the heritability of depression, few genes have been convincingly identified in genetic association studies. For example, a polymorphism in the human serotonin transporter gene has been linked to unipolar depression *(20)*. In other studies, linkage analysis identified a region on chromosome 2 that exhibited significant evidence of linkage to mood disorders among women, but not men *(21)*. Cyclic AMP response element binding protein 1 (CREB1) lies within this region and sequence variation in its promoter and intron eight have been detected that cosegregate with unipolar depression and mood disorders in women *(22)*. As depression affects women twice as often as men, these data would seem to implicate CREB as a gender-specific susceptibility gene for unipolar depression. Part of the difficulty in identifying specific genes for unipolar depression is likely the result of the complex nature of this disease, which results from multiple and overlapping causes.

8. ANIMAL MODELS OF DEPRESSION

Animal models are essential for identifying potential neurobiological causes for depression and for developing improved treatments. A number of animal models of depression have been proposed, but the most widespread ones are those that screen for new antidepressant treatments. Their utility rests on their ability to predict which treatments will be efficacious or have low side-effect liability in humans. Another approach is to reproduce in laboratory animals particular symptoms of depression. Such models, which have face validity, are used to study the biological mechanisms underlying specific symptoms. The ideal model would reproduce etiological factors that cause depression resulting in a full range of symptoms. Such a model is said to have construct validity. Unfortunately, no such model for depression has been identified, because the core etiological factors that cause the illness are unknown and are likely to involve a mixture of environmental and genetic influences. The most commonly used predictive animal models of depression are discussed here.

8.1. Forced Swim and Tail Suspension Tests

The forced swim test, also known as the Porsolt test, is the most widely used animal model in depression research. It is not a true model of depression; rather it is used more as a screen for antidepressant treatments. It is based on a behavioral trait that has been shown to be sensitive to changes in affective state. The test involves placing a rat or mouse in a tank filled with water, and measuring the amount of time the animal is immobile when it stops struggling. Acute treatment or short-term treatment with most antidepressants increases the latency to immobility and decreases the amount of immobility time, and in most cases this occurs at drug doses that do not increase locomotor activity on their own. The interpretation is that antidepressants reinstate active coping mechanisms and decrease the passive immobility evoked by stress. Although false-positives in the test include drugs that are stimulants (and hence decrease immobility) rather than antidepressants, such false-positives can be detected with an additional locomotor activity test. A modified version of the test in rats measures other behaviors in the tank that enables more specific identification of antidepressants. For example, NE reuptake blockers increase climbing behavior, whereas selective serotonin reuptake blockers increase swimming.

A variant of the forced swim test used with mice is the tail suspension test. Here, mice are suspended by their tails and time until they become immobile is measured and acute administration of most antidepressants decreases immobility. A major advantage of the tail suspension test or forced swim test is that they are relatively easy to perform and amenable to high throughput. Most antidepressants decrease immobility after acute or short-term treatment making these tests good screens for novel antidepressant compounds. However, a problem for the validity of these tests is that antidepressant drugs must be administered for several weeks to achieve a maximal clinical effect in humans.

8.2. Chronic Stress-Induced Depression Models

Several tests based on exposure of animals to uncontrollable stress, have been utilized in rats. In the learned helplessness paradigm, animals that are first exposed to inescapable shock subsequently fail to escape from a situation in which escape is possible. The attraction of the learned helplessness model is that it is based on a plausible theory of depression that links exposure to uncontrollable stress to the cognitive, affective, and motoric deficits observed in major depression. Remarkably, animals that have developed learned helplessness show several changes that are reminiscent of depression, such as alterations in rapid eye movement sleep, reduced body weight, diminished sexual behavior, and altered secretion of stress hormones. Repeated treatment with antidepressants reduces the latency to escape and decreases the number of animals that display the learned helplessness behavior. However, because the exposure to stressors is extreme, it is unclear whether the learned helplessness model might be more appropriate for PTSD.

In the chronic mild stress paradigm, rodents are exposed to a variety of relatively mild stresses (e.g., isolation housing, disruption of light–dark cycles, brief food or water deprivation, tilting of home cages) intermittently for relatively prolonged periods of time (e.g., several weeks). The advantage of these tests is their face and construct validity, because they involve chronic exposure of rodents to more naturalistic stressors. Chronic mildly stressed animals also exhibit another core symptom of depression, anhedonia, as inferred from a reduction in sucrose drinking. This model is not as widely employed, however, as it is extremely difficult to replicate these abnormalities, and the palliative effects of antidepressants are difficult to demonstrate.

8.3. Selective Breeding

Selective breeding has been used to generate animals with larger differences in depression-like phenotypes. This approach is based on the realization that most rodent models of depression involve the use of normal, healthy individuals, whereas depression in most humans requires a genetic vulnerability that interacts in an exaggerated manner with environmental provocation. Rats and mice have been selectively breed for high or low levels of swimming activity in the forced swim test. Breeds with inherently low swimming activity show increased activity after antidepressant administration. Furthermore, continued breeding paradigms have led to the identification of quantitative trait loci or gene regions that are associated with differential performance. Such selectively breed animals may be valuable research tools for identifying homologous genetic components that underlie depression in humans.

9. ANTIDEPRESSANT TREATMENTS

9.1. Pharmacotherapies

Antidepressant drugs are the most common treatment for clinical depression, and they relieve symptoms in approx 60% of those who use them as prescribed *(23)*. Until the 1980s, tricyclic antidepressants (TCAs), which are named for their chemical structure, were the primary drug treatment for major depression. TCAs, including clomipramine and imipramine, act to increase NE and/or serotonin levels by blocking their reuptake through synaptic transporters. However, most of the early TCAs, like desipramine, function primarily as selective inhibitors of NE reuptake. Although effective in alleviating depressive episodes, treatment with TCAs is associated with significant toxicity and side effects owing to the high affinity these compounds have for adrenergic α_1 receptors, histamine H_1 receptors, and muscarinic receptors.

The second class of antidepressants developed has no structural similarities to the TCAs, but they also act at monoamine reuptake sites and are highly selective blockers of the serotonin transporter. These selective serotonin reuptake inhibitors (SSRIs) include escitalopram, citalopram, fluoxetine, paroxetine, and sertraline. These drugs act to increase 5-HT levels but they have low affinity for neurotransmitter G protein-coupled receptors. Additionally, metabolites of some of the antidepressants bind directly to serotonin receptors, which may contribute to their therapeutic effectiveness. For instance, trazodone has an active metabolite (meta-chlorophenylpeperazine [mCPP]), which is a serotonin receptor ligand. On the other hand, some metabolites can be problematic, particularly when switching patients from one antidepressant drug class to another. For example, norfluoxetine is an active metabolite of fluoxetine, which has an exceptionally long half-life of 4 to 16 days. Hence, the presence of this metabolite must be carefully monitored to avoid a "serotonin syndrome" when switching from fluoxetine to another antidepressant medication. Serotonin syndrome results from an overactivation of central 5-HT receptors and may manifest with features such as abdominal pain, diarrhea, sweating, fever, tachycardia increased blood pressure, and an altered mental state *(24)*.

Monoamine oxidase inhibitors (MAOIs) are a third class of effective antidepressants. These drugs have a different mechanism of action from both TCAs and SSRIs in that they bind irreversibly to the active site of MAO, which is an enzyme responsible for the degradation of both NE and serotonin. Although most MAOIs are not used because of toxicity, three are still prescribed: phenelzine, tranylcypromine,

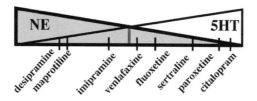

Fig. 1. Range of selectivity of some antidepressant drugs for inhibition of 5-HT and NE reuptake. Drugs such as desipramine and maprotiline have a greater selectivity for NE reuptake compared to drugs such as paroxetine and citalopram, which have a greater selectivity for 5-HT reuptake *(26,28)*.

and isocarboxazid. These drugs are often effective in those depressed patients that do not respond to the other classic pharmacotherapies mentioned above. Additionally, MAOIs are especially effective in treating atypical depression, which is depression with a greater expression of anxiety or agitation. One disadvantage of MAOIs is the need for dietary restrictions, in order to prevent a hypertensive crisis. However, recently developed reversible MAOIs, such as moclobemide, can be especially advantageous for patients because of a more favorable side-effect profile and the rapid elimination of effects after the drug is discontinued *(25)*.

More recent classifications are based on acute pharmacological effects of antidepressant drugs and their affinities for serotonin and NE transporters *(26–28)* (Fig. 1). New classes include selective norepinephrine reuptake inhibitors (NRIs), such as reboxetine and desipramine, and dual-action serotonin–norepinephrine reuptake inhibitors (SNRIs), such as venlafaxine and duloxetine. In a recent review of several clinical trials, the rates of response with SSRIs and NRIs were not significantly different, that is, 61.4 and 59.5%, respectively *(23)*. Although equally effective during the treatment phase, combining a SSRI with a NRI produces a greater protection from relapse *(29)*.

Although preclinical studies confirm that SSRIs increase extracellular levels of 5-HT, the maximal effects caused by the acute systemic administration of SSRIs are restricted to only a two- to fourfold increase *(30)*. This minimal level of increase is the result of a restraining effect exerted by the activation of 5-HT autoreceptors that inhibit neurotransmitter synthesis and release. Pharmacological blockade or genetic disruption of inhibitory somatodendritic 5-HT$_{1A}$ and terminal 5-HT$_{1B}$ autoreceptors, for example, augments the magnitude of 5-HT increase produced by acute administration of fluoxetine or paroxetine *(31)*.

Although all classes of antidepressants demonstrate varying degrees of clinical efficacy, the majority of patients do not respond to therapy for 2 to 4 weeks after the initiation of treatment. Chronic administration of SSRIs cause diminished responsiveness of 5-HT autoreceptors: somatodendritic 5-HT$_{1A}$ receptors or 5-HT$_{1B}$ autoreceptors located at nerve terminals *(32)*. Additionally, chronic administration of SSRIs causes a downregulation of serotonin transporters and a prolongation of 5-HT clearance in the CA3 region of the hippocampus *(33)*. These changes following chronic administration would help to further enhance 5-HT neurotransmission, which is important, because a persistently elevated synaptic level of 5-HT is required for the maintenance of antidepressant effects *(34)*.

9.2. Natural Product Treatments

Hypericum perforatum, commonly called St. Johns Wort, is used extensively in Europe to treat mild to moderate depression. Despite its widespread use, recent randomized, double-blind, placebo-controlled clinical studies indicate no significant antidepressant effect *(35)*.

9.3. Electroconvulsive Therapy

Electroconvulsive therapy (ECT) has been used as a treatment for mental disorders for the last half of the century. Although ECT can be highly effective for patients with severe depression, concerns regarding its safety and efficacy are prevalent. Briefly, the procedure involves pretreatment with a short-duration anesthetic, followed by medications to relax the muscles. Electrodes are placed on the patient's scalp and a current is passed through them, producing a seizure lasting 30 to 45 seconds. Generally, ECT treatments are applied two to three times a week. Following complete recovery or no further improvement, maintenance ECT is given periodically or antidepressant medication is administered, in order to prevent relapse. The most common side effects of ECT include headache and transient memory disturbances, which are dependent to some extent on details of the treatment (electrode placement, current, frequency) and patient status (age, history of brain injury, or brain disease). In a recent review of the literature, ECT was found to be significantly more effective than pharmacotherapy, as a short-term treatment for depression *(36)*.

9.4. Transcranial Magnetic Stimulation

Transcranial magnetic stimulation (TMS) is a noninvasive treatment that directly stimulates cortical neurons through electromagnetic induction. The procedure involves the discharge of a large current (up to 5000 amps) through a copper-wire coil. When the coil is held up to the head of a subject, the magnetic field produced penetrates the scalp and skull and induces a small current in the brain parallel to the plane of the coil. Once sufficient current has penetrated the brain (several mA/cm^2), depolarization of neuronal membranes occurs and action potentials can be generated *(37)*. TMS is becoming increasingly popular for a number of applications as a result of its ease of use and relatively few side effects. Although TMS is certainly less established than pharmacotherapy or ECT, some evidence for its effectiveness as an antidepressant has accumulated. Both low- and high-frequency TMS results in antidepressant effects greater than those of placebo.

9.5. Exercise

Strong correlations in animal and human studies have emerged suggesting an important role for exercise in mediating the therapeutic benefits of antidepressant treatment. In animal models, long-term physical activity has been shown to increase the expression of brain-derived neurotrophic factor (BDNF) and induce neurogenesis. The effects of exercise combined with antidepressant drugs are additive *(38)*. The therapeutic benefit of exercise also has been demonstrated in patients with major depression, with exercise alone eliciting similar changes in the Hamilton Rating Scale for Depression as sertraline therapy, or a combination of exercise and sertraline *(39)*. In a recent pilot study, patients who exercised at least 30 minutes a day for most days significantly decreased symptoms of depression in people already taking SSRIs or venlafaxine *(40)*. Although neurogenesis cannot be identified as a causal factor in these clinical studies, the evidence from animal studies suggests that the effects of exercise and antidepressant drugs can converge at the cellular level to potentially improve depression treatment.

10. MOLECULAR MEDIATORS OF ANTIDEPRESSANT ACTIVITY

The need for chronic treatment with antidepressant drugs has led to research efforts aimed at understanding the long-term molecular mechanisms that underlie depression and antidepressant treatments. The regulation of key signaling pathways downstream of the serotonin and norepinephrine receptors involved in gene transcription, as well as changes in cell proliferation and survival, have become a primary focus in depression research. Evidence associating depression, stress, and antidepressant action suggest that depression may result from an impairment of neuronal adaptations and/or disruption of neuronal plasticity. Antidepressant treatments are hypothesized to reverse dysfunctional neuronal adaptations that can occur in response to stress, which then contribute to depression. These neuronal adaptations, including neuronal activity, gene expression, and cell survival are under the control of intracellular signaling cascades. Long-term adaptations in these intracellular signal transduction cascades may underlie the efficacy of chronic antidepressant treatment (Fig. 2). Among the second messenger cascades that mediate the effects of antidepressant treatments is the cAMP pathway, which can be regulated by both serotonin and norepinephrine. Regulation of G proteins by antidepressants has been shown both at the level of enhanced coupling of Gsα to adenylyl cyclase and as increased adenylyl cyclase activity. cAMP elevation results in the activation of cAMP-dependent protein kinase (PKA) and PKA activity is reported to increase following chronic antidepressant administration *(41)*. Among the many substrates of PKA in the brain, is the family of cAMP-sensitive transcription factors, consisting of CREB (cAMP response element binding protein), and CREM (cAMP response element modulator protein). These proteins are related by their ability to bind a cAMP response element (CRE), which are present in the regulatory regions of most cAMP-responsive genes. CREB has been shown to be regulated by chronic, but not acute antidepressant treatment. Chronic administration of the selective serotonin reuptake inhibitor fluoxetine increases phosphorylated CREB levels in the mouse in several brain regions, including the amygdala, cortex, dentate gyrus,

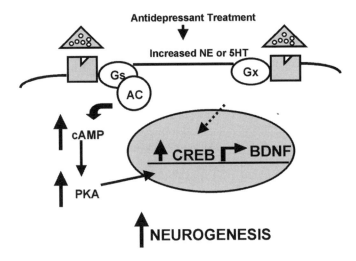

Fig. 2. Overview of the molecular mechanisms associated with antidepressant treatments. Current therapies lead to increases in synaptic 5-HT or NE, which activate postsynaptic receptors that then alter levels of intracellular cAMP or Ca^{++}. Antidepressant drugs have been shown to increase levels of CREB, BDNF, promote neurogenesis, and alter behaviors in animal models that predict antidepressant efficacy in humans.

and hypothalamus, although desipramine increases CREB phosphorylation only in the dentate gyrus *(42)*.

CREB is hypothesized to regulate the expression of BDNF, which is a peptide that is involved in neuronal plasticity and differentiation and that more recently has been implicated as a mediator of antidepressant action *(43)*. BDNF infusion into the midbrain of rats induces antidepressant-like behaviors in both the learned helplessness paradigm and the forced swimming test *(44)*. Furthermore, postmortem studies indicate increased levels of BDNF expression in the dentate gyrus, hilus and supragranular regions in depressed patients treated with antidepressant medications as compared with untreated subjects *(45)*.

Clinical and preclinical studies have focused on the interactions between stress and depression and their effects on the hippocampus *(46)*. Hippocampal volume is reduced in patients with stress-related psychiatric illnesses, such as clinical depression and PTSD. In animal models, physiological and psychosocial stress also induces hippocampal atrophy and cell loss.

The hippocampus is a unique brain region that supports the production of new neurons throughout life *(47)*. The birth of new neurons, or neurogenesis, is a dynamic process regulated by environmental, endocrine, and pharmacological stimuli. For example, stress suppresses hippocampal granule cell formation in mammals, and both acute and chronic stress paradigms decrease cell proliferation *(48)*. Together, these data suggest that the stress-induced hippocampal atrophy and concomitant reduction of hippocampal neurogenesis may be associated with the loss of hippocampal volume observed in depressed patients.

Recent studies have explored the potential for antidepressants to attenuate or even reverse the effects of stress on hippocampal cell proliferation. BDNF promotes neuronal differentiation and survival throughout development and into adulthood. Stress can downregulate BDNF expression in the hippocampus and this effect can be reversed by chronic antidepressant administration. Because the regulation of BDNF is hypothesized to mediate alterations in hippocampal neurogenesis *(49)* and chronic antidepressant treatment increases neurogenesis in the hippocampus *(50)*, antidepressants are hypothesized to oppose the dystrophic effects of stress through a BDNF-dependent mechanism.

GLOSSARY OF MEDICAL TERMINOLOGY

Anhedonia: The lack of enjoyment or interest in activities that were once pleasurable.

Construct validity: A criterion for evaluating animal models that examines whether animal models measure factors that could contribute to the etiology of a disease in humans.

Dysthymic depression: A neuropsychiatric illness similar to major depression, often with an onset beginning at an early age. The illness is often less severe than unipolar depression involving symptoms that do not disable, but are pervasive and keep individuals from functioning well or feeling good.

Face validity: A criterion for evaluating animal models that assesses whether responses measured in animals are similar to symptoms exhibited by patients.

Serotonin syndrome: An overactivation of central serotonin receptors resulting in abdominal pain, diarrhea, sweating, fever, tachycardia, hyptenison, and altered mood state. Risk of serotonin syndrome is increased when SSRIs are administered temporally with a second serotonin-enhancing agent (MAOI).

Unipolar depression: A neuropsychiatric illness manifested by a combination of symptoms that interfere with the ability to work, study, sleep, eat, and enjoy once pleasurable activities.

REFERENCES

1. Murray CJ, Lopez AD. Alternative projections of mortality and disability by cause 1990–2020: Global Burden of Disease Study. Lancet 1997;349:1498–1504.
2. Kessler RC, McGonagle KA, Zhao S, et al. Lifetime and 12-month prevalence of DSM-III-R psychiatric disorders in the United States. Results from the National Comorbidity Survey. Arch Gen Psychiatry 1994;51:8–19.
3. DSM-IV. Diagnostic and Statistical Manual of Mental Disorders. Fourth ed. Washington, DC: American Psychiatric Association; 2000.
4. Olsson GI, Nordstrom ML, Arinell H, von Knorring AL. Adolescent depression: social network and family climate—a case-control study. J Child Psychol Psychiatry 1999;40:227–237.
5. Kessler RC. The effects of stressful life events on depression. Annu Rev Psychol 1997;48: 191–214.
6. Sapolsky RM. Glucocorticoids and hippocampal atrophy in neuropsychiatric disorders. Arch Gen Psychiatry 2000;57:925–935.
7. Holsboer-Trachsler E, Hemmeter U, Hatzinger M, Seifritz E, Gerhard U, Hobi V. Sleep deprivation and bright light as potential augmenters of antidepressant drug treatment—neurobiological and psychometric assessment of course. J Psychiatr Res 1994;28:381–399.

8. Manji HK, Duman RS. Impairments of neuroplasticity and cellular resilience in severe mood disorders: implications for the development of novel therapeutics. Psychopharmacol Bull 2001;35:5–49.

9. Sheline YI, Wang PW, Gado MH, Csernansky JG, Vannier MW. Hippocampal atrophy in recurrent major depression. Proc Natl Acad Sci U S A 1996;93:3908–3913.

10. Czeh B, Michaelis T, Watanabe T, et al. Stress-induced changes in cerebral metabolites, hippocampal volume, and cell proliferation are prevented by antidepressant treatment with tianeptine. Proc Natl Acad Sci U S A 2001;98:12796–12801.

11. Sheline YI, Gado MH, Kraemer HC. Untreated depression and hippocampal volume loss. Am J Psychiatry 2003;160:1516–1518.

12. Davidson RJ. Anxiety and affective style: role of prefrontal cortex and amygdala. Biol Psychiatry 2002;51:68–80.

13. Placidi GP, Oquendo MA, Malone KM, Huang YY, Ellis SP, Mann JJ. Aggressivity, suicide attempts, and depression: relationship to cerebrospinal fluid monoamine metabolite levels. Biol Psychiatry 2001;50:783–791.

14. Gershon ES, Hamovit J, Guroff JJ, et al. A family study of schizoaffective, bipolar I, bipolar II, unipolar, and normal control probands. Arch Gen Psychiatry 1982;39:1157–1167.

15. Winokur G, Tsuang MT, Crowe RR. The Iowa 500: affective disorder in relatives of manic and depressed patients. Am J Psychiatry 1982;139:209–212.

16. Weissman MM, Gershon ES, Kidd KK, et al. Psychiatric disorders in the relatives of probands with affective disorders. The Yale University—National Institute of Mental Health Collaborative Study. Arch Gen Psychiatry 1984;41:13–21.

17. McGuffin P, Katz R, Watkins S, Rutherford J. A hospital-based twin register of the heritability of DSM-IV unipolar depression. Arch Gen Psychiatry 1996;53:129–136.

18. Allen MG, Cohen S, Pollin W, Greenspan SI. Affective illness in veteran twins: a diagnostic review. Am J Psychiatry 1974;131:1234–1239.

19. Bertelsen A, Harvald B, Hauge M. A Danish twin study of manic-depressive disorders. Br J Psychiatry 1977;130:330–351.

20. Ogilvie AD, Battersby S, Bubb VJ, et al. Polymorphism in serotonin transporter gene associated with susceptibility to major depression. Lancet 1996;347:731–733.

21. Zubenko GS, Hughes HB, 3rd, Maher BS, Stiffler JS, Zubenko WN, Marazita ML. Genetic linkage of region containing the CREB1 gene to depressive disorders in women from families with recurrent, early-onset, major depression. Am J Med Genet 2002;114:980–987.

22. Zubenko GS, Hughes HB, 3rd, Stiffler JS, et al. Sequence variations in CREB1 cosegregate with depressive disorders in women. Mol Psychiatry 2003;8:611–618.

23. Nelson JC. A review of the efficacy of serotonergic and noradrenergic reuptake inhibitors for treatment of major depression. Biol Psychiatry 1999;46:1301–1308.

24. Ener RA, Meglathery SB, Van Decker WA, Gallagher RM. Serotonin syndrome and other serotonergic disorders. Pain Med 2003;4:63–74.

25. Bonnet U. Moclobemide: evolution, pharmacodynamic, and pharmacokinetic properties. CNS Drug Rev 2002;8:283–308.

26. Owens MJ, Morgan WN, Plott SJ, Nemeroff CB. Neurotransmitter receptor and transporter binding profile of antidepressants and their metabolites. J Pharmacol Exp Ther 1997;283:1305–1322.

27. Sanchez C, Hyttel J. Comparison of the effects of antidepressants and their metabolites on reuptake of biogenic amines and on receptor binding. Cell Mol Neurobiol 1999;19:467–489.

28. Frazer A. Antidepressants. J Clin Psychiatry 1997;58 Suppl 6:9–25.

29. Nelson JC. Managing treatment-resistant major depression. J Clin Psychiatry 2003;64(Suppl 1):5–12.

30. Fuller R. Uptake inhibitor increase extracellular serotonin concentration measured by brain microdialysis. Life Science 1994;55:163–167.

31. Hjorth S, Bengtsson HJ, Kullberg A, Carlzon D, Peilot H, Auerbach SB. Serotonin autoreceptor function and antidepressant drug action. J Psychopharmacol 2000;14:177–185.

32. Blier P, de Montigny C. Current advances and trends in the treatment of depression. Trends Pharmacol Sci 1994;15:220–226.
33. Benmansour S, Owens WA, Cecchi M, Morilak DA, Frazer A. Serotonin clearance in vivo is altered to a greater extent by antidepressant-induced downregulation of the serotonin transporter than by acute blockade of this transporter. J Neurosci 2002;22:6766–6772.
34. Heninger GR, Delgado PL, Charney DS. The revised monoamine theory of depression: a modulatory role for monoamines, based on new findings from monoamine depletion experiments in humans. Pharmacopsychiatry 1996;29:2–11.
35. Shelton RC, Keller MB, Gelenberg A, et al. Effectiveness of St John's Wort in major depression: a randomized controlled trial. Jama 2001;285:1978–1986.
36. Group tUER. Efficacy and safety of electroconvulsive therapy in depressive disorders: a systematic review and meta-analysis. Lancet 2003;361:799–808.
37. Maeda F, Pascual-Leone A. Transcranial magnetic stimulation: studying motor neurophysiology of psychiatric disorders. Psychopharmacology (Berl) 2003;168:359–376.
38. Russo-Neustadt AA, Beard RC, Huang YM, Cotman CW. Physical activity and antidepressant treatment potentiate the expression of specific brain-derived neurotrophic factor transcripts in the rat hippocampus. Neuroscience 2000;101:305–312.
39. Babyak M, Blumenthal JA, Herman S, et al. Exercise treatment for major depression: maintenance of therapeutic benefit at 10 months. Psychosom Med 2000;62:633–638.
40. Trivedi MH, Greer TL, Grannemann BD, et al. Exercise as an augmenting treatment for major depressive disorder: a pilot study. In: Society for Neuroscience; 2003; Washington, D.C.; 2003.
41. Perez J, Tardito D, Mori S, Racagni G, Smeraldi E, Zanardi R. Abnormalities of cAMP signaling in affective disorders: implication for pathophysiology and treatment. Bipolar Disord 2000;2:27–36.
42. Thome J, Sakai N, Shin K, et al. cAMP response element-mediated gene transcription is upregulated by chronic antidepressant treatment. J Neurosci 2000;20:4030–4036.
43. Duman RS, Heninger GR, Nestler EJ. A molecular and cellular theory of depression. Arch Gen Psychiatry 1997;54:597–606.
44. Siuciak JA, Lewis DR, Wiegand SJ, Lindsay RM. Antidepressant-like effect of brain-derived neurotrophic factor (BDNF). Pharmacol Biochem Behav 1997;56:131–137.
45. Chen AC, Shirayama Y, Shin K, Neve RL, Duman RS. Expression of the cAMP response element binding protein (CREB) in hippocampus produces an antidepressant effect. Biol Psychiatry 2001;49:753–762.
46. McEwen BS. Protective and damaging effects of stress mediators: central role of the brain. Prog Brain Res 2000;122:25–34.
47. Eriksson PS, Perfilieva E, Bjork-Eriksson T, et al. Neurogenesis in the adult human hippocampus. Nat Med 1998;4:1313–1317.
48. Gould E, McEwen BS, Tanapat P, Galea LA, Fuchs E. Neurogenesis in the dentate gyrus of the adult tree shrew is regulated by psychosocial stress and NMDA receptor activation. J Neurosci 1997;17:2492–2498.
49. Duman RS, Malberg J, Nakagawa S, D'Sa C. Neuronal plasticity and survival in mood disorders. Biol Psychiatry 2000;48:732–739.
50. Malberg JE, Eisch AJ, Nestler EJ, Duman RS. Chronic antidepressant treatment increases neurogenesis in adult rat hippocampus. J Neurosci 2000;20:9104–10.

11

Bipolar Disorder

Leonardo Tondo, Matthew J. Albert, Alexia E. Koukopoulos, Christopher Baethge, and Ross J. Baldessarini

Summary

The 19th-century concept of manic-depressive illness was separated into the distinct syndromes of bipolar disorder (BPD) and recurrent major depression in the mid-20th century. BPD is an episodic illness characterized by acute depressive, manic, or mixed states of variable frequency, duration and severity, and often with psychotic features, with intervals of full or partial recovery. Modern diagnostic systems recognize three forms: *bipolar I* (mania and usually also depression), *bipolar II* (recurrent depression and hypomania), and *cyclothymia* (moderate, continuous mood swings). BPD is associated with variable dysfunction and excess mortality, with a 20-fold increased risk of suicide. Lifetime prevalence of type I BPD is approx 1.2%, but including type II, cyclothymia, juvenile variants, and proposed "bipolar spectrum" disorders yields total rates at least 5%. Heritability of risk for BPD is supported by family, twin, and some adoption studies, but specific genetic factors are not firmly identified. Biological investigations in BPD have documented disturbed biorhythms; knowledge of actions of mood-altering medicines has encouraged speculation about biochemical factors, and brain-imaging technologies are being applied intensively to seek structural or functional differences unique to patients with BPD. However, a BPD-specific pathophysiology has not been defined. Clinical care of patients with BPD is complex and challenging. Risks are associated with under- or overtreating with mood-altering agents. Treatment of bipolar depression remains particularly unsatisfactory. Overuse of antidepressants can induce mixed states, mania, or rapid-cycling, and the adverse sedative, neurological, and metabolic effects of some antipsychotic agents and anticonvulsants can be intolerable. Modern therapeutic management is based on *long-term* efforts to stabilize mood, optimize functioning and quality of life, and reduce risks of premature mortality with combinations of mood-stabilizing medicines and supportive psychosocial care.

Key Words: Anticonvulsants; antidepressants; antipsychotics; bipolar disorder; depression; disability; lithium; mania; manic-depressive illness; mortality; psychoeducation; psychosis; suicide.

From: *Current Clinical Neurology: Neurological and Psychiatric Disorders:
From Bench to Bedside*
Edited by: F. I. Tarazi and J. A. Schetz © Humana Press Inc., Totowa, NJ

1. INTRODUCTION

Bipolar disorder (BPD) or as it was called earlier, *manic-depressive illness,* is characterized by an episodic course of major changes in mood, thinking, and behavior of variable severity. Phases of the disorder range from depression, through dysphoric-agitated, *mixed states* of simultaneous depression and mania, to hypomania or mania, often with psychotic features *(1).* Three forms of the disorder are now recognized *(2): bipolar I* disorder with mania, and usually severe depression, *bipolar II* disorder with severe recurrent depression and hypomania, and *cyclothymia* with relatively moderate and more continuous mood swings. Introduction of modern psychopharmacological treatments since the 1950s has markedly improved short-term clinical care of acute mania and bipolar depression, and supportive and psychosocial treatments and long-term prophylactic treatment have substantially limited long-term morbidity in BPD *(1,2).*

Even with sustained treatment, intervals between acute episodes of BPD may still be characterized by at least mild and fluctuating symptoms and varying levels of dysfunction; prolonged and full recovery (euthymia) may not occur in some cases *(1,3,4).* The prominent and difficult-to-treat depressive component of the illness appears to limit or slow treatment response, and contributes importantly to disability and premature mortality. Early deaths occur not only with extraordinarily high rates of suicide, but also from excess mortality associated with cardiovascular, pulmonary, endocrine, and other medical disorders, many of which are probably worsened by the stress associated with BPD illness *(1,5,6).* Anxiety and dysphoric mood may worsen the course and prognosis and are also likely to contribute to high rates of comorbid abuse of alcohol and other substances by patients with BPD, with additional contributions to mortality owing to intoxication, accidents, and medical complications *(1).*

2. HISTORICAL BACKGROUND

Ancient physicians (Hippocrates 5th century BC) were familiar with states of depression (melancholia) and agitated exaltation (mania) and some also recognized their occurrence in the same persons at different times (Aretæus of Cappadocia, second century AD) *(7).* However, the modern concept of BPD did not evolve until the 19th and 20th centuries. Emil Kraepelin (1856–1926) distinguished "manic-depressive insanity" as a group of episodic mood disorders with a relatively benign prognosis from more chronic and primarily psychotic disorders, which he labeled *dementia præcox,* later termed *schizophrenia.* Clear separation of bipolar mood disorders from unipolar major depression did not occur until the mid-20th century. Broad international acceptance of lithium and chlorpromazine as innovative treatments for mania, effective medical treatments for major depression, and later use of lithium to prevent recurrences of mania and bipolar depression in the 1960s–1970s further helped to establish BPD as a relatively treatment-responsive form of severe mental illness *(3).*

Four issues were addressed to arrive at the modern conceptualization of BPD, and still remain under discussion: (a) distinguishing it from other forms of psychotic illness; (b) including or excluding predominantly depressive disorders; (c) clarifying the significance of mixed states, rapid-cycling, and residual symptoms in BPD; and (d) determining the significance of BPD in children and the elderly. Current scientific controversy centers around widening the BPD concept to a spectrum of bipolarity, to include a growing proportion of cases of depression with mild or brief forms of hypomania, recognizing pediatric and geriatric forms of BPD, shifting diagnosis toward BPD from some personality disorders, and generally increasing recognition of bipolarity in a growing proportion of the general population.

3. EPIDEMIOLOGY

3.1. Incidence, Prevalence, and Onset

Owing to the preceding definitional uncertainties and to ascertainment problems, the epidemiology in BPD is in flux, and reported rates remain tentative. Currently estimated international *incidence* of type I BPD is about 0.02% per year, with 1.2% lifetime prevalence *(1,8)*. These rates are at least twice higher with type II BPD cases included, and may be 5% or more of the general population if cyclothymia and other proposed "bipolar spectrum" disorders are added *(8,9)*. These higher rates than former estimates may reflect a real trend toward rising incidence of major affective illness in Western countries over the past century or simply reflect wider recognition of mood disorders. Unlike major depression, which is much more prevalent among women than men, the lifetime risk of BPD is probably only moderately greater in women who do have higher rates of type II BPD, somewhat more depression than mania, and more rapid-cycling *(10)*. Given that many BPD patients, especially type I, have psychotic features during acute episodes of mania, and sometimes in depression, BPD, and psychotic forms of major depression probably represent the most prevalent forms of idiopathic psychotic illness *(8)*. Salient findings in the epidemiology of BPD are summarized in Table 1.

The reported median age at onset of symptoms of BPD is about 20 years *(1,11)*. Many adults with BPD have had psychiatric symptoms before age 20, although it is unclear whether BPD or precursor states can be diagnosed reliably in juveniles, and particularly in young children *(11)*. Behavioral and mood changes in childhood are often considered to represent attentional, conduct, anxiety, or depressive disorders, and the diagnosis of BPD is often delayed until a more familiar, adult-like, symptomatic picture evolves, or until mania is induced by treatment with an antidepressant or stimulant for another presumed disorder. Prevalence of mania before adulthood has been reported to be as high as 1% in the United States, whereas in the United Kingdom childhood mania is very rarely diagnosed *(1,9,11,12)*, indicating that the diagnosis of BPD in juveniles remains to be clarified.

Table 1
Epidemiology of Bipolar Disorder

Annual incidence	
Bipolar I	0.02%
Lifetime prevalence	
Bipolar I	1.2%
Bipolar II	~2%
Cyclothymia	~2%
Juvenile	≤1%
Bipolar spectrum	~5%
Female/male risk ratio	
Bipolar I	~1.3
Bipolar II	≥1.5
Rapid cycling	
Women	15–25%
Men	10–15%
Median onset age (years)	20 (with skewing toward 30–50)
Recurrence risk	
Recurrences after first mania	~90%
More than 10 lifetime recurrences	10–15%
Recurrence rate, untreated	~1 per year
Recurrence rate, treated	~1/1–2 years (briefer, milder)
Risk or concordance rates	
First-degree relatives	10–20%
Dizygotic twin	20%
Monozygotic twin	40–70%
Episode duration (untreated vs treated)	
Mania	4–12 vs 2–4 months
Mixed	similar to mania
Depressive	6–9 vs 2–4 months
Morbidity (% of time with modern treatment)	
Mania/hypomania	5–15%
Depression/dysthymia	25–35%
Major dysfunction	30–40%
Psychiatric comorbidity	10–30%
(panic, obsessive-compulsive disorder)	
Substance use comorbidity	30–60%
Suicide	
Among causes of death	6–18%
Annual suicide rate	0.3%
Annual attempt rate	~1.5%
Attempt/suicide ratio	~5 (15–20 in general population)
Lifetime attempt risk	20–40%

3.2. Mortality

Mortality rates are greatly elevated with BPD. They are at least three times higher than in other patients with general medical disorders, and BPD patients experience increased mortality from accidents associated with intoxication, dangerous driving, and other risk-taking behaviors, as well as medical complications of highly prevalent, comorbid substance use disorders *(5,6)*. However, by far, the greatest increase of mortal risk results from suicide, rates of which are higher than in other psychiatric disorders, including major depression, particularly when milder cases of depression that do not involve psychiatric hospitalization are considered (Table 1).

Estimated rates of *completed suicide* in patients with BPD average about 0.3% per year, untreated, or more than 20 times above those in the general population (approx 0.015% per year). Suicide accounts for 6 to 18% of causes of death among BPD patients, and this disorder is associated with more than half of *all* suicides *(1,5)*. Suicide *attempts* occur in 20 to 40% of patients with BPD *(1,5)*. Moreover, their potential lethality of intent or means appears to be much greater than in the general population because the ratio of attempts/suicides is only about 5 to 1 among patients with BPD, compared to estimates of 15 or 20 to 1 in the general population *(5)*.

The depressive phase of a BPD carries the highest suicide risk and accounts for about 75% of all attempts and fatalities in the disorder; most of the remaining risk is accounted for by mixed states of dysphoric agitation *(5)*. Other specific risk factors include previous attempts, frequent and severe previous bipolar depressive episodes, early onset of illness and older current age, a family history of suicidal behavior, and co-occurring substance abuse *(5)*. Women as well as men with BPD are at high risk for suicide, whereas the risk is much higher for men in the general population *(1)*. Suicidal risk arises early in the illness, often before BPD is diagnosed, and typically long before adequate long-term treatment is established.

4. BIOLOGY

4.1. Genetics

Genetic factors in the transmission of BPD are supported by family, twin, and some adoption studies *(9,13)*. Risks of BPD itself, or of depression, psychosis or suicide in first-degree relatives of index cases of BPD have ranged from 10% to as high as 60%, but typically are 10 to 20%. Rates in dizygotic (DZ) twins (like other siblings) also have been in the range of 10 to 20%, compared to 40 to 70% in monozygotic (MZ; identical) twins, to provide MZ/DZ concordance ratios of 3 or 4 to 1 that further support a genetic transmission hypothesis *(13)*. Rare adoption studies in BPD have found more affective illness and suicides, but not necessarily more BPD, in biological relatives than in adopting families *(13)*. In addition to contributing to risk of BPD, genetic factors are also strongly implicated in suicidal behavior, possibly independent of mood disorders *per se (14)*.

Attempts to define molecular genetic linkages to BPD or to associate specific candidate genes (such as those for enzymes, transporter proteins, or receptors essential to the cerebral metabolism of monoamine neurotransmitters) with the disorder have not yet led to consistently replicated findings. Neither a specific mode of inheritance nor a discrete genetic marker for BPD has yet to be firmly identified *(15)*. Even within the same pedigrees, linkage may occur on different chromosomes *(16,17)*. Such findings are consistent with the emerging view of that BPD, particularly when broadly diagnosed, is a complex condition involving multifactorial inherited risk factors with interactions among genetic factors and their modified expression by environmental influences.

4.2. Neurochemistry

Biochemical or metabolic abnormalities associated with BPD, specifically, and likely to have a pathophysiological or etiological role remain to be elucidated. Based on current neuroscientific understanding of characteristic emotional and autonomic manifestations of BPD, brain regions and mechanisms of obvious interest for a pathophysiology of the disorder include limbic, striatal, and frontal cerebral cortical neuronal circuits and their neurotransmitter and receptor-effector mechanisms. Indeed, the interacting cerebral catecholaminergic, serotonergic, and cholinergic systems of limbic forebrain have been studied for four decades in search of candidate abnormalities. These systems are strongly implicated in functions that are characteristically disturbed in BPD patients (motility and sleep–wake rhythms, sexual activity, appetite, emotions, and systemic responses of stress-hormone systems, including corticosteroids). Some of these biological manifestations of BPD (endophenotypes), such as altered circadian rhythms, may be more tractable targets for genetic studies than the range of clinical conditions currently diagnosed as BPD *(18)*. Interest in the biology of these systems also has been given strong indirect encouragement by partial knowledge of the action mechanisms of antimanic, antidepressant, and mood-stabilizing drugs that are clinically effective in managing symptoms of BPD, as a route to pathophysiology *(3,19)*. Pharmacocentric speculations arising in this process include proposals that mania may involve excessive dopaminergic functioning because most antipsychotic-antimanic agents block dopamine (DA) receptors and lithium can inhibit release of DA from nerve terminals, and that bipolar depression may reflect a functional deficiency of norepinephrine or serotonin because most effective antidepressants enhance these functions *(3)*.

Indeed, changes in the metabolism of monoamines based on assays of body fluids, are found, and are often qualitatively opposite, in bipolar depression and mania, whereas stress-hormone responses occur in both states *(19,20)*. Many of these findings are likely to represent coincidental molecular manifestations of profound excitement and overactivity in mania or of being psychomotorically, and probably metabolically, inhibited in bipolar depressive states, or to represent nonspecific stress responses *(19)*. Moreover, many molecular measurements pertaining to neurotransmitters or neurohormones are nonspecific by diagnosis. In short, none of these pharmacocentric hypotheses has led to a compelling pathophysiological theory that is specific to BPD. This circumstance is hardly surprising because most psychotropic drugs are not specific to particular diagnoses, and moreover, because actions of drugs are typically remote from pathophysiological or etiological factors in most disorders *(3,19)*.

A recent trend in this kind of research is to focus on the molecular and cellular physiology of neurotransmitter and neurohormone systems for additional leads, if not to pathophysiology, at least to innovative targets for development of novel treatments for BPD patients *(21,22)*. This strategy has proved quite successful in defining apparently shared mechanisms of action of dissimilar antimanic or mood-stabilizing agents, particularly lithium and valproic acid, with a greatly expanded understanding of the actions of these agents. Such insights include evidence that lithium, and often valproate as well, can alter the functioning of a growing number of critical and ubiquitous intercellular signaling pathways. These include: (a) changes in the GTP-associated (G) proteins that regulate receptor functions; (b) decreasing the activity of protein kinase C (PKC) and reducing levels of second messengers diacyl glycerol (DAG) and inositol 1,4,5-trisphosphate (IP_3) in pathways that mediate the functions of receptors for neurotransmitters and neurohormones; (c) decreasing the abundance of myrisoylated, alanine-rich C-kinase substrate (MARCKS), the major protein substrate for PKC; (d) activating *ras*-mitogen-activated protein (MAP) kinase signaling processes; (e) increasing the abundance of the cyclic-AMP (3',5'-*cyclic*-adenosine-monophosphate) response element binding protein (CREB) and cell-protective factors such as the antiapoptotic oncoprotein *bcl-2* and brain-derived neurotrophic factor (BDNF); (f) inhibiting glycogen synthase kinase-3 (CSK-3); and (g) promoting the accumulation of β-catenin, which has anti-apoptotic, cell-sparing, effects.

In addition to stimulating searches for novel mood-stabilizing agents *(21,22)*, such findings have renewed exploration of biological differences of BPD patients and their responses to mood-stabilizing treatments. Interesting findings include: (a) suggestive evidence for altered distribution of calcium and other cations in cells, (b) possibly increased expression of $G\alpha_s$ proteins, (c) subtle changes in PKC, and (d) emerging evidence for possible neuroprotective effects of long-term treatment with lithium and perhaps also valproate.

Finally, some of the findings arising from the preceding molecular neuro-pharmacodynamics of mood-stabilizing agents might lead to plausible laboratory models that may predict novel treatments. To date, however, efforts to model the cyclic nature of BPD in the behavioral responses of animals subjected to various drug treatments or brain lesioning or stimulation have not proved useful in providing correlations or predictions of clinically effective treatments.

4.3. Biological Rhythms

The episodic or cyclic nature of BPD and the tendency to shift from manic-excited to depressive-withdrawn states of mood and behavior have encouraged interest in physiological rhythms. Many cases of BPD, and especially type II, show seasonal mood shifts, sometimes with striking regularity. Typically such seasonal affective disorders involve fall-winter depression and spring-summer mania, but in some patients, the opposite pattern is found. The tendency toward major shifts in mood, energy, and behavior approximately every 6 months is considered a *hemicircannual* rhythm, and may be a fundamental feature of the psychobiology of BPD *(23)*.

Additionally, shorter biological rhythms may be altered in BPD patients. Daily or *circadian* rhythms of motor activity, temperature, and cortisol secretion tend to show a peak (acrophase) earlier in the day (phase-advanced) in patients with BPD *(24)*. Alterations in shorter *(ultradian)* rhythms include earlier onset of rapid eye-movement (REM) sleep associated with dreaming in both depression and mania *(24)*. Some of these changes are illness-related and tend to normalize during periods of relative euthymia (so-called "state" rather than "trait" indicators), and their specificity to BPD or indication of a primary central pathophysiology is far from clear.

4.4. Brain Imaging

Modern computed brain-imaging technologies, including structural, functional, and chemical magnetic resonance imaging (MRI), positron emission tomography (PET), and single-photon emission computed tomography (SPECT) are being applied intensively to compare patients with BPD and other human subjects. Structural changes include increases in the volume of the fluid-filled cerebral ventricles, minor changes in estimated volume or relative abundance of gray and white matter in specific brain regions, and functional characteristics include changes in local cerebral blood flow or glucose utilization rates. Some changes appear to correlate with specific neuropsychological defects in patients with BPD; others are diagnostically nonspecific, inconsistent, or poorly replicated *(25)*. Neurochemical studies based on magnetic resonance spectroscopy (MRS) suggest altered cerebral levels of an important neuronal metabolite, *N*-acetyl-aspartate, and of membrane phospholipids in specific forebrain regions *(25)*.

5. CLINICAL FEATURES

5.1. Acute Illness

Clinical features of BPD are summarized in Table 2.

5.1.1. Mania

Episodes of *mania* are the hallmark of bipolar I disorder *(1,2)*. They are characterized by profound changes in emotions, cognition, and motor activity. Typically, mood is elevated or irritable, but highly characteristic of severe mania are rapid shifts in mood (lability) from extreme excitement and grandiosity, through irritability or anger, to profound dejection or tearfulness, that may suggest a mixed manic-depressive state. Activity can be markedly increased and, untreated, may lead to exhaustion. The need for sleep is decreased, and sex drive increased. Speech is rapid and pressured and the content of thinking usually is marked by excessive and unrealistic optimism, grandiose expansiveness, and may turn to excited but dysphoric and paranoid preoccupations. Cognitive disturbances include rapid, over-productive thinking, with rapid shifts in topics that can be hard to follow ("flight-

Table 2
Typical Symptoms of Manic and Depressive Episodes

	Mania	Depression
Mood	Elevated, intolerant, easily irritable	Depressed, anhedonic, "dead" or exquisite suffering, anxiety
Drive	Hyperactive	Decreased, lack of interest
Thinking		
Form	Pressured speech, overtalkativeness, associative thinking, clang associations Flight-of-ideas	Slowed, often quiet, impaired attention and memory
Content	Ideas of power and grandiosity (sometimes delusional)	Ideas of guilt, illness, financial distress, nihilism (sometimes delusional)
Perception	Hallucinations when severe	Hallucinations uncommon
Sleep	Decreased need (not tired)	Early or slow awakening, hypersomnia
Sexuality	Increased interest or activity	Decreased libido, lack of arousal
Appetite	Lack of interest	Variable: anorexia with weight loss or overeating with carbohydrate craving
Vigor	Inexhaustible to latter collapse	Somatic complaints (aches, gastrointestinal, fatigue)
Psychomotor activity	Acceleration	Retardation
Behavior	Disinhibition, risk-taking, spending	Withdrawal, decreased social contacts isolation
Suicidality	Rare unless mixed-dysphoric (reckless accidents)	Suicidal thoughts common, high risk of attempts and deaths

of-ideas") or appear only semi-logical (with "clang associations"), and a tendency to easy distractibility. The patient is poorly able to modulate speech, behavior, or interactions with others, with a low tolerance to frustration, and irritability or anger, particularly if facing opposition or restricted freedom.

Severe acute mania can include prominent, and diagnostically nonspecific, *psychotic features* that can include grandiose, religious, persecutory-paranoid, or sexual delusions, and even hallucinations. Behavior can be extremely disinhibited, intrusive, impulsive, or reckless, and sometimes dangerously aggressive. Risk-taking is common, and may include impulsive and unrealistic plans or business initiatives, reckless driving, excessive spending, imprudent sexual activity, and substance abuse. Judgment and self-appraisal are severely impaired, so that manic patients often require protective interventions.

Hypomania can arise in both type I and II BPD *(1)* and usually presents with features that are similar, but less intense than in mania and with lesser degrees of social and occupational impairment. Hypomania typically is not recognized as abnormal by the patient during or after an episode, and discussion with a relative or friend may be required to verify the occurrence of such episodes. Even milder upswings of mood and energy occur in *cyclothymia*, which involves more or less continuous cycling between mild depression and mild hyperthymia or euphoria *(1,2)*. Sustained high energy, with elevated mood or excessive emotionality can be considered a "hyperthymic" temperament or personality type, sometimes with striking social and occupational success and accomplishment.

5.1.2. Bipolar Depression

The depressive phase in BPD shares clinical features with major depressive disorder, and indeed, recurring severe forms of depression (melancholia) were originally included by Kraepelin in his broad concept of manic-depressive insanity *(1,7)*. Bipolar depression presents with depressed mood, sometimes characterized as emotional emptiness or "deadness" rather than sadness. Nevertheless, suffering can be extreme, with despair and suicidal ideation or behavior. Some patients may be quite irritable or agitated, and may raise the diagnostic question of a mixed state.

Vegetative signs and symptoms include characteristic psychomotor retardation, with a profound lack of energy, interest or pleasure, lassitude, and decreased sexual drive. Appetite can be decreased or increased (sometimes with carbohydrate-craving) with consequent weight variations. Sleep disturbances are routine, and can include insomnia or hypersomnia. Lethargy and anergy can be either sustained or more profound early in the day. Thinking is slow, attention and memory impaired, reaction times prolonged, problem solving strategies limited, and feelings of guilt, worthlessness, self-blame, despair, hopelessness may be present. Self-esteem is low with unrealistic, negative, and pessimistic self-assessments.

Somatic complaints such as headaches, muscular aches, gastrointestinal, respiratory, cardiac, and other vegetative symptoms, may be present and even more prominent than psychic symptoms, and may consume the patient's attention or seem psychotic in their exaggeration or irrational interpretation. Psychotic features may include extreme pessimism to the level of nihilism, with gross exaggerations of social isolation, financial failure, self-blame, and guilt. Persecutory preoccupations and delusions may stem from the idea of receiving a just punishment. Perceptual disturbances and hallucinations occur infrequently, with content similar to the delusional thoughts. Bipolar depression can severely impair social, interpersonal, and occupational functioning, as well as judgment, and can be lethal.

In addition to full episodes of major depression, depressed mood in BPD can include a relatively high proportion of time in *subsyndromal* or *dysthymic* states, and milder depressive phases are characteristic of cyclothymia.

5.1.3. Mixed States

Depressive and manic symptoms occurring at the same time or in rapid alternation or transition between manic and bipolar depressive states are considered a "mixed" manic-depressive episode *(2)*. Classic descriptions of such complex mood states were provided by German authors in the 1890s and may have encouraged Kraepelin's shift toward a more broadly inclusive manic-depressive concept. Common forms of mixed states are dysphoric mania and agitated depression *(26–28)*. Both states include prominent depression or dysphoric feelings along with agitation, irritability, and anger, with variable inclusion of crowded or rapid thoughts. Bipolar mixed states probably are often misdiagnosed and considered a form of depression, with the risk of potentially dangerous worsening if standard antidepressant treatment is pursued.

5.1.4. Juvenile and Geriatric Bipolar Disorder

Pediatric forms of BPD, particularly in preadolescent children, can be difficult to diagnose because they often lack features considered typical of more familiar adult forms of the condition *(11)*. Pediatric BPD usually is less clearly episodic and more rapidly or continuously cycling, with prominent dysphoric irritability and outbursts of angry, aggressive, and potentially destructive behavior that differ from ordinary tantrums in their intensity and duration. Psychotic features may be associated, and anxiety and insomnia are common features. BPD-like conditions in children were described a century ago, but until recently had been largely ignored or ascribed to other psychiatric disorders of childhood, including attentional and behavioral disorders as well as depressive or anxiety syndromes *(1,29,30)*.

A small proportion of cases of BPD begin in later life. Such syndromes may be associated with early phases of degenerative brain diseases, tend to follow an unstable or chronic course, respond relatively poorly to treatment, and often end in early death, probably by worsening the course of commonly comorbid general medical disorders of older ages *(29,31,32)*.

5.2. Diagnosis

The diagnosis of adult BPD is made when one or more major depressive episodes are preceded or followed by one or more manic or hypomanic episodes *(1,2)*. Differential diagnoses include other mood disorders and other psychotic illnesses, particularly acute forms of psychosis. Formerly, psychotic forms of BPD were commonly misdiagnosed as schizophrenia. It is important to recognize that BPD is a syndrome and not necessarily a disease. As such, it can emerge in response to treatment with certain mood-elevating agents including psychostimulants or corticosteroids, as well as infectious, inflammatory, metabolic, traumatic, and degenerative brain diseases. In the pre-antibiotic era, mania as a manifestation of tertiary syphilis of the brain ("general paresis of the insane") was very common. The extent to which specific individual proclivities or vulnerabilities are also required in such apparently "secondary" forms of mania or BPD remains unclear *(32)*.

Type II BPD is easily misdiagnosed as a nonbipolar form of depression. Diagnosis can be improved by seeking evidence from a family member or friend of hypomania not recognized as such by the patient. Several depressive episodes may occur before hypomania emerges, but late diagnoses of bipolarity are rare after three or more depressive episodes *(1)*. Personality disorders with prominent emotional instability and hyper-reactivity to minor stressors can be confused with BPD, which instead requires discrete and sustained episodes of mania or depression.

5.3. Comorbidity

Patients with BPD often show features of, or may meet diagnostic criteria for, other psychiatric syndromes, especially anxiety disorders such as panic with or without agoraphobia, and obsessive-compulsive disorders *(1,2,31)*. Many children with possible BPD may also meet criteria for a diagnosis of attention deficit hyperactivity disorder (ADHD), although BPD is uncommon among children with ADHD *(29)* (*see also* Chapter 6). Co-occurrence with substance use disorders is found in 40 to 60% of patients with BPD who have been ill for several years. There are cultural and regional differences in choices of specific substances, but alcohol and stimulants are often encountered *(1,31)*. Substance-use comorbidity is also a major contributor to risk of suicide in patients with BPD *(5)*. Among somatic disorders, patients with BPD have an excess risk of migraine syndrome and may have an increased risk of insulin-independent diabetes mellitus *(33,34)*. Complex clinical presentations of comorbidly ill patients with BPD can complicate diagnosis and challenge the planning of comprehensive and well-tolerated treatments.

6. ILLNESS COURSE

6.1. Episode Frequency

BPD may not be easily recognized very early in its development, with an average delay of several years to appropriate diagnosis and treatment. There is an approximately equal probability of manic or depressive first episodes, with some sex bias toward early and more frequent depressive episodes, and of the mainly depressive type II syndrome, in women *(1)*. In some patients with BPD, the diagnosis arises with an initial hypomanic or manic episode soon after starting treatment with an antidepressant for depression or anxiety symptoms, or a stimulant for an attention disorder *(3)*. Women with BPD are at high risk for depressive, manic, or psychotic episodes in the early postpartum period, when their first episode of illness may occur *(35)*.

Single episodes of mania, or recurrences of mania-only are very unusual. By definition, bipolar depression requires at least two lifetime episodes of illness (at least one depression and a mania or hypomania). Recurrent episodes are to be expected and, in most patients, an episode of mania is either preceded or followed by an episode of depression within several months. Shifts between mood states can be gradual or rapid (the "switch process"). Type I BPD, and especially type II and juvenile cases, can follow a *rapid-cycling* course (no less than four episodes within 12 months) that continues for varying periods.

Untreated episodes of mania average about 6 to 9 months in duration, and depressive episodes are somewhat longer. Treated episodes are shorter, although full symptomatic recovery may still require 2 to 3 months for mania and 3 to 4 months for depression *(4)*. Curiously, average recurrence rates of illness episodes in untreated BPD are not much higher than in large samples of patients maintained on mood-stabilizing treatments, and major benefits of long-term mood-stabilizing treatment are in limiting the severity and duration of episodes *(1,36)*.

Kraepelin initially reported a tendency for progressive shortening of periods of relative wellness between recurrences of BPD episodes. This tendency toward cycle-acceleration or a worsening course has been compared to the "kindling" phenomenon in animal models of experimental epilepsy, and has been supported by the efficacy of anticonvulsant treatments *(24)*. However, the finding of a progressive course in BPD has not been replicated consistently, probably occurs in a minority of cases, and can arise from a sampling artifact unless patients are matched for episode counts or analyzed for within-subject trends *(37)*. In general, the course of BPD is highly variable and largely unpredictable within and between patients.

Overall, patients with bipolar I disorder spend much more time in depressive and subsyndromal dysthymic states than in mania, and in bipolar II syndrome, depression is the predominant, clinically relevant polarity *(1,2)*. Major and minor depression accounts for about one-third of days during follow-up of patients with bipolar I disorder, both early and later in the illness course, despite ongoing, clinically determined treatment, and patients with bipolar II disorder spend an even higher proportion of time in depressive-dysthymic states *(36,38)*. In contrast, mania or hypomania typically accounts for less than 10% of days during long-term treatment of patients with bipolar I disorder.

Even with modern treatment, highly unfavorable long-term outcomes, with more-or-less chronic illness or highly unstable mood and substantial disability, occur in a minority of patients with BPD, particularly of type I *(1,4)*. A very small proportion of patients with BPD, at late stages of the illness, may present sustained psychotic features, cognitive impairment, and severe disability. Without knowledge of their earlier clinical history, a cross-sectional assessment might suggest a diagnosis of a schizoaffective disorder in such cases. As noted above, unfavorable outcomes and premature mortality also are common among geriatric-onset cases of BPD *(29,32)*.

7. CLINICAL MANAGEMENT

7.1. General Considerations

Clinical care of patients with BPD is a complex and challenging undertaking, with risks associated with under- and overtreating. Overuse of antidepressants can induce mixed states, mania, or rapid-cycling, and the adverse sedative, neurological, and metabolic effects of some antipsychotic agents can be intolerable. Pharmacological management has moved beyond relatively short-term interventions into acute episodes with lithium or neuroleptic drugs for mania or antidepressants for depression, usually during hospitalization. Modern treatment is based on *long-term*, prophylactic efforts at stabilizing mood and optimizing functioning and quality of life, as well as improving longevity in this typically complex and lifelong illness.

Treatment programs increasingly include psychosocial interventions and rehabilitation efforts as well as medication, and many patients with BPD can be managed on an ambulatory basis most of the time. Optimal use of the broadening array of pharmacological treatment options requires detailed knowledge of the illness, treatment-response history of individual patients, and a long-term therapeutic collaboration among patient, family, and one or more experienced clinicians working in minimally restrictive settings.

Manic, psychotic, and suicidally despondent patients with BPD may require protection from excessively stimulating environments, impulsive and potentially self-damaging actions or unwise decisions, and risks of being taken advantage of sexually or financially. Required interventions can also include voluntary or court-ordered hospitalization, or guardianship for very uncooperative and dangerously disturbed patients. Impaired judgment and lack of insight into having a major mental illness is a very common accompaniment of BPD that can limit cooperation and acceptance of treatment. This pattern is especially common among young patients early in their experience with the illness. Moreover, judgment and cooperation tend to decline with re-emerging symptoms, often leading to treatment discontinuation with rapid worsening of illness, further impairment of self-care, and risk of accidents or suicide.

Patients and their families can benefit from education about the illness and its treatment, its potential personal impact, and effects on work, finances, and the family *(39)*. Specific genetic counseling regarding risks to offspring can be offered, and advice provided about the major risks of an unplanned pregnancy or of continuing or discontinuing treatment during pregnancy *(35)*. Close clinical monitoring is required to optimize medical treatment and its potential adverse effects under changing conditions over time, as well as to detect early signs of impending mood changes. Such comprehensive programs of care are important to achieve optimal outcomes in the clinical management of this complex illness.

7.2. Medical Treatment

7.2.1. Short-Term Treatment

Treatment of acute episodes of mania in BPD typically relies on rapidly acting antimanic and sedating agents that can be administered vigorously and rapidly *(3)*. Accordingly, treatment usually involves use of either an antimanic-antipsychotic agent or an antimanic-anticonvulsant, typically supplemented briefly with sedating doses of a potent benzodiazepine such as lorazepam or clonazepam. Virtually all antipsychotic drugs are highly effectively antimanic, although only chlorpromazine, olanzapine, quetiapine and risperidone currently are approved by the US Food and Drug Administration (FDA) specifically for mania, although others may follow (Table 3). Among anticonvulsants, use of loading doses of valproate (10–20 mg/kg body weight in the first 24 hours) is a powerful, rapidly effective, and well-tolerated antimanic treatment *(40)*. Lithium is effective and FDA-approved for mania, but is slower acting and can be toxic if dosed aggressively.

Table 3
Treatments for Bipolar Disorder

Agents (generic and trade names)	Clinical applications
FDA-approved applications	
Antipsychotics	
Chlorpromzaine (Thorazine® and others)	Antimanic
Olanzapine (Zyprexa®)	Antimanic, may be mood-stabilizing
Risperidone (Risperdal®)	Antimanic
Anticonvulsants	
Divalproex (Depakote®)	Antimanic, probably mood-stabilizing
Lamotrigine (Lamictal®)	Mood-stabilizing (depression > mania)
Mood-stabilizer	
Lithium carbonate or citrate	Antimanic, mood-stabilizing
Antidepressants	
Tricyclics	Variable efficacy, high switch risk, antipanic
Monoamine oxidase inhibitors	Relatively effective, switch risk, antipanic
Serotonin reuptake inhibitors	Low doses tolerated, variable efficacy, anxiolytic, switch risk
Bupropion (Wellbutrin® and others)	Low doses tolerated, variable efficacy, switch risk
Benzodiazepines	Sedative, anxiolytic
Off-label indications	
Other antipsychotics	Antimanic
Anticonvulsants:	
Carbamazepine (Tegretol® and others)	Antimanic, mood-stabilizing
Gabapentin (Neurontin®)	Weakly antimanic, anxiolytic-sedative
Oxcarbazepine (Trileptal®)	Inadequately tested; relatively well tolerated
Topiramate (Topamax®)	Antimanic?; weight control
Zonisamide (Zonegran®)	Inadequately tested; weight control
Benzodiazepines (potent)	Antimanic, sedative, anxiolytic

The optimal treatment of acute bipolar depression remains much less well studied than in other forms of major affective illness. Trials of modern antidepressants have systematically excluded bipolar, psychotic, suicidal, or substance use-comorbid subjects, leaving major gaps in research-based treatment options. Traditionally, antidepressants have been used freely, even though their safely and efficacy for the short- or long-term treatment of bipolar depression remains largely unproved and increasingly in doubt *(3,41)*. Modern practice is shifting toward reliance on mood-stabilizing agents even for acute bipolar depression, and particularly when new episodes emerge despite ongoing treatment. If a mood-stabilizing treatment is unable to prevent new depression, treatment options include addition of a second mood-stabilizer, or temporary and cautious addition of an antidepressant in moderate doses. Plausible choices include lithium if not already in place and lamotrigine, recently FDA-approved for long-term treatment in BPD, with research support for efficacy in bipolar depression and little risk of inducing mania. Electroconvulsive treatment (ECT) is also a powerful option for manic and severe mixed states, and especially for psychotic and acutely suicidal forms of bipolar depression, with limited risk of inducing mania *(1)*.

7.2.2. Long-Term Treatment

The greatest therapeutic challenge in the care of BPD patients is to minimize the frequency, severity, and duration of recurrences of mania and depression over many years. Treatments with evidence of ability to limit long-term morbidity in BPD include lithium, several anticonvulsants, and some modern antipsychotic drugs *(3)*. As noted above, the symptoms in many patients with BPD are not fully controlled with any individual long-term treatment option. Accordingly, modern practice has tended toward use of more than one mood-stabilizing agent at once, sometimes with intermittent supplementation with an antipsychotic, anxiolytic-sedative, or antidepressant agent, as required by changing symptoms. These complex practices, although plausible, remain almost entirely empirical, and systematic research to support them is needed.

The decision to undertake indefinitely prolonged prophylactic treatment with medicines that carry substantial burdens of adverse effects, subjective discomfort, inconvenience, and rising acquisition costs is never a simple one. Current practice usually includes continuation of treatment for at least several months or a year following an acute episode of mania. It is usual to recommend indefinitely prolonged prophylactic treatment after two episodes within 5 years, especially if one is a suicidal depression, but sometimes even following a single, severe manic episode. Many patients are reluctant to continue such treatment for more than a few months at a time. When a patient has been relatively stable for many months, and continues to suffer from adverse effects of medication, acceptance of prolonged treatment can be particularly difficult.

Recent research supports the important generalization that discontinuing any long-term treatment with a psychotropic medicine is not equivalent to not treating. Indeed, abrupt discontinuation of mood-stabilizing agents such as lithium leads to sharp increases in early recurrences of both mania and depression, with markedly increased risk of suicide *(42)*. This response is not merely a manifestation of re-emergence of untreated illness, but almost certainly an iatrogenically produced, pharmacodynamic, stress effect. Support for this conclusion is that gradual discontinuation of treatment over weeks or even longer not only delays recurrences, but actually reduces risk *(42)*.

As discussed above, mechanisms of action of mood-stabilizing agents are probably associated with the interference with cellular signaling processes that include molecular pathways that mediate the actions of neurotransmitter reception (second-messengers) and intracellular regulatory processes (including those mediated by protein kinases and phosphorylated proteins that regulate the functioning, genetic expression, and survival of neurons *(22)*. Several of these mechanisms are common to the actions of lithium and valproic acid *(21)*.

7.2.2.1. LITHIUM SALTS

By the mid-1970s, abundant evidence had accumulated to support the concept that sustained treatment of manic-depressive patients (with BPD or recurrent severe depression) with lithium following recovery from an index episode of acute illness could reduce long-term morbidity *(3,43)*. This highly innovative approach to the care of such patients was modeled after earlier use of long-term treatment with neuroleptic agents to minimize long-term morbidity in schizophrenia and other chronic psychotic illnesses.

Preventive, long-term treatment with lithium is effective in reducing recurrences of both mania and depression, and in lessening the intensity of manic and depressive recurrences in about two-thirds of patients with BPD over many years without evidence of loss of benefits over time *(3)*. For safety, serum concentrations of lithium (and the status of other electrolytes, as well as renal and thyroid functioning) are assayed regularly. Lithium (and most mood-stabilizing agents) appear to be somewhat more effective against recurrences of mania than depression, but long-term benefits in both phases are substantial, and reductions of time in bipolar II depression is about as great as in bipolar I mania *(36)*. Moreover, lithium is the only psychiatric treatment with clear evidence of major reductions in risk of suicides (by about 80%), as well as attempts *(44)*.

Clinically useful predictors of long-term responses to mood-stabilizing treatment are not well established, but patients who present first in mania and later become depressed may benefit more from lithium than those with the opposite course-pattern *(45)*. It is also likely that delay of treatment, even for years, and a greater number of pretreatment illness-episodes or cycles do not limit benefits of long-term treatment with mood-stabilizers *(46,47)*.

7.2.2.2. ANTICONVULSANTS

Several drugs developed primarily to treat and prevent epileptic seizures also have proved antimanic efficacy *(3)* (Table 3). Initially, *carbamazepine* was commonly used; it appears to have secure antimanic, and considerably less secure long-term mood-stabilizing actions, and little evidence of reducing risk of suicide *(3,48)* (Table 3). Its congener, *oxcarbazepine*, was introduced recently. It is somewhat simpler to use than carbamazepine, particularly in having less risk of inducing the hepatic metabolism of itself or other drugs. Neither of these agents is FDA-approved for the treatment of BPD.

The *valproic acid* salt, sodium divalproex, has compelling evidence of a rapid antimanic effect, and it is FDA-approved for that indication *(4,40,48)*. Evidence for its long-term protective effects against recurrences of mania and especially of bipolar depression, as well as of reducing risk of suicide, is less secure. Nevertheless, it became the most widely employed mood-stabilizing agent the United States in recent years, in part owing to the relative simplicity of its clinical use and acceptability by many patients.

Lamotrigine was recently FDA-approved as the only mood-stabilizing agent that is *not* indicated for acute mania. It appears to have beneficial effects against bipolar depression with little risk of inducing mania or rapid-cycling. However, its lack of convincing evidence of acute antimanic effects, and the need to increase doses very slowly to avoid potentially severe dermatological complications, particularly in combination with valproic acid salts, preclude its use in acute episodes, and even limit its use as a primary long-term mood-stabilizing treatment, and may require combination with other agents *(3,48)*.

Potential antimanic or mood-stabilizing effectiveness of other anticonvulsants is unproved. However, *topiramate* and *zonisamide* are being studied currently. Both are of interest because they are rare among antimanic or mood-stabilizing agents in having little risk of weight gain *(3,48)*.

7.2.2.3. ANTIPSYCHOTICS

All effective antipsychotic agents appear to have useful antimanic effects. Among early agents, only *chlorpromazine* is FDA-approved for mania in the United States. Some of the older neuroleptics, including haloperidol, although powerfully antimanic, are suspected of worsening bipolar depression, and they produce uncomfortable and potentially serious adverse extrapyramidal neurological effects. These properties limit their utility in comparison to a series of newer antipsychotic agents *(3)* (Table 3). Currently *olanzapine*, *quetiapine*, and *risperidone* are FDA-approved for the treatment of mania, and olanzapine has a growing body of research to support long-term mood-stabilizing effects that may include protection against bipolar depression *(49)*. Long-term adverse effects of olanzapine, and perhaps quetiapine, include weight gain, and possibly increased risk of insulin-independent diabetes mellitus and hyperlipidemia. Those of risperidone include extrapyramidal neurological effects at even moderate doses, as well as major increases in circulating concentrations of prolactin, with uncertain long-term medical implications. These adverse risks may limit indefinitely prolonged use of these drugs, but they also appear to have clinically useful benefits when used for short periods as adjuncts to lithium or anticonvulsants. Risperidone is available in a long-acting injectable form that may be useful for treatment-nonadherent patients.

Clozapine appears to be quite effective in the treatment of type I BPD as well as schizoaffective disorder patients. It also has some evidence of reduced risk of suicide attempts in schizophrenia patients. However, its safe use requires regular monitoring of white blood cell counts to limit risk of leukopenia or agranulocytosis, and it has a dose-dependent risk of inducing epileptic seizures, as well as metabolic complications associated with weight gain. These shortcomings have limited its use to the empirical, off-label treatment of otherwise poorly treatment-responsive BPD cases *(49)*.

7.2.2.4. ANTIDEPRESSANTS

As stated above, modern and older antidepressant agents are very poorly studied in either the short-or long-term treatment of bipolar depression and dysthymia, despite their status as the major, and potentially lethal, morbidity of bipolar I and II patients *(2)* (Table 3). All types of antidepressants appear to be less effective in acute bipolar than nonbipolar depression, tend to lose effectiveness over time, and may dose-dependently increase risk of switching into mixed states or a rapid-cycling course, particularly when used without a mood-stabilizing agent. More-over, their long-term effectiveness and safety compared to a mood-stabilizing regimen alone, is not secure *(3,41)*.

7.3. Nonpharmacological Treatments

7.3.1. Biological Rhythms and Hygienic Measures

The cyclic nature of BPD and its frequent presentation as a seasonal disturbance of mood and behavior have suggested interventions aimed at adjusting or correct-ing disturbances in biological rhythms, particularly daily (circadian) rhythms. Timed exposure to intense daylight-mimicking artificial light is a proposed option, but remains an unproved treatment for severe BPD. Additionally, comprehensive clinical management of patients with BPD includes attention to sleep hygiene and maintaining regular daily rhythms of activity, meals, and rest, as well as avoidance of alcohol and stimulants including caffeine.

7.3.2. Psychosocial Interventions

Psychosocial components of comprehensive care of patients with BPD and their families are much less well developed and studied than for other major psychiatric disorders *(39,50)*. Nevertheless, there is growing interest in this approach, and emerging evidence of combined benefits that exceed those of treatment with mood-stabilizing agents alone. Methods that have received particular clinical and research attention include *interpersonal psychotherapy*, aimed at improving coping strate-gies for social and interpersonal relationships; *cognitive–behavioral therapy*, which attempts to modify ineffectual, self-detrimental, or exaggerated concepts by encouraging more flexible schemas, and rehearsal of new cognitive and behavioral responses; *interpersonal and social rhythm therapy*, which helps to re-organize everyday life, and improve sleep-activity rhythms and social relationships; *family-focused therapy* aims at reducing distress levels within the patients' families. Edu-cational psychotherapies that include family members, and other group therapies appear to improve interpersonal communication, recognition of early symptoms with earlier interventions, and improved knowledge of the illness and its treatments. Moreover, a controlled trial of group psychoeducation was recently found to decrease recurrence rates of bipolar I and II disorder *(50)*.

All of these supplemental interventions appear to improve treatment-adherence, add protection against illness recurrences, support coping skills, and avoid demor-alization. These methods require further research, but they appear to be cost-effec-tive as well as clinically useful for adults and children with BPD, and to enhance the effectiveness of mood-stabilizing medical treatment.

8. CONCLUSIONS

Bipolar disorder, one of the most recently defined major mental illnesses is characterized by discrete recurrences of depressive, manic, or mixed states that vary in their frequency, duration, and severity. BPD is associated with high rates of substance abuse, variable disability, and premature mortality, with very high suicide rates. Subtypes differ in the severity of their manic phases. Lifetime prevalence varies from about 1% for bipolar I disorder (with mania), to perhaps 5% if bipolar II (with hypomania), cyclothymia, and juvenile forms are included. BPD is highly heritable, but specific genetic factors and a coherent pathophysiology remain uncertain. Treatment of patients with BPD has advanced greatly in recent years, but treatment of bipolar depression and mixed dysphoric-agitated states is less well studied than the treatment of mania. Lithium and several newer medicines, supplemented with supportive psychosocial measures, provide long-term prophylactic benefits by reducing long-term morbidity in BPD, limiting disability and substance abuse, and prolonging life.

GLOSSARY OF MEDICAL TERMINOLOGY

Antidepressants: Drugs effective in treating depressive and some anxiety disorders; they risk inducing mania in vulnerable bipolar disorder patients

Bipolar disorder: A prevalent major psychiatric illness marked by *mania* or *hypomania*, almost always recurrent and alternating with *major depressive* or *mixed* states.

Circadian rhythms: Daily fluctuations of motor activity, temperature, cortisol secretion and other biological activities over an approximate 24-hour time course.

Dysphoria: A type of depressed mood, usually with a degree of anguish, tension, or irritability.

Electroconvulsive treatment (ECT): Controlled, electrically induced epileptic convulsive seizures as a highly effective treatment for severe and difficult to treat depression or mania.

Euthymia: More-or-less stable mood, especially intervals between major recurrent episodes of bipolar disorder or major depression.

Kindling: Phenomenon in animal models of experimental epilepsy whereby initially focal abnormal irritability of brain tissue spontaneously becomes more widespread, and seizure activity more generalized.

Limbic system: A neuroanatomical-neurophysiological concept of a large component of the forebrain involved in the management of emotional aspects of behavioral responses.

Manic-depressive illness: A group of recurring major psychiatric disorders marked by mania or severe depression, alone or in various combinations.

Mood stabilizers: Drugs (including lithium salts, certain anticonvulsants, and some modern antipsychotic agents) that reduce the frequency, severity, or duration of recurrences of mania and depression in bipolar disorder with low risk of switching mood states.

Rapid-cycling: A course specifier in DSM-IV for bipolar disorders, requiring at least four distinct episodes of mania, hypomania, or major depression within 12 months of assessment

Seasonal affective disorders (SADs): Usually involve fall-winter depression and spring-summer hypomania, or the opposite pattern, and are common among patients with bipolar disorders.

Ultradian rhythms: Changes in biological functioning shorter than 24 hours, including phases of sleep, attention, and many others.

ACKNOWLEDGMENTS

This work was supported, in part, by awards from the National Alliance for Research on Schizophrenia and Depression (NARSAD) and the Stanley Medical Research Institute (LT), the Max Kade Foundation (CB), the Bruce J. Anderson Foundation, and the McLean Private Donors Neuropsychopharmacology Research Fund (RJB).

REFERENCES

1. Goodwin FK, Jamison, KR. Manic-Depressive Illness. New York: Oxford University Press, 1990, and in press.
2. American Psychiatric Association (APA). Diagnostic and Statistical Manual of Mental Disorders, fourth edition, text revision (DSM-IV-TR). Washington, DC: American Psychiatric Press, 2000.
3. Baldessarini RJ, Tarazi FI. Drugs and the treatment of psychiatric disorders: Antipsychotic and antimanic agents. Chapts 19 and 20. In: Hardman JG, Limbird LE, Gilman AG, eds. Goodman and Gilman's The Pharmacological Basis of Therapeutics, 10th ed., New York: McGraw-Hill Press, 2001, pp. 447–520.
4. Tohen M, Zarate CA Jr, Hennen J, et al. The McLean-Harvard First-Episode Mania Study: Prediction of recovery and first recurrence. Am J Psychiatry 2003;160:2099–2107.
5. Tondo L, Isacsson G, Baldessarini RJ. Suicidal behavior in bipolar disorder: Risk and prevention. CNS Drugs 2003;17:491–511.
6. Sharma R, Markar HR. Mortality in affective disorder. J Affect Disord 1994;31:91–96.
7. Angst J, Marneros A. Bipolarity from ancient to modern times: conception, birth and rebirth. J Affect Disord 2001;67:3–19.
8. Tsuang MT, Tohen M, eds. Textbook in Psychiatric Epidemiology, 2nd edition. New York: John Wiley & Sons, 2002.
9. Angst J, Gamma A, Benazzi F, Ajdacic V, Eich D, Rössler W. Toward a re-definition of subthreshold bipolarity: Epidemiology and proposed criteria for bipolar-II, minor bipolar disorders and hypomania. J Affect Disord 2003;73:133–146.
10. Arnold LM. Gender differences in bipolar disorder. Psychiatr Clin No Am 2003;26:595–620.
11. Lish JD, Dime-Meenan S, Whybrow PC, Price RA, Hirschfield RM. National Depressive and Manic-Depressive Association (NDMDA) survey of bipolar members. J Aff Disord 1994;31: 281–294.
12. Harrington R, Myatt T. Is preadolescent mania the same condition as adult mania? A British perspective. Biol Psychiatry 2003;53:961–999.
13. Craddock N, Jones I. Genetics of bipolar disorder. J Med Genet 1999;36:585–594.
14. Baldessarini RJ, Hennen J. Genetics of suicide: An overview. Harvard Rev Psychiatry 2004; in press.
15. Berrettini W. Review of bipolar molecular linkage association studies. Curr Psychiatry Rep 2002;4:124–129.
16. Ewald H, Flint T, Kruse TA, Mors O. A genome-wide scan shows significant linkage between bipolar disorder and chromosome 12q24.3 and suggestive linkage to chromosomes 1p22-21, 4p16, 6q14-22, 10q26 and 16p13.3. Mol Psychiatry 2002;7:734–744.
17. Dick DM, Foroud T, Flury L, et al. Genome scan meta-analysis of schizophrenia and bipolar disorder, part III: Bipolar disorder. Am J Hum Genet. 2003;73:49–62.

18. Lenox RH, Gould TD, Manji HK. Endophenotypes in bipolar disorder. Am J Med Genet (Neuropsychiatr Genet) 2002;114:391–406.
19. Baldessarini RJ. American biological psychiatry and psychopharmacology 1944–1994, Chapter 16. In: Menninger RW, Nemiah JC, eds. American Psychiatry After World War II (1944–1994), Washington, DC: American Psychiatric Press, 2000:371–412.
20. Arana GW, Baldessarini RJ, Ornsteen M. The dexamethasone suppression test for diagnosis and prognosis in psychiatry. Arch Gen Psychiatry 1985;42:1193–1204.
21. Manji HK, Zarate CA. Molecular and cellular mechanisms underlying mood stabilization in bipolar disorder: Implication for the development of improved therapeutics. Mol Psychiatry 2002;7(Suppl):S1–S7.
22. Manji HK, Quiroz JA, Payne JL, et al. The underlying neurobiology of bipolar disorder. World Psychiatry 2003;2:137–146.
23. Faedda GL, Tondo L, Teicher MH, Baldessarini RJ, Gelbard HA, Floris GF. Seasonal mood disorders: Patterns of seasonal recurrence in major affective disorder. Arch Gen Psychiatry 1993;50:17–23.
24. Post RM, Ballenger JC, eds. Neurobiology of Mood Disorders. Baltimore, MD: Williams & Wilkins, 1984.
25. Soares JC. Contributions from brain imaging to the elucidation of pathophysiology of bipolar disorder. Int J Neuropsychopharmacol 2003;6:171–180.
26. Salvatore P, Baldessarini RJ, Centorrino F, et al. Weygandt's On the Mixed States of Manic-Depressive Insanity: Translation and commentary on its significance in the evolution of the concept of bipolar disorder. Harvard Rev Psychiatry. 2002;10:255–275.
27. Koukopoulos A and Koukopoulos A. Agitated depression as a mixed state and the problem of melancholia. Psychiatr Clin No Am 1999;22:547–564.
28. Cassidy F, Carroll BJ. Frequencies of signs and symptoms in mixed and pure episodes of mania: implications for the study of manic episodes. Progr Neuropsychopharmacol Biol Psychiatry 2001;25:659–665.
29. Shulman KI, Tohen M, Kutcher S, eds. Mood Disorders Across the Life Span. New York, NY: John Wiley & Sons, 1996.
30. Biederman J, Mick E, Faraone SV, Spencer T, Wilens TE, Wozniak J. Current concepts in the validity, diagnosis and treatment of pediatric bipolar disorder. Int J Neuropsychopharmacol 2003;6:293–300.
31. McElroy SL, Altshuler LL, Suppes T, et al. Axis I psychiatric comorbidity and its relationship to historical illness variables in 288 patients with BPD. Am J Psychiatry 2001;158:420–426.
32. Krauthammer C, Klerman GL. Secondary mania: Manic syndromes associated with antecedent physical illness or drugs. Arch Gen Psychiatry 1978;35:1333–1339.
33. Cassidy F, Ahearn E, Carroll BJ. Elevated frequency of diabetes mellitus in hospitalized manic-depressive patients. Am J Psychiatry 1999;156:1417–1420.
34. Low NC, Du Fort GG, Cervantes P. Prevalence, clinical correlates, and treatment of migraine in bipolar disorder. Headache 2003;43:940–949.
35. Viguera AC, Cohen LS, Baldessarini RJ, Nonacs R. Managing bipolar disorder in pregnancy: Weighing the risks and benefits. Can J Psychiatry 2002;47:426–436.
36. Tondo L, Baldessarini RJ, Floris G. Long-term clinical effectiveness of lithium maintenance treatment in types I and II bipolar manic-depressive disorders. Br J Psychiatry 2001;178 (Suppl40): S184–S190.
37. Oepen G, Baldessarini RJ, Salvatore P. On the periodicity of manic-depressive insanity, by Eliot Slater (1938): Translated excerpts and commentary. J Affect Disord. 2004;78:1–9.
38. Judd LL, Akiskal AS, Schettler PJ, et al. The long-term natural history of the weekly symptomatic status of bipolar I disorder. Arch Gen Psychiatry 2003;59:530–537.
39. Huxley NA, Parikh SV, Baldessarini RJ. Effectiveness of psychosocial treatments in bipolar disorder: State of the evidence. Harvard Rev Psychiatry 2000;8:126–140.
40. Keck PE Jr, McElroy SL, Bennett JA. Pharmacologic loading in the treatment of acute mania. Bipolar Disord. 2000;2:42–46.

41 Ghaemi SN, Ko JY, Rosenquist KJ, Balassano CF, Kontos NJ, Baldessarini RJ. Effects of antidepressant treatment in bipolar vs. unipolar depression. Am J Psychiatry 2004;161:163–165.

42. Baldessarini RJ, Tondo L, Viguera AC. Effects of discontinuing lithium maintenance treatment. Bipolar Disord 1999;1:17–24.

43. Baldessarini RJ, Tondo L, Hennen J, Viguera AC. Is lithium still worth using? An update of selected recent research. Harvard Rev Psychiatry 2002;10:59–75.

44. Tondo L, Hennen J, Baldessarini RJ. Reduced suicide risk with long-term lithium treatment in major affective Illness: A meta-analysis. Acta Psychiatr Scand 2001;104:163–172.

45. Kukopulos A, Reginaldi D, Laddomada P, Floris G, Serra G, Tondo L. Course of the manic-depressive cycle and changes caused by treatment. Pharmakopsychiatr Neuropsychopharmakol 1980;13:156–167.

46. Baethge C, Baldessarini RJ, Bratti IM, Tondo L. Effect of treatment-latency on outcome in bipolar disorder. Can J Psychiatry 2003;48:449–457.

47. Bratti IM, Baldessarini RJ, Baethge C, Tondo L. Pretreatment episode count and response to lithium treatment in manic-depressive illness. Harvard Rev Psychiatry 2003;11:245–256.

48. Bowden CL. Acute and maintenance treatment with mood stabilizers. Int J Neuropsychopharmacol 2003;6:269–275.

49. Ertugrul A, Meltzer HY. Antipsychotic drugs in bipolar disorder. Int J Neuropsychopharmacol 2003;6:277–284.

50. Colom F, Vieta E, Martinez-Aran A, et al. A randomized trial on the efficacy of group psychoeducation in the prophylaxis of recurrences in bipolar patients whose disease is in remission. Arch Gen Psychiatry 2003;60:402–407.

12

Attention Deficit Hyperactivity Disorder

Kehong Zhang, Eugen Davids, and Ross J. Baldessarini

Summary

Attention deficit hyperactivity disorder (ADHD) is a highly prevalent, heterogeneous syndrome of cognitive and behavioral features including inattention, impulsivity, deficient behavioral inhibition, and hyperactivity. Prevalence is about 4%, with a moderate excess of a mainly inattentive subtype, and fewer mixed or mainly hyperactive/impulsive cases. Comorbid conditions include conduct, learning, and mood disorders. ADHD can be found at any age, but the diagnosis is more common in boys than girls or adults, and in the United States than in Europe. Risk is 35% to 40% among first-degree relatives, and more than twice greater in identical twins; heritability is high. Polymorphisms of the dopamine neuronal transporter gene (DAT1) and D_4 receptor gene (DRD4) have been associated with ADHD. Diagnosis remains essentially clinical and there are no specific diagnostic tests. Prominent deficits occur in executive functions, including response inhibition, sustained attention, and working memory, all suggesting dysfunction of prefrontal cerebral cortex that is tentatively supported by some brain-imaging studies. A precise neuropathophysiology remains undefined. Laboratory animal models of ADHD include genetic (spontaneously hypertensive rat, DAT-knock-out mouse, coloboma mouse) and neurotoxin models (neonatal 6-hydroxy-dopamine-lesioned rodents). Most models emphasize hyperactivity rather than specific cognitive dysfunctions, and vary in their neuropharmacological congruence with the clinical therapeutics of ADHD. Empirically employed treatments with research support for cognitive as well as behavioral benefits include most stimulants, and antidepressants with noradrenergic actions; these treatments are best combined with comprehensive behavioral and educational interventions.

Key Words: ADHD; antidepressants; attention; attention deficit hyperactivity disorder; cognition; dopamine; hyperactivity; norepinephrine; prefrontal cerebral cortex; receptors; serotonin; transporters.

1. INTRODUCTION AND HISTORY

Attention deficit hyperactivity disorder (ADHD) is a highly prevalent, heterogeneous syndrome consisting of both cognitive and behavioral features, notably, inattention, impulsive behavior, and hyperactivity *(1,2)*. It has been recognized in

From: *Current Clinical Neurology: Neurological and Psychiatric Disorders:*
From Bench to Bedside
Edited by: F. I. Tarazi and J. A. Schetz © Humana Press Inc., Totowa, NJ

some form for at least a century, particularly in children and adolescents. The first well-documented clinical description was in a series of 20 pediatric patients reported by physician George Still in London in 1902. His cases were characterized by excessive motor activity, inattention, and poor self-control. Still also found a large excess of boys, as well as a frequent family history of depression, alcoholism, or antisocial behavior.

In the early decades of the 20th century, there was a great interest in behavioral disorders of children who had experienced encephalitis or other coarse brain diseases. Clinical phenomena associated with residual states of neurological diseases were later extended to similar behavioral abnormalities without obvious neurological disease, leading to the concept of "minimum brain dysfunction." By the late 1950s, there was more specific interest in deficits in attention or in hyperactivity as noteworthy clinical elements in some children with learning and conduct disorders but no evidence of neurological illness.

Interest in these conditions was advanced in the late 1930s through systematic clinical observations by physician Charles Bradley in children and adolescents with behavioral disorders in Providence, Rhode Island. Based on contemporary findings that amphetamine produced beneficial effects on cognition and behavior in adults, he carried out a planned and partly blinded, 1-week, intervention with D,L-amphetamine sulfate (Benzedrine®, at 10–30 mg per day). In all but 2 of the 30 patients in his sample, amphetamine reduced overactivity, and improved attention as well as school performance, with striking benefits in about half of the cases.

2. CLINICAL FEATURES AND DIAGNOSIS

2.1. Clinical Features

Clinical features of inattention, impulsivity, and overactivity, particularly in children, have been recognized in the Diagnostic and Statistical Manual (DSM) of the American Psychiatric Association since its second edition of 1968, initially as "hyperkinetic disorder of childhood" or as the informal clinical concept, "minimum brain dysfunction." The concept of hyperkinetic disorder has been sustained up to the most recent (1990) edition of the International Classification of Diseases (ICD-10) of the World Health Organization (WHO).

The third edition of the DSM (DSM-III) of 1980 included two subtypes of illness with either prominent inattention or hyperactivity. Excessive impulsivity was considered to be common in both forms, but greater emphasis was placed on cognitive deficits. This shift in emphasis was reflected in the new diagnostic term "attention deficit disorder" (ADD), based in part on influential studies by Douglas *(3)*. ADD subtypes were removed in the 1987 revision of DSM-III, and the diagnosis was modified to the collective term "attention deficit hyperactivity disorder" (ADHD). Subtypes reappeared in the fourth DSM edition (DSM-IV) of 1990 and continued in its latest revision in 2000. Subtyping was reconsidered based on additional observations of uneven distribution of specific clinical features in large samples of patients with ADHD *(4)*. The current DSM diagnostic term "attention deficit hyperactivity disorder" recognizes the subtypes proposed in DSM-III, and a third subtype with combined features of inattention and hyperactivity/impulsivity.

Continuing changes in American diagnostic terminology reflect the complexity and heterogeneity of ADHD. Clinical features vary greatly among individuals and this heterogeneity has been used to challenge the validity of ADHD as a discrete disorder. The heterogeneity of ADHD also contributes to dissimilar US and international diagnostic criteria, which in turn, complicate epidemiological and clinical comparisons among case samples ascertained by different criteria. Broadly defined, ADHD is largely an American phenomenon; WHO diagnostic criteria are considerably narrower. Moreover, in the United States, ADHD is widely considered a neuropsychiatric disorder with prominent cerebral dysfunction, whereas European experts tend to view it as a developmental behavioral abnormality.

2.2. Diagnosis and Assessment

The current American DSM diagnostic criteria for ADHD and its subtypes are summarized, and compared to the international criteria of ICD-10 in Table 1. Whether the three DSM subtypes represent variable forms of a single disorder, or separate clinical entities is unknown. By definition, greater impairment of selective attention and sluggish information processing are characteristic of the predominantly inattentive type. The hyperactive/impulsive and combined types are characterized by prominent hyperactivity, excessive impulsive behavior, as well as distractibility.

As of 2004, diagnosis of ADHD remains essentially descriptive, and more heavily dependent on secondary reports from parents and teachers than on direct clinical observation. Indeed, evaluation of behavior by direct observation in most clinical settings is of limited value owing to unrepresentativeness of behavior at home or school. Applications of specific psychological testing methods can be of some help. Beneficial effects of stimulant treatment do not confirm a diagnosis of ADHD, because similar effects can occur in normal boys or men.

Efforts to define specific features in ADHD by analyses of symptom clusters have met only limited success. Psychological studies have identified many deficits in ADHD, as described below. However, it is important to point out that none of these abnormalities is specific to, or diagnostic of ADHD. Psychological testing methods used to support the diagnosis of ADHD have included the Delay Aversion Task, Continuous Performance Task, Go/No-Go, and Stop-Signal tests. In these tasks, highly variable and slower reaction times are characteristic of subjects diagnosed with ADHD. This finding contrasts with the common belief that ADHD subjects respond more quickly than normal. Additionally, rates of errors-of-omission (failure to respond when given a signal to do so) are increased among ADHD subjects, suggesting either lack of motivation or poor attention. Errors-of-commission (responding when given a signal not to do so) also are frequent, suggesting lack of inhibitory control. There is some indication that ADHD subjects are more easily distracted from tasks. Use of electronic devices to detect body motion has indicated

Table 1
Standard American Diagnostic Criteria
for Attention Deficit Hyperactivity Disorder

A. Fulfills six or more of either of the following conditions that have persisted for at least 6 months:

1. *Inattention*
   a. Lacks close attention to details or makes careless mistakes at school, work, or other activities.
   b. Shows difficulty in attention to tasks at play or work.
   c. Does not listen when addressed directly.
   d. Does not follow through on instructions or fails to complete tasks (not due to oppositional behavior or lack of comprehension).
   e. Has difficulty in organizing tasks or activities.
   f. Avoids, dislikes, or is reluctant to engage in tasks requiring sustained mental effort.
   g. Loses materials required for tasks or activities.
   h. Easily distracted by extraneous stimuli.
   i. Forgetful in daily activities.

2. *Hyperactivity–Impulsivity*
   a. Fidgets with hands or feet and does not sit still.
   b. Leaves seat during a task.
   c. Overactive and may feel restless.
   d. Has difficulty in engaging quietly in leisure activities.
   e. On the go as if driven.
   f. Talks excessively.
   g. Blurts out answers before question is completed.
   h. Has difficulty in waiting a turn.
   i. Interrupts others or intrudes socially.

B. Onset before age 7 years.

C. Symptoms and some impairment in at least two settings (e.g., home and school or work).

D. Clear evidence of clinically significant dysfunction (social, academic, occupational).

E. Absence of a pervasive developmental or psychotic disorder, and not better accounted for by diagnosis of a mood, anxiety, or personality disorder.

The tabulated criteria are based on the most recent revision of the American Psychiatric Association Diagnostic and Statistical Manual of Mental Disorders (fourth edition, DSM-IV, text-revised) of 2000. DSM-IV considers three subtypes: Inattentive (I), Hyperactive-Impulsive (HI), or Combined (C; with both attentional and motor features), based on predominant clinical features for the preceding 6 months, with no upper age-limit. The World Health Organization's most recent edition of the Manual of the International Statistical Classification of Diseases, Injuries, and Causes of Death (tenth revision, ICD-10) of 1990 includes the narrower diagnosis of *Hyperkinetic Disorder*, which is very similar to the combined type of ADHD in DSM-IV, except for requiring onset before age 6 years and IQ greater than 50, with no subtypes, and direct observation of the patient's behavior by the diagnostician.

that children with ADHD are indeed more active than normal controls, particularly during tasks requiring sustained attention.

3. EPIDEMIOLOGY OF ADHD

Estimates of the prevalence of ADHD in general population, as well as in age- and gender-specific groups vary widely with the diagnostic and case-finding methods employed. Surveys of relatively large samples of school-age children have indicated lifetime prevalence in excess of 10%—an extraordinarily large proportion of the population. However, DSM-IV estimates of the prevalence of ADHD are lower, at about 4%, probably owing partly to the requirement of meeting full diagnostic criteria in two dissimilar settings. For comparison, the rate of prescription for methylphenidate—the most commonly prescribed medical treatment for ADHD in the United States in the 1990s—ranged from 1.5% to 10% of school-aged children, involving several million children in the United States alone *(5)*.

Prevalence of specific DSM-IV subtypes ranks: inattentive type ≥ combined type ≥ hyperactive-impulsive type, with a total of nearly 10% of youngsters aged 7 to 18 years *(6)*. Diagnosis of ADHD is made at least 2.5 times more often among boys or men than girls or women, but such gender differences probably are confounded by several factors *(7)*. First, girls or women with ADHD often display minimal features of hyperactivity and disruptive behaviors, and so tend to be overlooked. Second, symptoms of the hyperactive/impulsive type of ADHD may appear at an earlier age, and tend to diminish with maturation. Third, reported estimates in children may not reflect prevalence of ADHD in late adolescence and adulthood, especially in adult women, in whom syndrome definitions and diagnostic criteria are even less well established than in children or men.

The clinical similarity, or co-occurrence, of ADHD to other behavioral, cognitive, and emotional disorders of childhood presents a particular problem for diagnosis, as well as for effective and safe clinical management. For example, many symptoms of mild or moderate mental retardation or pervasive developmental disorders (such as Asperger's syndrome and autism) resemble those of ADHD. Other confusing conditions include oppositional-defiant disorder (ODD) of childhood, diagnosed in nearly half of children considered to have ADHD, and other conduct disorders reported to occur in about 14% of children diagnosed with ADHD *(8)*. Comorbidity of ADHD with anxiety disorders also is common, at about 25%, and rates of specific learning disabilities vary greatly, but average about 23%.

The diagnostic overlap or comorbidity of ADHD with mood disorders is an especially challenging phenomenon. Mood disorders, including severe depression and bipolar (manic-depressive) disorder, have long been recognized among children *(9)*, even though their clinical presentations may differ from classic syndrome descriptions based on observations of adult patients. Both clinical depression (nearly one-third) and bipolar disorder (approx 10%) have been reported in samples of children diagnosed with ADHD, and first-degree relatives of patients with ADHD have increased rates of mood disorders *(10)*. Bipolar disorder in children with comorbid or misdiagnosed ADHD can be particularly problematic because use of stimulants and antidepressants can induce potentially dangerous agitated-aggressive manic or mixed manic-depressive reactions, with the potential for violent behavior *(11)*.

4. HERITABILITY AND GENETICS

ADHD has a strong familial, and presumably genetic component, with an estimated heritability of 0.60 to 0.85 *(12)*. First-degree biological relatives of probands diagnosed with ADHD, have 5 to 10 times greater risk for ADHD (35–40%) than adoptive relatives or the general population. These rates do not differ in families identified with male or female probands. Family risk studies also provide opportunities to test for separate heritability of specific components or subtypes of ADHD, as well as to separate heritability of ADHD from commonly comorbid conditions, but the results have not been consistent so far. In twin studies, concordance averages about 83% for identical or monozygotic (MZ) twins, and 38% for fraternal or dizygotic (DZ) twins, as among other first-degree relatives. These rates yield a modest, 2.2-fold, difference in relative risk in MZ/DZ twins.

Molecular genetic studies have provided interesting, but generally scattered and poorly replicated leads in families with identified ADHD patients *(13)*. Some genes that encode proteins required for central monoaminergic neurotransmission have been implicated. These include polymorphisms of genes for the DA transporter (DAT1) and DA D_4 receptor (DRD4) *(14)*. The DA transporter is a cell membrane protein uniquely expressed in dopaminergic neurons; it provides the most important physiological mechanism for inactivating DA released into the synaptic cleft by transporting it back to the nerve terminals. Some support for abnormality of this transporter in ADHD patients is also provided by brain-imaging studies based on use of DAT-selective radioligands. The D_4 receptor membrane protein is a member of the D_2-like receptor family that inhibits the formation of cyclic AMP, an important second messenger that mediates intracellular molecular actions of DA and other transmitters and hormones.

The DAT1 allele associated with ADHD is more effective than other alleles in transporting or inactivating DA. The D_4 allele associated with ADHD is less efficient in transducing synaptic DA signals into an intracellular adenylyl cyclase response. These associations, consistent with the beneficial actions of DA-facilitating stimulant drugs, suggest that dopaminergic functioning in the brain may be decreased in ADHD patients. However, caution must be exercised in interpreting these findings because statistical association or linkage of a genetic polymorphism to a disorder does not necessarily imply a cause–effect relationship. Moreover, the magnitude of genetic linkage of ADHD to both the DA transporter and the D_4 receptor has been small *(14)*.

Other candidate genes related to cerebral neurotransmitters include those for the DA D_2, D_3, and D_5 receptors, the monoamine (catecholamines or serotonin) metabolizing enzymes monoamine oxidase (MAO) and catechol-*O*-methyltransferase (COMT), the α_{1C} and α_{2C} adrenoceptors for norepinephrine, as well as the α_4 nicotinic acetylcholine receptor, and the synaptosomal-associated protein of molecular weight 25 kDa (SNAP-25).

In general, efforts in identifying susceptibility genes in ADHD have yielded largely inconsistent results, with the possible exception of the DA D_4 receptor. Recent trends in genetics research on ADHD include use of intermediate phenotypes ("endophenotypes") instead of the complex ADHD syndrome itself as targets for genetic association *(15)*, and a genome-wide approach supported by powerful new technical innovations developed largely to support the human genome project *(16)*. An intermediate phenotype is a heritable, quantifiable trait of the disorder (such as response in a specific neurocognitive test) that may underlie or contribute to its pathophysiology and clinical features. Use of such intermediate targets should limit heterogeneity of samples and perhaps increase the statistical power of genetic associations. Genome-wide scanning compares large numbers of DNA markers in close relatives who share or do not share a disorder, and assumes that susceptibility genes reside within regions of the genome that display high degree of similarity between affected family members.

In the first genome-wide search for ADHD susceptibility genes, Ogdie and colleagues *(16)* recruited 270 ADHD sibling pairs, and identified chromosomes 5, 6, 16, and 17 as prime sites for candidate genes. Some of the same regions have also been implicated in genetic contributions to autism and dyslexia, suggesting that ADHD may share some common pathophysiological features with these clinically dissimilar neurobehavioral disorders.

5. NEUROIMAGING

Recent advances in clinical neuroimaging techniques have provided means of unprecedented power for probing the structure and functioning of the living human brain. These techniques have helped to identify several candidate brain structures as playing a critical role in ADHD. Most of the available evidence implicates structural and functional changes in the frontal cerebral lobe, but changes in the basal ganglia, corpus collosum, and cerebellum also have been reported. This complex, highly technical, and rapidly evolving topic has been reviewed elsewhere *(2)*.

In normal human subjects, the right frontal lobe is slightly larger than the left. In subjects diagnosed with ADHD, this asymmetry is reduced owing to a decrease of right frontal volume *(17)*. Moreover, the degree of reduction of right frontal volume correlated with decreased response inhibition, a characteristic feature of ADHD *(18)*. Consistent with these structural abnormalities, regionally selective decreases in cerebral blood flow and glucose utilization have been reported in ADHD subjects compared to normal controls during the performance of a continuous performance task (CPT; a test for sustained attention). The regions most strongly implicated are the premotor and prefrontal cerebral cortex (PFC). Functional magnetic resonance imaging (fMRI) studies of the brain during the performance of other cognitive tasks that require frontal lobe functioning also demonstrated subnormal activation of PFC and anterior cingulate cortex in ADHD patients *(19)*.

It is important to emphasize that not all imaging studies have found structural or functional changes in the PFC *(2)*. Additionally, uncertainties surround the interpretation of functional brain-imaging data obtained during cognitive testing. In particular, it is often very difficult to ascertain whether abnormalities revealed by imaging methods are primary or causal, or if they merely reflect deficits in cognitive functioning in ADHD. Despite limitations of reported studies based on modern neuroimaging techniques, there is a growing consensus that the frontal lobes represent a brain region of especially great interest for understanding the neurobiological basis of ADHD. This conclusion is consistent with neuropsychological models of ADHD discussed in the next section, because the cognitive functions described in these models require integrity of the frontal lobes, and especially the PFC and anterior cingulate cortex.

6. EXPERIMENTAL MODELS OF ADHD

6.1. Animal Models

More than a dozen animal models representing specific components of clinical ADHD have been studied in efforts to advance knowledge of the pathophysiology and therapeutics of the clinical disorder *(20)*. Animal models of ADHD generally fall into two categories: genetic variants or neurotoxin exposures in early neurodevelopment. Such models allow greater experimental control of suspected contributing factors, and avoid confounding factors such as comorbidity and drug exposure than are possible in clinical studies. Particularly extensively studied models include three genetic models, the spontaneously hypertensive rat, the DA transporter knock-out mouse, the coloboma mutant mouse with defective SNAP-25 protein, and a neurotoxin model involving juvenile rats with neonatal lesions of central dopaminergic neurons.

The earliest animal model proposed to represent some features of ADHD is the *spontaneously hypertensive rat* (SHR). SHR was selected for hypertension from the Wistar-Kyoto rat (WKY). High motor activity co-segregated unexpectedly with hypertension. However, substrains that selectively express either hyperactivity or hypertension have subsequently been developed *(21)*. SHR bears several similarities to patients diagnosed with ADHD, including motor hyperactivity and learning deficits. SHR is also more sensitive to immediate but smaller rewards than to larger, delayed rewards. Sagvolden and colleagues argue that preference for immediate rewards is a key feature of ADHD, and that SHR particularly faithfully represents ADHD in domains of behavior under control of reinforcers. The stimulant drug methylphenidate, *increases* motor activity in SHR, albeit less than in the wild-type WKY rat, suggesting a *hypo*-dopaminergic state. However, the fact that stimulants increase rather than decrease motor activity in SHR is inconsistent with the hyperactivity-decreasing effects of these drugs in ADHD patients.

A recent ADHD model is a genetically engineered knock-out mouse (*DAT-KO* or *DAT*$^{-/-}$ *[22]*) that lacks functional DA transporters in neuronal membranes. Motor hyperactivity in this model parallels dramatically reduced clearance of DA from the synaptic cleft. This behavioral hyperactivity can be attenuated by various stimulants, but this effect may not be directly relevant to their effectiveness in ADHD because the drug effects in the mutant mouse appear to be mediated through activation of 5-HT, and not DA neurotransmission. Because selective serotonin reuptake inhibitors (SSRIs) are essentially ineffective in the treatment of ADHD, the usefulness of the DAT-KO mice as an ADHD model remains uncertain. The DAT-KO mouse also displays learning deficits, the pharmacology of which requires further study.

The *Coloboma mutant mouse* was produced by neutron irradiation *(23)*. These mice display robust and highly variable motor hyperactivity and developmental delays. Their hyperactivity can be inhibited by moderate doses of amphetamine, but methylphenidate paradoxically increases activity to limit the validity of this preparation as a model of ADHD. This mutant mouse carries a mutation in the gene that encodes protein SNAP-25, which contributes to the fusion of synaptic vesicles with presynaptic membranes. The mutation impairs release of monoamine neurotransmitters by exocytosis. Genetic linkage of polymorphisms for the SNAP-25 protein has been suggested in clinical ADHD, as mentioned previously, but the specific mutation associated with the coloboma mouse mutation is not known to be involved.

Juvenile rats and mice with selective dopaminergic lesions induced by the neurotoxin 6-hydroxydopamine shortly after birth is another extensively studied laboratory model of ADHD *(24)*. These rodents do not develop bradykinesia and other features of the parkinsonism syndrome as is found with adult lesioning. Instead, they display paradoxical motor hyperactivity during youth that inexplicably disappears in adulthood despite persistent loss of DA innervation to forebrain. Their hyperactive behavior is inhibited by both stimulants and tricyclic antidepressants, as in clinical ADHD, but also by SSRIs, thus limiting its value as a model of ADHD. Encouraged by the findings of genetic linkage of DA D_4 receptor polymorphisms with ADHD, we found that the magnitude and timing of motor hyperactivity in this model correlated well with abnormal expression of D_4 receptor in forebrain, and several selective D_4 receptor antagonists inhibited the hyperactivity *(25)*.

Although there are many laboratory models for ADHD, none is entirely satisfactory. Their limitations as models of clinical ADHD include use of experimental manipulations that are not relevant to the clinical disorder, variable concordance between the neuropharmacology of the models and of the disorder, and heavy reliance on hyperactivity or lack of habituation to a novel environment as a primary measure that is only one component of ADHD, and probably one that is less essential than its cognitive manifestations.

6.2. Neuropsychological Models

Many attempts have been made to devise theoretical constructs for ADHD that account for clinical symptoms as well as experimental findings. One influential model emphasizes the importance and primacy of deficient inhibition of behavioral responses *(26)*. Other proposals emphasize the importance of working memory and attention *(27,28)*.

6.2.1. Response Inhibition

Deficient behavioral response inhibition is a measure of impulsivity *(29)*. Impulsivity is a characteristic feature of ADHD, and deficient response inhibition may underlie some of its symptoms. Barkley *(26)* suggested that impaired response inhibition leads to dysfunctions of other executive cognitive functions in ADHD, including attention, motivation, working memory, and behavioral synthesis, although probably not in the predominantly inattentive subtype.

Empirical evidence supporting this theory mainly comes from human studies using tests sensitive to behavioral inhibition, particularly the "Stop-Signal" task *(30)*. In this procedure, subjects engaged in a primary task are required to respond to a stimulus (go signal) as fast as possible. In a small proportion of randomly selected trials, a "stop" signal is presented at a specified delay after the "go signal," and subjects are required to refrain from responding. The basic assumption in this testing paradigm is that outcome is determined by the race between a "go" process and a "stop" process. A shorter stop-signal reaction time (SSRT) is a primary index of response inhibition, indicating more efficient inhibitory control. Studies using this paradigm have consistently found that ADHD patients have longer and more variable SSRT, and that stimulant drugs decrease SSRT *(31)*.

Despite a critical role of response inhibition in ADHD, there was little information about the basic neurobiology of this executive cognitive function until the recent development of a behavioral testing method applicable to laboratory animals *(32)*. In this paradigm, rats are engaged in a primary task, and must stop the "go" response and perform an alternative response when a "stop" signal is presented at a certain delay after the "go" signal. In rats with long baseline SSRT, *d*-amphetamine significantly decreased the SSRT. In rats with short baseline SSRT, however, stimulants had no effect. This finding provides the first direct evidence in experimental animals that stimulants can improve response inhibition.

6.2.2. Attention

Attention is a broad cognitive construct with multiple dimensions. Depending on the context, it may refer to: (a) initial selection of a stimulus to which to allocate neurocognitive processing resources, (b) sustaining these resources to a relevant stimulus (sustained attention), (c) inhibition of irrelevant stimuli (selective attention), and (d) shifting of the same resources when other stimuli become relevant. Problems with attention in ADHD subjects typically include short attention span and distractibility, which are suggestive of impaired sustained attention and deficient selective attention, respectively.

The most widely used test for sustained attention is the continuous performance task (CPT). In its original version, subjects are presented a series of visual stimuli (typically, letters A–Z), with a rarely occurring stimulus (e.g., the letter X) designated as a target stimulus. Subjects are required to respond by pressing a lever when a target stimulus occurs, and to withhold response otherwise. Response accuracy (the proportion of correct responses relative to the number of target presentations) is used as the primary index of sustained attention.

Many studies using the CPT have demonstrated decreased response accuracy and slower responding in subjects with ADHD compared to normal controls *(33)*. Slow responses are inconsistent with Barkley's model in which deficient response inhibition should result in decreased, not increased, response latency. This inconsistency suggests that attention deficit and deficient response inhibition are separate features of ADHD.

In laboratory animals, sustained attention has been studied extensively using a 5-choice serial reaction time task (5-CSRTT), developed by Robbins and colleagues *(34)*. This behavioral paradigm has basic elements of the CPT, and measures ability to sustain attention over a large number of trials. Choice accuracy is used as a primary index for sustained attention. Several neurotransmitter systems are implicated in sustained attention as reflected in responses in the 5-CSRTT, including dopamine, norepinephrine, γ-aminobutyric acid (GABA), and others. Alternatively, sustained attention can be examined with a method developed by Sarter and colleagues that indicates paramount importance of acetylcholine to this function *(35)*. Whereas the 5-CSRTT has a component of spatial attention (rats must monitor events in several different locations), Sarter's method emphasizes the importance of nonsignal trials that are analogous to components of the human CPT.

The mesocortical DA pathway projecting from the ventral tegmental area of midbrain to the PFC is important in maintaining choice accuracy in the 5-CSRTT paradigm. Rats with low baseline choice accuracy show improved sustained attention with direct infusion of the D_1 partial agonist SKF-38393 into PFC, whereas the selective D_1 antagonist SCH-23390 can reduce choice accuracy in rats with relatively high baseline performance. When given either systemically or directly into the nucleus accumbens (a primary mesolimbic dopaminergic projection site), stimulants usually increase overall responses and premature responding, with no change in choice accuracy at moderate doses. However, in rats with spontaneous poor performance, low doses of methylphenidate may enhance choice accuracy and decrease premature responding, suggesting that rats with naturally occurring poor performance in this task may serve as a model for ADHD.

Lesions of norepinephrine neurons that project from the brainstem to forebrain usually do not affect performance in the 5-CSRTT task. However, poor choice accuracy becomes evident when interfering stimuli are presented prior to salient stimuli under such conditions, suggesting that the central noradrenergic system may protect selective attention from distractions. Studies using selective noradrenergic drugs indicate further, that stimulation of postsynaptic α_1 adrenoceptors can improve choice accuracy, whereas stimulation of α_2 adrenoceptors impairs test performance, presumably by reducing overall noradrenergic activity through an autoreceptor mechanism. Effects of tricyclic antidepressants in this model have yet to be studied.

6.2.3. Working Memory

Working memory encodes and maintains newly acquired, task relevant information that is held "on-line" for a short time, and used to guide future response selection, and therefore is essential for the temporal organization of goal-directed behavior. Based on extensive testing of ADHD patients with relevant cognitive tasks, working memory appears to be a major area of deficit *(2)*. ADHD subjects perform poorly in tasks that require intact working memory (e.g., CPT, Stop-Signal, Go/No-Go, and digit span), but not in others with minimal demand for working memory (e.g., visuomotor, finger-tapping, pegboard, and others). One possibility is that "inability to maintain working memory representations may lead to an increased rate at which input is delivered to working memory so as to compensate for rapid fading of representations in working memory" *(2)*. Such considerations support the hypothesis that a deficit in working memory may underlie the rapid shifts of attention and the disorganized/hyperactive behavior in ADHD patients.

In laboratory animals, working memory is commonly assessed with delayed response/alternation tasks. Studies using such paradigms support a critical role of DA and norepinephrine innervation to the PFC in the regulation of working memory *(36)*. Removal of dopaminergic input to the PFC impairs working memory. These deficits can be reversed by treatment with a direct dopaminergic agonist, and optimal responses are supported at an intermediate level of stimulation of D_1 DA receptors in the PFC.

The DA D_4 receptor also may play a role in the regulation of working memory because deficits in working memory induced by the benzodiazepine inverse agonist FG-7142 in monkeys could be prevented by pretreatment with a selective D_4 antagonist *(37)*. Furthermore, we recently found in rats with poor baseline working memory, that this cognitive function was enhanced with low doses of the selective D_4 antagonist L-745,870, whereas high doses reversed this beneficial effect. In rats with good baseline performance, the D_4 antagonist had no effect at low doses, but disrupted working memory at high doses. Again, interest in D_4 receptor-mediated mechanisms in ADHD is supported by evidence of genetic linkage of the disorder to polymorphism of the D_4 receptor gene, as already discussed *(14)*.

In addition to DA, norepinephrine also plays an important role in working memory. Selective stimulation of the α_{2A} adrenoceptor ameliorates working memory deficits induced by depletion of catecholamines in the PFC of laboratory animals. Beneficial effects of α_2 receptor agonists such as clonidine are especially prominent when a working memory task is affected by competing stimuli. This observation is consistent with the findings in the 5-CSRTT testing paradigm that noradrenergic lesions decrease choice accuracy when interfering stimuli are present. Such effects of clonidine parallel the benefits of this direct α_2 receptor agonist in clinical ADHD, and may reflect actions on postsynaptic adrenoceptors in PFC rather than on autoreceptors that limit the production and release of norepinephrine.

6.2.4. Summary of Neuropsychological Models

In summary, neuropsychological studies demonstrate that executive functions (response inhibition, sustained attention, working memory, and others) are deficient or defective in persons diagnosed with ADHD. Experimental models for these cognitive domains provide a heuristic theoretical framework for future studies of ADHD, including further development of reliable diagnostic tools for clinical ADHD, potential endophenotypes for genetic analysis, and methods for predicting innovative treatments. The broad spectrum of ADHD symptoms is not adequately explained by any single model of response inhibition, attention, or working memory alone. Instead, such cognitive models should be viewed as complimentary to each other, as well as partly overlapping in their underlying mechanisms. For example, interference control, or resistance to distraction can be viewed as a component of response inhibition, as a manifestation of selective attention, or as an integral part of working memory.

Despite limitations of these models, they point to common neuroanatomical and neurophysiological substrates. Electrophysiological and lesioning studies have provided ample evidence indicating that certain cognitive processes found to be deficient in ADHD patients (e.g., response inhibition, attention, and working memory) are critically dependent on the integrity of neuronal circuitry in the frontal cerebral cortex, and particularly prefrontal cortex. This conclusion is consistent with the clinical observation that some features of ADHD are reproduced in human subjects with lesions or injuries of the frontal cortex.

The catecholamines DA and norepinephrine are implicated in response inhibition, attention, and working memory. This involvement is consistent with the clinical efficacy of stimulants and noradrenergic antidepressants, and adds strong support to the validity of these cognitive measures as targets of experimental modeling as well as clinical investigation. Moreover, they may serve as important intermediate phenotypes of ADHD and therefore useful experimental targets in future studies of the genetics and neuropharmacology of the clinical disorder.

7. TREATMENT

Patients diagnosed with ADHD, especially children, require comprehensive interventions that include use of appropriate medication. Various elements of special education, behavior therapy, psychotherapy, and family therapy are also essential parts of the intervention, but are beyond the scope of the present discussion. The clinical management of ADHD is complicated by comorbidity with other disorders. A matter of particular concern is that the syndrome of bipolar disorder is often undiagnosed or misdiagnosed among patients considered to have ADHD, and especially children. In such patients, use of stimulants or antidepressants can produce adverse behavioral responses including manic or mixed manic-depressive states, psychosis, aggression, self-injury, or suicide *(11)*. Treatments with evidence of effectiveness in clinical ADHD are summarized in Table 2.

Table 2
Pharmacological Treatments for Attention Deficit Hyperactivity Disorder

Agents	Brand Names	FDA status for ADHD	FDA-approved ages (years)	Typical doses (mg/day)	Dose Range (mg/day)
Mixed DAT/NET inhibitors (stimulants)					
Amphetamines[a]	Adderall®	Approved (controlled: II)	6–17	5–20	2.5–40
d-Amphetamine	Dexedrine®, etc.	Approved	≥3	5–20	2.5–40
d,l-Amphetamine[b]	Benzedrine®, etc.	Not marketed			—
Bupropion	Wellbutrin®, etc.	Off-label	≥18	100–300	75–450
GW-320659		Experimental	—		—
d-Methylphenidate[c]	Focalin®	Approved (controlled: II)	6–17	5–10	2.5–20
d,l-Methylphenidate[d]	Concerta®, Ritalin®, etc.	Approved (controlled: II)	≥6	20–30	10–60
Pemoline magnesium[e]	Cylert®	Limited approval (controlled: IV)	≥6	37.5–75	18.75–112.5
R-Dinorsibutramine[f]		Experimental	—	(10)	(5–15)
Mixed NET/SERT inhibitors (antidepressants)					
Atomoxetine	Strattera®	Approved (ADHD, not depression)	unrestricted	60–80	20–100
Desipramine	Norpramin®, etc.	Off-label	>12	50–200 (ca. 2.5–5 mg/kg)	25–300
Imipramine	Tofranil®, etc.	Off-label	>12	100–200 (ca. 2.5–5 mg/kg)	25–300
Nortriptyline	Aventyl®, etc.	Off-label	>12	50–150 (ca. 2 mg/kg)	25–200
Venlafaxine[g]	Effexor®	Off-label	≥18	100–225	50–375

MAO inhibitors[h]					
Tranylcypromine	Parnate®	Off-label	≥16	10–30	5–60
Selegiline (l-deprenyl)[i]	Eldepryl®	Off-label	adults	10–15	5–30
Antihypertensives[j]					
Clonidine	Catapres®, etc.	Off-label	>12	0.2–0.6	0.2–2.4
Guanfacine	Tenex,® etc.	Off-label	>12	1–2	0.5–3.0
Pindolol	Generic	Off-label	adults	40	20–60
Miscellaneous[j]					
Carbamazepine	Tegretol®, etc.	Off-label	≤6	400–600	50–800
Donepezil	Aricept®	Off-label	adults	5–10	5–10
GT-2331	Perceptin®	Experimental	—	—	—
Modafinil	Provigil®	Off-label	≥16	200	100–400

Footnotes:

Abbreviations: etc. implies that other brands, including generics are available in the US; *Controlled:* considered by the US Drug Enforcement Administration (DEA) a drug of potential abuse, with limited distribution under controlled conditions (e.g., some stimulants are in DEA category II [amphetamines, methylphenidate] or the lesser category IV [pemoline]); *FDA:* U.S. Food and Drug Administration ("approval" is specific for the indication ADHD, otherwise use in ADHD is "off-label"; *MAO:* monoamine oxidase; *NET:* norepinephrine transporter (some NET inhibitors can also inhibit neuronal uptake of serotonin, as well as cortical uptake of DA), contrasted to stimulants that decrease transport or neuronal storage of both norepinephrine and dopamine; *Off-label:* FDA-approved for other indications (such as depression, high blood pressure, epilepsy, narcolepsy, or dementia) but not specifically for ADHD; *SERT:* serotonin transporter; *SR:* slow-release.

[a]This product is a mixture of d,l- and d-amphetamine sulfate, d,l-amphetamine aspartate, and d-amphetamine saccharate in approximately equimolar proportions.

[b]Racemic d,l-amphetamine sulfate (Benzedrine®, and other generics) was the first stimulant used to treat pediatric patients with what later was conceptualized as ADHD, but is no longer marketed as such (in the US currently only in the mixed amphetamine preparation Adderall® includes racemic amphetamine).

[c]d-Methylphenidate is the isolated d-threo- or R,R-[+]-isomer, which is more than twice as potent as the racemate, since the l-isomer can inhibit the more active d-isomer.

[d]Racemic d,l-methylphenidate is available as tablets, including slow-release and delayed-release forms, a multilayered oral form that releases three increasingly graded doses during the day to provide sustained delivery and to avoid rapid-tolerance (tachyphylaxis), and a transdermal skin patch delivery system is in advanced clinical trials.

[e]Pemoline is FDA-approved for ADHD, but not as a first-line agent (limited to when other agents have failed), owing mainly to its relatively high risk of liver toxicity. It is considered to have relatively low abuse-liability.

(continued)

Table 2 (*continued*)

Footnotes:

*f*An experimental compound that is the active, isolated R-isomer of the *N,N*-di-desmethyl metabolite of *d,l*-sibutramine [Meridia®] a diet-control agent with mild stimulant-like properties and ability to inhibit transporters for dopamine, norepinephrine, and serotonin, but itself is not used to treat ADHD).

*g*Venlafaxine may be active in ADHD, perhaps owing to its NET-antagonism at high doses, whereas other more selective SERT (selective serotonin transport inhibitors) appear to have little therapeutic effect in ADHD.

*h*Tranylcypromine also has amphetamine-like structure and stimulant-like actions; *selegiline* is relatively selective for MAO type B, at least at daily doses less than 20 mg, but at higher doses it also inhibits MAO-A and may produce hypertensive crises in the presence of tyramine or other sympathomimetic amines; it may be metabolized in part to methamphetamine or other amphetamine-like agents (as may also occur with bupropion). The experimental, selective, irreversible MAO-A inhibitor *clorgyline* also has been found effective in ADHD but is not available for clinical use.

*i*Clonidine and *guanfacine* are centrally active α₂-adrenoceptor agonists with (autoreceptor-mediated) antihypertensive action and probable postsynaptic actions in cerebral cortex (Catapres® is available as a transdermal skin patch as well as tablets); *pindolol* is a centrally active β-adrenoceptor antagonist that may also block presynaptic serotonin (5-HT) autoreceptors to enhance release of serotonin.

*j*Carbamazepine is an anticonvulsant with mood-stabilizing effects; *donepezil* is a centrally active, reversible anticholinesterase agent used primarily for early dementia; *GT-2331* is a centrally active histamine H₃ receptor antagonist; *modafinil* is an nonstimulant agent of uncertain neuropharmacology that selectively suppresses sleep in narcolepsy.

Note that none of these agents is specifically FDA-approved for long-term use (more than about 6 weeks), though standard care requires indefinitely prolonged use in ADHD; tentatively proposed doses of non-FDA-approved agents are based on literature reports and may change with further experience.

244

7.1. Stimulants

Stimulants have been used to treat both behavioral and cognitive features of ADHD since the 1930s, when Bradley introduced *d,l*-amphetamine for the treatment of a range of behavioral disorders in children and adolescents. Indeed, amphetamines and other stimulants have become the cornerstone of medical treatment for ADHD. This group of drugs includes several amphetamines, racemic or *d*-methylphenidate, pemoline, the antidepressant bupropion, and an emerging group of experimental agents that share some neuropharmacological features of typical stimulants, notably their ability to release or prevent the inactivation of catecholamines by neuronal reuptake.

The pharmacology of stimulants, which facilitate release of both norepinephrine and DA, overlaps that of many antidepressants that act by inhibition of norepinephrine transport and also have proved to be effective in the treatment of ADHD. Agents that act selectively to block neuronal transport of DA, or use of stimulants in combination with selective antagonists of DA receptors, have not been tested experimentally in ADHD patients, leaving considerable uncertainty about the relative importance of norepinephrine and DA in mediating clinically useful effects of stimulants in ADHD.

The only drugs that are Food and Drug Administration (FDA)-approved specifically for the treatment of ADHD are amphetamines, methylphenidate, pemoline (under limited circumstances), and the new antidepressant-like agent atomoxetine (Table 2). All other treatment options represent empirical, "off-label" applications of agents approved for other indications, such as depression or hypertension. Moreover, use of many agents found to be effective in the treatment of ADHD in children is considered "off-label" as a result of specific FDA-approval for treatment of adults only, notably including the tricyclic antidepressants. Additionally, FDA-approved recommendations for the duration of treatment are typically as brief as 4 to 6 weeks, even although ADHD typically requires indefinitely prolonged treatment.

By far, the most commonly employed treatment for ADHD in the United States has been racemic *d,l-threo*-methylphenidate (Ritalin®), a diasteriomeric compound with four possible conformations (*d-* and *l-, threo* or *erythro*). Methylphenidate is available in a wide range of preparations, including ordinary and slow-release tablets, as well as a multicompartment oral preparation (Concerta®) that releases the drug in rising amounts over at least 12 hours, with minimized risk of rapid tolerance or *tachyphylaxis* that can limit the action of ordinary long-acting preparations *(38)*. A transdermal skin patch delivery system also is available. Finally, the pure *d-threo*-isomer of methylphenidate (Focalin®) was recently FDA-approved for treatment of ADHD.

Pemoline is recommended only when other stimulants fail to alleviate symptoms or are poorly tolerated, owing to an increased risk of liver damage. Bupropion appears to be somewhat less consistently effective than other stimulants, and is associated with a risk of epileptic seizures at higher doses. Other stimulant-like agents remain experimental, including an active metabolite of the anorexic agent sibutramine, and the new agent GW-329659, that inhibits both DA and norepinephrine transporters.

Despite their status as a treatment of choice for ADHD at all ages, stimulants continue to draw criticism for their alleged overuse and potential for abuse or illicit diversion. Some stimulants (amphetamines and pemoline, but not methylphenidate, bupropion, or sibutramine) are categorized as controlled substances by US Drug Enforcement Administration regulations. A recent study of a sample of nearly 6000 children and adolescents suggested that overuse of stimulants may not be as widespread as once thought *(39)*. In that study, the prevalence of "definite" ADHD across all ages was 7.4%, and 86.5% of youths so diagnosed were treated with a stimulant at some time. However, among those without ADHD, only 0.2% was ever given a stimulant, with intermediate rates for those with less certain diagnostic status.

7.2. Antidepressants

Antidepressants that selectively block norepinephrine reuptake, or both norepinephrine and serotonin transport, are effective in the treatment of ADHD, whereas SSRI antidepressants are not *(1,40)*. Beneficial effects of adrenergic antidepressants have been demonstrated with both older tricyclic antidepressants (e.g., imipramine, desipramine, and nortriptyline), which are relatively toxic in overdoses and the newer, safer agent atomoxetine *(41)*. These agents may also have beneficial effects in suppressing tics in children with a primary tic disorder such as Gilles de la Tourette's syndrome, or those induced by stimulants. Monoamine oxidase inhibitors (MAOIs; e.g., tranylcypromine and selegiline), which potentiate catecholamines and serotonin, also have been reported to be of benefit in ADHD.

The potential toxicity of the tricyclic antidepressants and MAOIs has limited clinical enthusiasm for their use except when stimulants prove to be ineffective or poorly tolerated. Newer agents that block the norepinephrine transporter, such as atomoxetine and duloxetine, have a much improved safety profile, and are emerging as plausible alternatives to the older antidepressants and even the stimulants.

7.3. Miscellaneous Agents

The α_2 adrenoceptor agonists clonidine and guanfacine have some evidence of clinical utility in ADHD although their primary indication is hypertension. Mechanisms by which these drugs alleviate ADHD symptoms remain unknown. An autoreceptor mechanism seems unlikely because activation of the presynaptic α_2 autoreceptor reduces noradrenergic neurotransmission, and so, a direct postsynaptic action is more likely. There is some evidence that centrally active β-adrenergic blockers including pindolol may also be helpful in ADHD, through unexplained mechanisms.

Finally, several agents developed mainly for other purposes may be useful in the treatment of ADHD. These include the anticonvulsant carbamazepine, the cholinesterase inhibitor donepezil, the antinarcolepsy agent of uncertain mechanism of action, modafinil, as well as the experimental histamine H_3 receptor antagonist GT-2331 (Perceptin®). However, experimental trials of these agents remain limited and mainly anecdotal.

8. CONCLUSIONS

ADHD is a highly prevalent and heterogeneous syndrome consisting of cognitive and behavioral deficits, notably, inattention, impulsivity, deficient behavioral inhibition, and hyperactivity that can be comorbid with conduct, learning, and mood disorders. ADHD can be found at any age, but is more often diagnosed in boys than girls or adults, and in the United States more than Europe. Compared to the general population, risk of ADHD is 5 to 10 times greater among first-degree relatives of index cases, and more than twice greater in identical than fraternal twins. Heritability of ADHD is high and there are suggestive associations with specific genetic polymorphisms of neuronal proteins essential to cerebral dopaminergic neurotransmission. Diagnosis remains essentially clinical, based on multiple sources of information. There are no specific psychological or other diagnostic tests, but objective measures of body motility during sustained attention tasks are promising.

Prominent deficits in executive functions suggest dysfunction of the prefrontal cerebral cortex. This theory is tentatively supported by some brain-imaging studies, although a specific pathophysiology is unknown. Laboratory animal models of ADHD include genetic and neurotoxin models, and paradoxically, include states of either dopaminergic excess or deficiency. These models vary in their similarity to clinical ADHD, and emphasize behavioral hyperactivity rather than specific cognitive dysfunctions. Newer approaches to laboratory modeling include use of relatively specific cognitive testing methods that are applicable to animal and human subjects. These models of specific cognitive deficits (including response inhibition, sustained attention, working memory, and others) may also represent endophenotypes appropriate for genetic and pharmacological study instead of the more complex and heterogeneous clinical syndrome of ADHD.

Effective treatment of ADHD includes most stimulants (with dopaminergic and noradrenergic actions), and antidepressants with noradrenergic, but not selective serotonergic, actions, along with comprehensive behavioral and educational interventions. Interest in developing innovative treatments for ADHD has increased greatly in recent years following decades of heavy reliance on the use of stimulants.

GLOSSARY OF MEDICAL TERMINOLOGY

Allele: Any one of a series of two or more different genes that occupy the same locus on a chromosome.
Attention: The ability to attend to a specific stimulus. Notice the contrast to alertness in which a person can response to any stimulus.
Comorbidity: A concomitant but separable disease.
Polymorphism: Occurrence of multiple discrete alleles.
Prevalence: The number of cases of a disease relative to a given population at a specific time or period of time.

Proband: The patient carrying a specific disease.

Relative risk: The ratio of the risk of a disease among those exposed to a specific factor, to the risk among those not exposed.

Stimulant: An agent that increases motor activity, decreases fatigue, or promotes a sense of well-being.

ACKNOWLEDGMENTS

This work was supported, in part, by the Fred Corneel Research Fellowship (KZ), and by the Bruce J. Anderson Foundation and the McLean Private Donors Neuropsychopharmacology Research Fund (RJB).

REFERENCES

1. Barkley RA. Attention-Deficit Hyperactivity Disorder: A Handbook for Diagnosis and Treatment. New York, NY: Guilford Press, 1998.
2. Solanto MV, Arnsten AFT, Castellanos FX, ed. Stimulant Drugs and ADHD. New York, NY: Oxford University Press, 2001.
3. Douglas VI. Stop, look, and listen: The problems of sustained attention and impulse control in hyperactive and normal children. Can J Behav Sci 1972;41:259–283.
4. Lahey BB, Applegate B, McBurnett K, et al. DSM-IV field trials for attention deficit hyperactivity disorder in children and adolescents. Am J Psychiatry 1994;151:1673–1685.
5. Zito JM, Safer DJ, DosReis S, et al. Psychotropic practice patterns for youth: 10-year perspective. Arch Pediatr Adolesc Med 2003;157:17–25.
6. McBurnett K, Pfiffner LJ, Willcutt E, et al. Experimental cross-validation of DSM-IV types of attention deficit/hyperactivity disorder. J Am Acad Child Adolesc Psychiatry 1999;38:17–24.
7. Biederman J, Faraone SV, Mick E, et al. Clinical correlates of ADHD in females: Findings from a large group of girls ascertained from pediatric and psychiatric referral sources. J Am Acad Child Adolesc Psychiatry 1999;38:966–975.
8. Ishii T, Takahashi O, Kawamura Y, Ohta T. Comorbidity in attention deficit-hyperactivity disorder. Psychiatry Clin Neurosci 2003;57:457–463.
9. Faedda GL, Baldessarini RJ, Suppes T, Tondo L, Becker I, Lipschitz DS. Pediatric-onset bipolar disorder: A neglected clinical and public health problem. Harvard Rev Psychiatry 1995; 3:171–195.
10. Wozniak J, Biederman J, Kiely K, et al. Mania-like symptoms suggestive of childhood onset bipolar disorder in clinically referred children. J Am Acad Child Adolesc Psychiatry 1995; 34:1577–1583.
11. Faedda GL, Baldessarini RJ, Glovinsky IP, Austin NB. Mania in pediatric bipolar illness associated with antidepressant and stimulant treatment. J Affect Disord 2004; in press.
12. Smidt J, Heiser P, Dempfle A, et al. [Formal genetic findings in attention-deficit/hyperactivity-disorder]. Fortschr Neurol Psychiatr 2003;71:366–377.
13. Galili-Weisstub E, Segman RH. Attention deficit and hyperactivity disorder: Review of genetic association studies. Israeli J Psychiatry Relat Sci 2003;40:57–66.
14. Faraone SV, Doyle AE, Mick E, Biederman J. Meta-analysis of the association between the 7-repeat allele of the dopamine D_4 receptor gene and attention deficit hyperactivity disorder. Am J Psychiatry 2001;158:1052–1057.
15. Castellanos FX, Tannock R. Neuroscience of attention-deficit/hyperactivity disorder: The search for endophenotype. Nature Rev Neurosci 2002;3:617–628.
16. Ogdie MN, Macphie IL, Minassian SL, et al. A genome-wide scan for attention-deficit/hyperactivity disorder in an extended sample: Suggestive linkage on 17p11. Am J Human Genet 2003;72:1268–1279.

17. Castellanos FX, Giedd JN, Marsh WL, et al. Quantitative brain magnetic resonance imaging in attention-deficit hyperactivity disorder. Arch Gen Psychiatry 1996;53:607–616.
18. Casey BJ, Castellanos FX, Giedd JN, et al. Implications of right frontostriatal circuitry in response inhibition and attention-deficit/hyperactivity disorder. J Am Acad Child Adolesc Psychiatry 1997;36:374–383.
19. Schweitzer JB, Faber TL, Grafton ST, Tune LE, Hoffman JM, Kilts CD. Alterations in the functional anatomy of working memory in adult attention deficit hyperactivity disorder. Am J Psychiatry. 2000;157:278–280.
20. Davids E, Zhang K, Tarazi FI, Baldessarini RJ. Animal models of attention-deficit hyperactivity disorder. Brain Res Rev 2003;42:1–21.
21. Sagvolden T. Behavioral validation of the spontaneously hypertensive rat (SHR) as an animal model of attention-deficit/hyperactivity disorder (ADHD). Neurosci Biobehav Rev 2000;24:31–39.
22. Giros B, Jaber M, Jones SR, Wightman RM, Caron MG. Hyperlocomotion and indifference to cocaine and amphetamine in mice lacking the dopamine transporter. Nature 1996;379:606–612.
23. Hess EJ, Jinnah HA, Kozak CA, Wilson MC. Spontaneous locomotor hyperactivity in a mouse mutant with a deletion including the SNAP gene on chromosome 2. J Neurosci 1992;12:2865–2874.
24. Shaywitz BA, Klopper JH, Yager RD, Gordon JW. Paradoxical response to amphetamine in developing rats treated with 6-hydroxydopamine. Nature 1976;261:153–155.
25. Zhang K, Davids E, Tarazi FI, Baldessarini RJ. Effects of dopamine D_4 receptor-selective antagonists on motor hyperactivity in rats with neonatal 6-hydroxydopamine lesions. Psychopharmacology 2002;161:100–106.
26. Barkley RA. ADHD and the Nature of Self-Control. New York, NY: Guilford Press, 1997.
27. Douglas VI. Cognitive control processes in attention deficit/hyperactivity disorder. In: Quay HC, Hogan AE, ed. Handbook of Disruptive Behavior Disorders. New York, NY: Kluwer-Plenum, 1991:105–138.
28. Denckla MB. Biological correlates of learning and attention: What is relevant to learning disability and attention-deficit hyperactivity disorder? J Devel Behav Pediatrics 1996;17:114–119.
29. Evenden JL. Varieties of impulsivity. Psychopharmacology 1999;146:348–161.
30. Logan GD. On the ability to inhibit thought and action: A user's guide to the stop signal paradigm. In: Dagenbach D, Carr TH, ed. Inhibitory Processes in Attention, Memory, and Language. San Diego, CA: Academic Press 1994:189–239.
31. Aron AR, Dowson JH, Sahakian BJ, Robbins TW. Methylphenidate improves response inhibition in adults with attention-deficit/hyperactivity disorder. Biol Psychiatry 2003;54:1465–1468.
32. Feola TW, de Wit H, Richards JB. Effects of *d*-amphetamine and alcohol on a measure of behavioral inhibition in rats. Behav Neurosci 2000;114:838–848.
33. Riccio CA, Reynolds CR. Continuous performance tests are sensitive to ADHD in adults but lack specificity: Review and critique for differential diagnosis. Ann NY Acad Sci 2001;931:113–139.
34. Robbins TW. The 5-choice serial reaction time task: Behavioral pharmacology and functional neurochemistry. Psychopharmacology 2002;163:362–380.
35. Sarter M, Givens B, Bruno JP. The cognitive neuroscience of sustained attention: where top-down meets bottom-up. Brain Res Rev 2001;35:146–60.
36. Goldman-Rakic PS. Working memory dysfunction in schizophrenia. In: Salloway SP, Malloy PF, Duffy JD, ed. The Frontal Lobes and Neuropsychiatric Illness. Washington DC: American Psychiatric Press, 2001:71–82.
37. Arnsten AFT, Murphy B, Merchant K. The selective dopamine D_4 receptor antagonist, PNU-101387G, prevents stress-induced cognitive deficits in monkeys. Neuropsychopharmacology 2000;4:405–410.
38. Swanson J, Gupta S, Lam A, Shoulson I, Lerner M, Modi N, Lindemulder E, Wigal S. Development of a new once-a-day formulation of methylphenidate for the treatment of attention-deficit/hyperactivity disorder: Proof-of-concept and proof-of-product studies. Arch Gen Psychiatry 2003;60:204–211.

39. Barbaresi WJ, Katusic SK, Colligan RC, et al. How common is attention-deficit/hyperactivity disorder? Arch Pediatr Adolesc Med 2002:156:217–224.

40. Baldessarini RJ. Drugs and the treatment of psychiatric disorders: Antidepressant and antianxiety agents. In: Hardman JG, Limbird LE, Gilman AG, ed. Goodman and Gilman's The Pharmacological Basis of Therapeutics, tenth edition. New York, NY: McGraw-Hill Press, 2001:447–483, and Chapter 17, 2005, in press.

41. Kratochvil CJ, Vaughan BS, Harrington MJ, Burke WJ. Atomoxetine: Selective noradrenaline reuptake inhibitor for the treatment of attention-deficit/hyperactivity disorder. Expert Opin Pharmacother 2003;4:1165–1174.

Index